preservation and restoration of tooth structure

GJ Mount AM BDS(Syd) DDSc(Adel) FRACDS
General Dental Practice
Visiting Research Fellow
The University of Adelaide
Australia

WR Hume BDS(Adel) PhD DDSc FRACDS
Dean, Faculty of Dentistry
Center for the Health Sciences
University of California, Los Angeles
USA

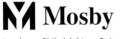 Mosby

London • Philadelphia • St Louis • Sydney • Tokyo

Copyright © 1998 Mosby International Ltd.
Published in 1998 by Mosby, an imprint of Mosby
International Ltd.
Printed by Grafos SA, Arte sobre papel, Barcelona, Spain.
ISBN 0 7234 3102 7

For full details of all Mosby titles, please write to Mosby
International, Lynton House, 7–12 Tavistock Square, London
WC1H 9LB, UK.
A CIP catalogue record for this book is available from the
British Library.
Library of Congress Cataloging-in-Publication Data applied
for.

Designer	Ian Spick
Illustration	Mike Saiz
Index	Anita Reid
Layout	Chris Read
Production	Siobhán Egan
Project Manager	Sarah Gray
Acquisitions Editor	Penny Rudolph
Publisher	John Schrefer

Contents

Introduction

The original concept for this book arose from discussions between the two principal authors, one of whom has had many years of general practice; the other has been in academia for most of his professional career. They are both well aware of the changes that are taking place in the practice of dentistry and the speed at which the changes are occurring. It is obvious to any thinking observer that it is increasingly difficult for the average practitioner to keep pace; it is also apparent that the student needs to have available a text including as many of the latest changes as possible. It is, in fact, unfair to allow a student to graduate at this time only to find that the outside world is different and has already moved far ahead. Similarly, the general practitioner is seriously in need of a consolidated text that combines most of the current principles of operative dentistry and obviates the need to read endless journals in an attempt to become up to date.

One of the problems with any text book is that it is rapidly outdated, because knowledge is being accumulated with such speed. It must also be acknowledged that, along with this exponential growth, there is a growing emphasis upon marketing and even the most experienced practitioner may become confused with the rapid changes and the plethora of advertising material that are posted daily through the letter box. Many of the new materials are promoted as if they had been under clinical scrutiny for years, when in fact there is too often a serious lack of relevant trials; the clinician must rely heavily upon personal judgement to make a choice.

An original set of principles for restorative dentistry was laid down by GV Black 100 years ago; it is only in recent years that they have been challenged to any extent. The advent of long-term adhesion in the oral cavity, as well as a more sophisticated understanding of the influence of fluoride in the demineralisation–remineralisation cycle of the cariously involved tooth, have made it possible to redefine the real meaning of 'conservative' dentistry. We have moved beyond the surgical approach to the elimination of the carious lesion, which required the removal of varying quantities of sound tooth structure to make room for the restoration. It is now possible to heal a carious lesion, at least in its early stages; as the cavity enlarges to the point where restoration is required, there will often be reasonable quantities of demineralised tooth structure that can be retained and remineralised. Such healing processes were not available to GV Black because fluoride and adhesion were not understood. The ultimate aim now must be preservation of remaining tooth structure which, of course, will lead to maintenance of physical properties as well as aesthetics.

But this demands a redefinition of the principles, otherwise it all becomes rather clumsy. So we have taken the plunge and redefined much of restorative dentistry on the grounds that there has been sufficient clinical experience gained over the last decade to justify what follows.

Two other decisions of considerable importance arose out of those early discussions. First, we agreed that there is sufficient expertise in this country to confine ourselves to Australian contributors only. Each of our co-contributors received their initial dental education here; much of the research upon which our thesis is based has been conducted by them. We are proud to call them experts.

The second decision was taken as the manuscript progressed. In this modern era of communication it is apparent that books alone are not sufficient. We are told that every home will have a CD-ROM player in the near future – even if it is in the children's playroom – and that putting illustrations on disc is far simpler and cheaper than having them printed. We have created a CD-ROM which can be purchased with the book as part of a package, and this includes over 600 full-colour illustrations, complete with explanations. All the illustrations that appear in the book are repeated on the disc and are supported by a further 340 pictures; we feel this will increase its educational value to a considerable extent. In fact, it is possible on the disc to give a far more detailed explanation for each picture and to show complete series in relation to restorative techniques where space constraints limit this in the textbook.

The disc is available only with the book because it does not make a great deal of sense without the book with its detailed reasoning. The program used is Adobe Acrobat and the disc can be played on either Apple Macintosh or IBM-compatible machines. The full instructions are included with the disc so that even a neophyte computer operator should have no difficulty.

We hope the text will be read and enjoyed by students as well as the practising profession. The proposed new classification of cavity designs is simple and uncomplicated, making it possible to include cavities that were not available before adhesion. It is designed to improve communication between dentists as well as between the profession and other authorities and it eases record keeping on a computer.

We look forward to comment and trust the book will be accepted for what it is meant to be – a redefinition of modern dentistry to suit our modern times.

Acknowledgements

It is not easy to acknowledge all those who have made a contribution to a work of this magnitude but of course Rory Hume and I must start by paying tribute to all those who have made a considerable contribution to the manuscript. I am grateful for their cooperation and tolerance. They have generally kept to time and, more importantly, they have put up with considerable editing of their work. This is not always well received by an author, but these people have been very tolerant. Hopefully, they will all agree that the end result flows adequately but at the same time has lost nothing in significance.

The generation of the original manuscript and its illustrations was all made possible through the expertise of Henny Poort, who came to Adelaide just in time to save the day. He is a skilled computer operator as well as a patient teacher; he has guided me through a number of programmes and did all the original setting up of the first layout. His guidance has been invaluable and is greatly appreciated.

The CD-ROM is, of course, a departure from the norm and, again, I needed a lot of support and encouragement before I accepted the value of this approach. Henny Poort first stimulated the thought and then Ray Marchant from Bridgehead Australia Pty Ltd, Adelaide, did all the hard work and helped to guide me through another new discipline. I think the concept is fine because it has doubled the number of illustrations and greatly increased the size of the legends available to the reader, thus enhancing the value of the final product. At the same time it has kept the final cost within reach of the average reader.

Most of the illustrations were supplied by the authors relative to their own chapters and most of the balance come from my own library. Several of the scanning electron micrographs were taken recently by Dr Hien Ngo, a general practitioner in Adelaide who continues to be a very keen student of progress in dentistry. He has considerable experience in handling the scanning electron microscope as well as the con-focal optical microscope; he can drive the new machines at the University of Adelaide with great dexterity. The best of the micrographs are his, and some of the inspiration for the new concepts arise from his studies.

The concept of the new classification for carious lesions was first published as an article in Quintessence International in 1997 (volume 28, pp.301–303), entitled '*A revised classification of carious lesions by site and size.*'

My good friend Michael Williams volunteered to proofread the entire original manuscript before I submitted it to Mosby. His dental knowledge made this contribution absolutely invaluable, because he not only looked for 'typos' but also for expressions of thought that were not put clearly enough. When an author has read a manuscript often enough, the meaning is entirely clear – to the author – but not necessarily to the reader! Another opinion is essential and is gratefully received.

As this is essentially an Australian book written by Australian authorities in the field, we have stayed entirely with Australian language, expressions and spelling. If this varies from the norm in other countries, we beg your indulgence. The meaning is, hopefully, still clear and the pronunciation, doubtless, remains the same.

The book, as you see it in its present form, was generated and edited in the London office of Mosby International. We, the contributors, are deeply grateful to Sarah Gray and all who worked with her for the end result. Proper interpretation of the thoughts of others, particularly in such a specialised discipline as dentistry, is not easy and requires endless patience. The Mosby team have been most supportive at all times, even when chased by an exacting timetable, but we are confident that the following pages are a tribute to their efforts.

Finally, as I reach the end of this task I recognise that I must have just about reached the limit of tolerance of my greatest supporter – my wife Margaret. At this point I think she is quite looking forward to getting me back as home-side company and will not be sorry to see the computer shut down.

Graham J Mount
Adelaide, 1998.

FIGURE CREDIT

I am grateful to Martin Dunitz at Martin Dunitz Publishers, London, for permission to include the following illustrations on glass–ionomers:

Chapter 8: Figs 1–12, 15–18, 23–28.
Chapter 11: Figs 1, 2, 9, 22–27, 37–40, 53, 54, 77–82, 91, 96, 97, 101–102, 104–106, 108–113.
Chapter 19: Figs 10, 11.

The illustrations, which appear both in Chapter 8, 11 and 19 on the disc, first appeared in '*An atlas of glass–ionomers: a clinician's guide*' which was published in 1989, with a second edition in 1994.

Contributors

RW Bryant BDS MDS PhD FRACDS
Professor and Head of Tooth Conservation
The University of Sydney
Australia

TM Gerzina BDS MDS PhD FRACDS
Lecturer, Tooth Conservation
The University of Sydney
Australia

JA Kaidonis BDS Bsc Dent PhD
Lecturer, Clinical Dentistry
The University of Adelaide
Australia

JW McIntyre BDS PhD
Visiting Research Fellow
The University of Adelaide
Australia

FE Martin BDS MDS FRACDS
Senior Lecturer, Tooth Conservation
The University of Sydney
Australia

WLK Massey BDS PhD
Senior Lecturer, Tooth Conservation
The University of Sydney
Australia

LC Richards BSc Dent. PhD
Senior Lecturer, Prosthodontics
The University of Adelaide
Australia

D Southan BDS, MDS, PhD, DDSc, FDSRCS, FRACDS
Private Practice in Prosthodontics
Sydney
Australia

GC Townsend BDS Bsc Dent. PhD DDSc
Professor, Oral Anatomy
The University of Adelaide
Australia

How to use the CD-ROM

You may have purchased this book with a CD-ROM.

On the CD-ROM which accompanies this book, you will find freely distributed software called Adobe Acrobat Reader. This is supplied in either a Macintosh or Windows format and is industry and worldwide standard. The software is available without cost, and opens files created using a range of Adobe products.

INSTALLING ADOBE ACROBAT READER

Simply click on the **Ar32e3o.exe** (Windows) or **Ardr3o1e.bin** (Macintosh) icons, depending on your computer system. Your system will install Adobe Acrobat Reader into a folder on your hard drive. You will then be able to open the CD-ROM by double clicking on the icon.

USING THE CD-ROM

If you already have Adobe Acrobat Reader installed on your computer, simply double click on the CD-ROM icon. When it is first opened, the image will fill the screen. Click on ESC to escape to smaller images with a menu bar. This includes the possibility of accessing thumbnail images which will appear down the left hand side of the screen.

As the thumbnails are not fully in sequence, normal navigation to move from one thumbnail to the next should be undertaken by using the red dots that appear in the lower left hand corner of each image. However, it is possible to scroll through the thumbnails using the left-hand scroll bar. Alternatively, it is also possible to move from one image to another, viewing one image at a time. You can move both up and down by using the scroll bar on the right-hand side of the screen. This is the preferred technique for comparing immediately adjacent images.

The program is set up in a chapter-by-chapter format. When you have completed viewing one chapter you will be automatically returned to the primary menu screen for the selection of the next chapter. Chapter 11 deals with the new classification system, and is therefore divided into sections that deal with each type of carious lesion, one series of lesions at a time. You may click on a number selected from the Chapter 11 primary menu screen to access the illustrations relevant to a particular lesion or cavity design.

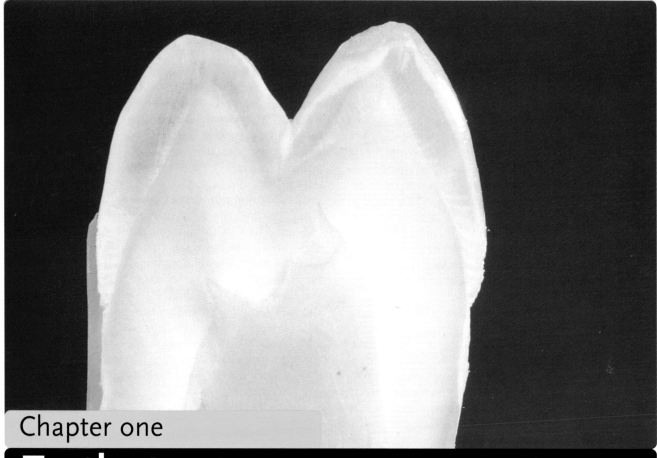

Chapter one

Tooth structure

W.R. Hume • G.C. Townsend

It is essential to have a good knowledge of tooth structure to understand the nature of both the defects and diseases that can occur and then to make rational decisions on prevention, treatment and repair.

Teeth are composed of four different tissues: enamel, dentine, dental pulp and cementum. Each of these is made up of structural elements found elsewhere in the body, but arranged in unique ways.

In the brief description that follows, a basic knowledge of the embryology and histology of the developing tooth is assumed. Readers interested in further information are referred to the reading list at the end of this chapter.

ENAMEL

Calcification

Ameloblasts differentiate from cells of the embryonic oral epithelium and receive metabolic support within the enamel organ via the stratum intermedium. During the process of amelogenesis, a mixture of enamel matrix proteins (amelogenins and enamelins) is secreted by the ameloblasts along their basal border (**Fig. 1.1**). Apatite begins to precipitate within the extracellular protein gel immediately adjacent to each ameloblast. It is likely that the amelogenin provides an ideal substrate for the precipitation of carbonated hydroxyapatite from the locally supersaturated environment of calcium and phosphate. As each apatite crystal grows, the amelogenin immediately adjacent to it and much of the enamelin go into solution. Crystal growth continues, leaving long apatite crystals stacked in arrays (enamel rods) corresponding to the parent ameloblasts, with an enamelin-rich boundary layer between the rods.

Modifications to calcification

During enamel formation, the rate of dissolution of matrix protein seems to be temperature dependent: episodes of fever during enamel formation cause defects in enamel structure. The rate of dissolution may also be dependent upon fluoride levels in the hydroxyapatite crystals: very high levels of fluoride cause defects in enamel mineralisation (mottling), whereas, at optimal levels, fluoride induces the formation of enamel of low solubility.

Process of calcification

The process of matrix protein secretion and its almost immediate replacement by hydroxyapatite, with ameloblast withdrawal, continues for a period of years. The ameloblasts leave behind stacks of crystals that are aligned to form long rods. There is a change in the crystal orientation at the rod boundaries, with individual rods being separated by varying amounts of inter-rod enamel.

Enamel prisms

Human enamel has a physical structure (**Fig. 1.2**), or grain, caused by the alignment of the enamel rods (also known as prisms). When enamel fractures it usually does so along the grain of these rods. However, the enamel rods in the regions of cusp tips and incisal edges are often arranged more irregularly; they are referred to as gnarled enamel and it is believed that this twisting increases strength. The innermost, and some parts of the outermost, layers of enamel are more homogeneously mineralised and are termed 'prismless'.

Pre-eruption maturation of enamel

After the ameloblasts have completed secreting matrix they take part in the process of pre-eruption enamel maturation, during which the hydroxyapatite crystals continue to grow, with protein and water being lost from the matrix. The process takes several years. By completion, the enamel is 96–98% apatite by weight (about 85% by volume); the remainder is protein, lipid and water. Pores exist between the crystals in enamel; by volume, the water space is about 12% in newly formed enamel. It is within this aqueous phase that the dynamics of enamel demineralisation and remineralisation take place, as is described below.

Reduced enamel epithelium

After matrix secretion is complete, the ameloblasts become part of the reduced enamel epithelium covering the tooth crown. When the tooth emerges into the oral cavity, most of the reduced enamel epithelium is shed, although some remnants may remain in occlusal grooves and some of the cells also contribute to the formation of the dentogingival attachment. On exposure to saliva, the coronal enamel becomes covered by a protective coating, or pellicle, that consists of strongly adsorbed salivary proteins and lipids.

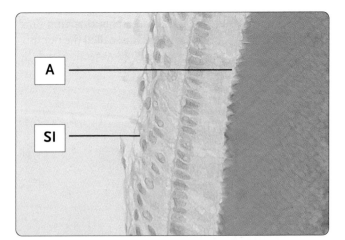

Fig. 1.1 Enamel. A photomicrograph of developing enamel with a layer of ameloblasts (A) beyond which are the cells of the stratum intermedium (SI) (×200).

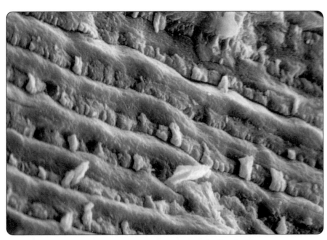

Fig. 1.2 Enamel prisms. A scanning electron micrograph of fractured enamel showing some enamel rods in longitudinal section with inter-rod enamel between layers.

Thickness of enamel and the effect on colour

The thickness of enamel varies in different parts of the crown, being thickest at the cusps and incisal edges and thinnest in the cervical region. The natural colour of the enamel is white or whitish-blue and this shows in the incisal region of teeth and the cusp tips where there is no under-lying dentine. As the enamel becomes thinner the colour of the dentine shows through and the enamel appears to be darker. The degree of mineralisation also influences its appearance with the result that hypomineralised areas appear more opaque than normally mineralised regions, which are relatively translucent.

Striae of Retzius

Enamel is formed in an incremental manner and the cross striations seen in the prisms may represent daily increments of matrix production, whereas the striae of Retzius are likely to reflect a 7–10 day rhythm. Where the striae of Retzius reach the surface, mainly in the cervical region, they produce distinct grooves or depressions, referred to as enamel perikymata. These run circumferentially around the crown giving it a rough surface texture (**Fig. 1.3**).

Posteruption mineralisation

Enamel is highly mineralised before the tooth erupts and calcium and phosphate deposition continues in crystallite defects after eruption because saliva is supersaturated with these ions.

The components by volume of mature enamel are approximately 85% inorganic, 12% water and the remaining 3% protein and lipid. Tooth mineral is highly substituted with various ions, including sodium, zinc, strontium and carbonate, which make it more reactive than pure hydroxyapatite.

The apatite crystals of enamel, particularly those at the surface and near the surface, are in dynamic equilibrium with the adjacent aqueous phase of saliva or dental plaque.

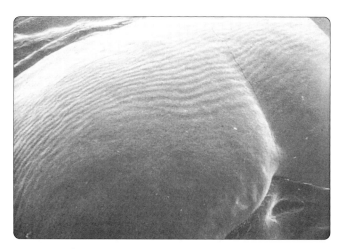

Fig. 1.3 Perikymata. A scanning electron micrograph showing the perikymata on the buccal surface of a molar tooth.

Extra fluoride may be taken into the crystal structure, depending on local fluoride concentration at the tooth surface. In time, the enamel surface becomes very well mineralised if the pH of its local environment is neutral or alkaline.

Continuing change in enamel

Almost all of the enamel matrix protein disappears as enamel forms. Enamel contains no cells, yet is far from an inert tissue. Ionic exchange of calcium, phosphate and fluoride in and out of enamel occurs continually, depending on local concentrations and pH. This is centrally important in many aspects of dental care.

Effect of ambient pH
- Below pH 5.5, mineral can be lost from the surface and the central core of enamel crystallite.
- Above pH 5.5, lost mineral can be regained from salivary calcium and phosphate.

Tissue fluid flow

Filtered tissue fluid moves very slowly outward through enamel in living, erupted teeth because the pressure inside the tooth is higher than outside. This tissue fluid is called ultrafiltrate and contains no protein, only water and inorganic ions. Ultrafiltrate has the potential to slowly hydrate the inner surface of restorative materials bonded to enamel.

DENTINE

Early formation

Concurrently with enamel formation, the ectomesenchyme-derived odontoblasts secrete both collagen and relatively complex mucopolysaccharides from their outer end to form the dentinal matrix. The collagen acts as a matrix for mineral-isation, both during tooth formation and throughout life.

Development of dentine tubules

Most of the odontoblast cell body withdraws towards the pulp as matrix secretion continues, but a thin and continuous tube of protoplasm remains, called the odonto-blastic process or Tomes' fibre. This phenomenon and the unique structure which develops because of it, the dentinal tubule, are central to the form and nature of dentine and determine many of its properties.

The complexity of dentine

The components of dentine are similar to those of bone, but the arrangement of the protoplasmic cell processes and the tubules in which they lie is unique (**Figs 1.4** and **1.5**). Unlike bone, dentine contains no blood vessels, nor does it undergo remodelling. The presence of collagen, mucopolysaccharide ground substance and odontoblastic processes in the formed tissue produces a relatively complex tissue.

The dentino–enamel junction

The junction between dentine and enamel, the dentino–enamel junction, is not a flat plane but is scalloped, especially in those areas subject to high occlusal stress. Dentine physically supports the overlying enamel and has some physical flexibility, which may help to prevent fracture of the highly mineralised brittle enamel.

Anatomy of dentinal tubules

The noncalcified tubule created by the presence of the odontoblastic process extends from the dentino-enamel junction to the odontoblastic cell body. When the dentine is completely formed this can be 5 mm or more in length. The dentinal tubules have unique characteristics. They are tapered, with the diameter near the pulp reducing by about one-half as it approaches the enamel. In adult dentine, the odontoblastic cell process may only occupy the inner one-third to one-half of the tubule but the entire tubule can remain patent. The nonprotoplasmic portion of the tubule is filled with tissue fluid.

Dentinal tubules are pathways through which fluid, chemicals and bacteria can move.

Continuing maturation of dentine

The calcification of the dentinal matrix is most rapid in the months following its secretion, but the process continues slowly throughout life. In particular, the dentine immediately adjacent to the tubule lumen becomes more heavily calcified and the tubule diameter itself decreases as more hydroxyapatite precipitates from the supersaturated dentinal fluid. The increasing thickness of the peritubular dentine increases the density of the whole tissue as the diameter of individual tubules decreases.

Odontoblasts

Odontoblasts normally remain during the life of the tooth, with their cell bodies on the inner surface of predentine and their processes extending into it (**Figs 1.6** and **1.7**). They retain their capacity to secrete matrix protein and to form additional dentine.

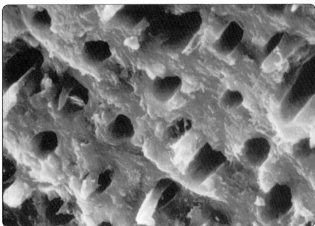

Fig. 1.4 Mature dentine. A horizontal cross section of mature dentine showing the tubules. This section is relatively close to the pulp, hence the frequency and size of the tubules (×1000).

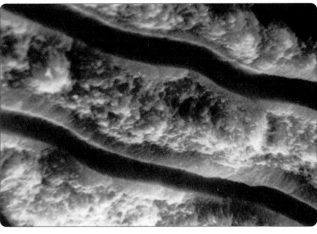

Fig. 1.5 Mature dentine. A longitudinal section of dentine in a similar area. Tubular diameter is approximately 2 μm (×1000).

Fig. 1.6 Histology of dentine. Low-power view of dentine showing from right to left: dentine, predentine, odontoblasts and dental pulp (×100).

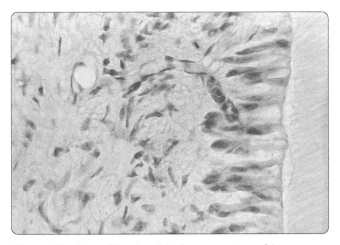

Fig. 1.7 Histology of dentine. A higher-power view of the odontoblast region (×400).

Secondary dentine

Dentine is slowly laid down throughout the life of the tooth, causing a reduction in the size of the pulp cavity. This so-called secondary dentine is laid down particularly on the roof and floor of the pulp chamber, producing a change in its size and shape.

Tertiary (reparative) dentine

Thickening of the dentine occurs more rapidly when the dentinal surface is exposed to the oral environment by accident or wear, or when the odontoblast comes into contact with the products of bacterial metabolism at levels below those which would kill the cell (i.e. in advancing caries or beneath a leaky restoration). In these circumstances, the odontoblasts can lay down additional dentine relatively rapidly. This tissue is termed 'tertiary reparative dentine'.

Irregular reparative dentine

If sufficient damage occurs to kill odontoblasts but the adjacent pulpal tissue survives, new dentine-forming cells can differentiate from the pulpal ectomesenchyme. The resultant tissue is called irregular reparative dentine and may lack the usual tubular structure but include cell bodies.

Dentine is wet

The odontoblastic tubules are full of fluid, some intracellular and some extracellular. The extracellular fluid moves outwards because of the pressure gradient between the extracellular fluid of the pulp and the inside of the mouth. In the normal erupted tooth, the movement is slow because of the very limited permeability of enamel; however, if the enamel is missing, fluid flow is much more rapid.

Factors affecting wetness

Dentinal wetness depends primarily on the size and number of tubules; so dentine is wetter closer to the pulp, where the tubules are larger in diameter and more closely packed. Dentine becomes less wet with age, because of continuing peritubular dentine deposition throughout life. If the pulp dies the dentine stays wet, but the outward flow rate is likely to be much lower.

Smear layer

If dentine is cut or polished during dental treatment the tubule orifices become, at least partially, occluded with debris called 'smear layer' (**Fig. 1.8**). This smear layer consists primarily of tooth debris but also contains other contaminants such as plaque, pellicle, saliva and possibly blood. Following fracture, the tubules may become blocked by natural deposition of salivary components. The smear layer can be removed by acids, as will be described in more detail in Chapter 8 (**Fig. 1.9**).

Diffusion through dentine

Chemicals can diffuse through the dentinal tubules just as they can through any water-based medium. Dentine behaves as if it is an impermeable solid traversed by water-filled tubules. The rate and amount of diffusion is dependent on the concentration gradient, the molecular size of the solute, the temperature, the thickness of dentine, the diameter and number of tubules, and whether or not the tubules are partially blocked with smear layer.

The natural wetness of dentine, the tubule structure and characteristics of the smear layer are all important factors to be considered when replacing missing tooth tissue.

DENTAL PULP

Development

The growth of dentine inwards from the epithelial cap (encompassing an area of tissue which is the dental pulp) slows dramatically as the tooth matures. The rate of dentine formation thereafter is sufficiently slow that the pulp usually remains throughout life, although it becomes progressively smaller in volume.

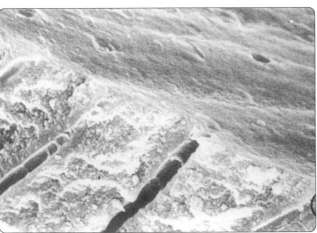

Fig. 1.8 Dentine with smear layer. Smear layer left on the surface of the dentine following cavity preparation. Note that the tubules are partially blocked (×800).

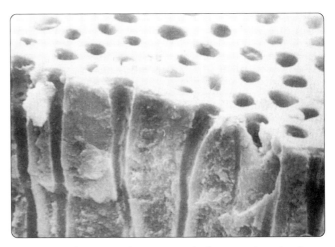

Fig. 1.9 Dentine: smear layer removed. The smear layer has been removed by etching. Note the tubules are partly funnelled open by the etchant (×800).

Constituents

The outer layer of the pulp, which is also the inner layer of dentine, is composed of odontoblastic cell bodies. Immediately beneath this layer is a relatively cell-free zone, rich in sensory nerve endings and blood capillaries. The great bulk of the remaining central pulp tissue is similar to connective tissue elsewhere, being made up of mesenchymal cells, defence cells and fibroblasts, collagen fibres, ground substance, blood vessel networks (from arterioles to capillaries to venules with accompanying sympathetic nerves), lymphatics, sensory nerve trunks and free sensory endings. This tissue provides metabolic support for the odontoblasts during rapid dentinal deposition, both in initial growth and during repair. If odontoblasts die but the remainder of the pulpal tissues survives then new odontoblasts can differentiate from the pulpal ecto-mesenchyme to lay down irregular reparative dentine.

Sensory innervation of the pulp

Bare sensory nerve endings are in intimate association with the odontoblastic cell bodies, and some extend short distances into dentinal tubules. Any stimulus that causes movement of these cell bodies may trigger action potentials within the sensory nerve network. Fluid movement within the dentinal tubules therefore elicits sensation, which is interpreted as pain. Cutting dentine, drying dentine, osmotically induced fluid flow in the tubules, heat and cold can all cause pulpal pain. Cell damage, inflammation or touch within the main body of the pulp also cause pain. The degree of stimulus necessary to bring about a pain response depends upon the sensitivity of the receptors and this will be substantially increased by inflammation within the tissue (see Chapter 5). It is reasonable to propose that the rich sensory innervation of the pulp serves a protective function for the mouth. It is also of great diagnostic value in dental practice, since reported pain symptoms can give a strong indication of the presence and nature of pathological processes in dentine and pulp.

The blood supply of the pulp

The blood supply of the pulp is particularly rich, with the rate of blood flow per mass of tissue being similar to that found in the brain. This probably reflects the high metabolic activity levels of the odontoblasts during dentine formation and repair. It also helps the tissue to overcome chemical and bacterial insult. The large number of capillaries present in the subodontoblastic layer are able to respond to local trauma by producing a hyperaemic response.

Effect of ageing

With advancing age a number of changes occur in the pulp, including a decrease in cellularity and an increase in the incidence of pulp stones and diffuse calcification. As the size of the pulp chamber decreases with continued deposition of dentine, the degree of vascularity decreases and so does the capacity of the pulp to withstand various insults.

TOOTH ROOT AND CEMENTUM

Root formation

After the crown has formed, the cellular events at the proliferating cervical loop of the enamel organ change and the cemento-enamel junction begins to form. The cells no longer differentiate into ameloblasts but continue to induce the formation of odontoblasts, and therefore dentine. The odontoblasts grow inwards, each leaving behind a cell process and matrix proteins, which mineralise to form root dentine.

Development of cementum

The outer surface of the root dentine becomes covered with the fourth tissue unique to teeth, cementum. This bone-like tissue is formed by the calcification of matrix protein secreted by cementoblasts, cells which are derived from adjacent ecto-mesenchyme of the dental follicle. Enmeshed in the cementum are the collagen fibres of the periodontal ligament, which connect the tooth root to the adjacent bone.

PERIODONTAL TISSUES

Formation of the periodontal ligament

By the time crown formation is complete, ossification of the maxilla and mandible is well advanced. As new bone is formed around the erupting teeth, collagen fibres link alveolar bone to the cementum of the tooth root and the periodontal ligament becomes organised. Although a detailed description of the development of periodontal tissues and the process of tooth eruption is beyond the scope of this book, it is relevant to note that by the time the tooth erupts, the oral mucosa overlying the dental arches has become keratinised to form gingivae, which then adapt closely to the enamel of the tooth crown. The healthy periodontium has periodontal ligament fibres connecting cementum to adjacent alveolar bone and, near the cemento-enamel junction, contains fibres connecting cementum to gingival tissue. The gingivae are supported by these fibres and by the alveolar bone to form a tight cuff of fibrous connective tissue covered with epithelium around the enamel of the tooth crowns. The epithelium that becomes closely adapted to the enamel at the dentogingival junction is composed of two parts:

- sulcular epithelium, related to the gingival sulcus or crevice around the neck of the tooth
- junctional epithelium, forming an attachment to the enamel via a laminar structure and a system of hemidesmosomes.

As long as it is in good health the closely adapted gingival tissue provides an effective barrier against bacterial movement from the oral cavity into the tissues around the tooth. The significance of the maintenance of gingival health is further described in Chapter 20.

FURTHER READING

Avery JK. *Essentials of oral histology and embryology: a clinical approach.* St Louis: Mosby; 1992.

Mjor IA, Fejerskov O. *Human oral embryology and histology.* Copenhagen: Munksgaard; 1986.

Pashley DH. Clinical correlations of dentine structure and function. *J Prosthet Dent* 1991; **66**:777–81.

Sasaki T. *Cell biology of tooth enamel formation.* Basel: Karger; 1990.

Ten-Cate AR. *Oral histology: development, structure, and function.* St Louis: Mosby; 1994.

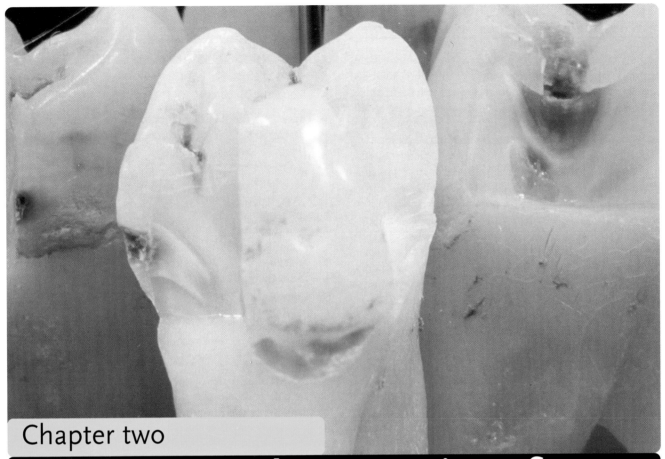

Chapter two

The nature and progression of dental caries

J. McIntyre

This chapter emphasises the modern concept of dental caries. For many years caries was thought to consist of a one-way progressive demineralisation of enamel crystallite followed by degradation of dentine, leading to cavity formation. Theories concerning the actual cause of the degradation have varied, but it has always been regarded as primarily of bacterial origin.

In the present concept, the emphasis is on a demineralisation–remineralisation cycle of the chemical reactions that occur on tooth structure. This model assists the dentist in guiding the patient to independently maintain a high level of control over the disease.

Caries is perceived to be a prolonged imbalance in the oral cavity such that factors favouring demineralisation of enamel and dentine overwhelm factors that favour remineralisation and repair of those tissues. Using such a model for a patient, the current status of the demineralisation–remineralisation balance can be determined and a caries management programme defined.

This approach is not inconsistent with models that focus on the concept of caries as an infectious disease. However, the 'demineralisation–remineralisation balance' approach places greater emphasis on the aspect of enhancement of the natural host protective factors, rather than simply the control of bacterial plaque infection.

THE MULTIFACTORIAL AETIOLOGY OF DENTAL CARIES

To assist patients in managing effectively a continuing caries problem, it is essential to consider the multifactorial aetiology of the disease. Frequency of carbohydrate intake is the major contributing factor in most cases; however, deficiencies in natural protective factors are still very important and must be fully understood and taken into account.

A high level of acid concentration and a high frequency of contact will lead to demineralisation of the tooth surface. However, natural protective factors and repair mechanisms can be enhanced for most patients and the problem controlled, at least to a degree. There is a delicate balance between health and disease, involving acid arising from bacteria-laden plaque competing with protective factors that are provided through normal salivary flow and good hygiene (**Fig. 2.1**). The most significant components contributing to this balance are shown in **Figure 2.2**.

In order to detect accurately the prime cause of an imbalance in a particular patient, it is essential to be familiar with the precise nature of each of the factors and the activity that occurs on the tooth surface.

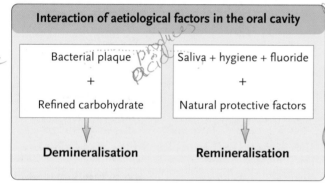

Interaction of aetiological factors in the oral cavity

Bacterial plaque + Refined carbohydrate	Saliva + hygiene + fluoride + Natural protective factors
Demineralisation	**Remineralisation**

Fig. 2.1 Interaction of aetiological factors in the oral cavity.

Main contributing factors to the demineralisation–remineralisation balance

Destabilising factors	Protective factors
Diet + plaque = plaque acids	Saliva Buffering capacity
Reduction in salivary flow	Ca^{2+} and PO_4^{3-} levels
Low buffering and oral clearance	Buffering and remineralisation
Acidic saliva Erosive acids	Oral clearance proteins/glycoproteins
	Fluoride contact developmental topical application

Fig. 2.2 Main contributing factors to the demineralisation–remineralisation balance.

Bacterial flora and plaque

Summary

Plaque and plaque pH

There are a number of factors to take into account:
- Bacterial flora – *streptococcus mutans*
- Plaque retention
  contact areas
  overhangs
  over-contour
  pits and fissures
  sticky foods
- Plaque content
  thickness
- Salivary buffering
  salivary flow
- Fluoride
  time in contact
- Carbohydrate intake frequency

Normally, many types of bacteria live in the oral cavity and some can colonise the tooth surface, forming plaque. Among these are adherent streptococci, such as *Streptococcus mutans*, which use dietary sucrose to assemble extracellular polysaccharides. Following cavitation in the enamel, the proportion of *Lactobacillus* will increase.

Plaque retention

Bacterial plaque causes fermentation of carbohydrates from food and beverages leading to production of acid ions at the tooth surface. The effectiveness of salivary buffering of this acid is inversely proportional to plaque thickness. Thick plaque is held in deep fissures and grooves, between interproximal surfaces, particularly in relation to those areas where teeth contact each other and around rough or overcontoured restorations. Mechanical oral hygiene procedures are not very effective in removing plaque from these sites, which are therefore the most common areas for caries initiation.

Effect of plaque on pH

Some of the fermentable carbohydrates entering the oral environment go into solution in saliva and become available to plaque micro-organisms, which metabolise them and cause an immediate 2–4 point drop in pH at the tooth surface (**Fig. 2.3**). The degree of fall depends on plaque thickness, the number and mix of plaque bacteria, the efficiency of salivary buffering and, perhaps, other factors. Recovery to normal resting pH takes from 20 minutes for the average patient to several hours for those with a high susceptibility to caries. A very high salivary flow rate may return the pH towards neutrality quite rapidly, but local retention of sticky foods may delay the rise in pH until the food is dissolved or removed.

Frequency of eating fermentable carbohydrate

The most significant patient behaviour factor leading to an increased risk of caries is the frequency of consumption of fermentable carbohydrate. There is good evidence that it is the frequency of eating fermentable carbohydrate that causes caries rather than the total quantity of fermentable carbohydrate consumed. The acids resulting from carbo-hydrate fermentation are weak organic acids and, in most cases, will cause only chronic low-grade caries, with progress initiating from a typical subsurface lesion. When high-frequency sugar consumption is maintained over a prolonged period, or if there is a serious deficiency of natural host protective factors, caries will progress more rapidly. In some circumstances the addition of highly erosive acids will exacerbate the problem considerably.

Other acid sources

Strong acids are available from a variety of extrinsic sources such as carbonated soft drinks, cordials, citrus fruit juices and gastric reflux or regurgitation. Frequent or prolonged exposure to these can lead to rapid demineralisation and can turn mild caries into a rampant attack. A common example is seen in infants who are allowed to sleep with a bottle of fruit juice being suckled. The pH will drop rapidly to a very low level and this may be sustained for long periods. Gastric reflux is another problem that is often not recognised by the patient, who may think it is normal or at least acceptable and not contributing to any oral health problems.

Protective dietary factors

Some foods contribute protective factors against demineralisation. Plaque is less able to attach to the tooth surface in the presence of fat. Milk products, especially cheese, and perhaps nuts fall in this category. Other foods may themselves act as buffers. Foods that require vigorous chewing can be considered protective, because such chewing markedly increases salivary flow and, therefore, buffering capacity. This factor alone can return pH in plaque to neutrality quite rapidly.

Saliva

Saliva plays a major role in protecting the teeth against acid challenge. The most convincing clinical evidence is the serious and rapid damage to tooth structure that can result from the sudden loss of saliva (xerostomia). This can result from the need to take certain prescription drugs, from irradiation of the salivary glands, from prolonged stress or from certain medical conditions.

Protective factors

The main protective factors of saliva are:

- The Ca^{2+} and PO_4^{3-} ions – usually the saliva is super-saturated when the enamel apatite is at neutral pH. The PO_4^{3-} ion also provides a significant buffering capacity at resting pH and in the early stages of acidic challenge.
- Pellicle, which arises from saliva, provides a high level of protection against an acid challenge. It acts as a barrier to diffusion of acid ions into the tooth, as well as to the movement of dissolution products from apatite out of the tooth. It may also inhibit mineralisation of apatite to form calculus from the supersaturated levels of Ca^{2+} and PO_4^{3-} ions in saliva.
- There is a very effective bicarbonate buffering system in stimulated salivary flow that contributes a high level of protection against both organic and erosive acids on the tooth surface.
- Salivary flow and oral clearance rate influence removal of food debris and microorganisms. Note that a high salivary flow may also remove topically applied fluoride resulting in the need to increase the amount required to maintain optimal levels for tooth protection.
- The fluoride ion content of saliva is low (0.03 p.p.m. or 1.6 μmol/l on average) but will still contribute to the overall protection and repair of the tooth mineral.

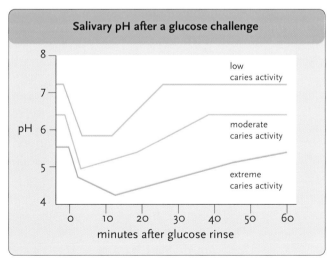

Fig. 2.3 Salivary pH after a glucose challenge. Note that with caries activity ranging from inactive to low activity the buffering capacity of saliva is adequate and the pH recovers within about 20 minutes. With moderate activity the pH is lower to begin with and recovers more slowly. In the presence of extreme activity the pH falls for a longer time and recovers much more slowly.

Summary

Salivary protective factors
- Ca^{2+} and PO_4^{3-} ions
- Pellicle
- Buffer with bicarbonates
- Salivary flow
- Oral clearance rate
- Fluoride ion content

Salivary flow

Both the quality and the quantity of saliva being secreted will vary throughout the day while awake and will be depressed during sleep. Unstimulated saliva contains little bicarbonate buffer, with fewer Ca^{2+} ions and more PO_4^{3-} ions than found in plasma. Reflex stimulation of salivary flow by chewing (such as chewing gum) or through the presence of acidic foods (such as citric acid) can increase the flow by a factor of more than ten (**Fig. 2.4**). Bicarbonate buffer concentrations can increase sixty times upon stimulation. Ca^{2+} ion levels also increase slightly, but PO_4^{3-} ions do not increase in proportion to flow rate.

Saliva provides the major source of natural protection of and repair to teeth following acid challenge. Reduction of maximum salivary flow to less than 0.7 ml/min may increase caries risk, although this depends on many other interacting factors.

Occasionally there may be a marked reduction in the resting pH of saliva not necessarily associated with a reduced flow. The cause is often not clear and the patient will then be susceptible to an increased caries rate.

Fluoride

Effect on enamel

Fluoride plays a highly significant role in the demineralisation–remineralisation process. In an acid environment, the fluoride ion reacts strongly with free Ca^{2+} and HPO_4^{2-} ions, forming fluorapatite crystals $Ca_{10}(PO_4)_6(OH.F)_2$, in which fluoride substitutes for some hydroxyl ions. Fluorapatite is less soluble than pure hydroxyapatite because of better subunit stacking. Fluorapatite crystals are unable to be dissolved by acid ions above pH 4.5 (the critical pH for fluorapatite), with the result that the mineral is more resistant to acid dissolution.

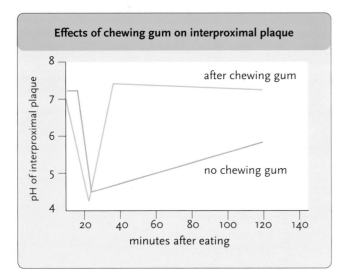

Effects of chewing gum on interproximal plaque

after chewing gum

no chewing gum

pH of interproximal plaque

minutes after eating

Fig. 2.4 Effects of chewing gum on interproximal plaque. Two hours after a meal, not followed by cleaning teeth, the interproximal plaque still shows a low pH. Chewing two pellets of sugared chewing gum for 20 minutes after eating is sufficient to raise the pH back to normal.

Fluoride ions are present within tooth structure in concentrations as high as 2500–4000 p.p.m (132–210 μmol/l). at the surface of enamel but the concentration in saliva may be as low as 0.03 p.p.m (1.6 μmol/l). The incorporation of fluorides into teeth during development, or the use of topical fluoride after eruption, enhances the availability of these ions, leading to increased inhibition of demineralisation and enhancement of remineralisation when acid ions interact with the tooth surface.

Daily consumption of water containing fluoride at 1 mg/l (52.6 μmol/l), for the whole of life, increases resistance to caries in all age groups from infancy to old age. Topical applications of fluoride can also help inhibit dental caries in those with a high caries rate.

Summary

Fluoride

Reacts directly with enamel and dentine and produces several effects.

- Forms fluorapatite, which is less soluble than hydroxyapatite
- Inhibits demineralisation
- Enhances remineralisation
- Inhibits bacterial metabolism
- Reduces 'wettability' of tooth structure
- Inhibits plaque formation

Inhibition of caries

Fluoride inhibits the development of caries by:

- inhibiting the demineralisation process and enhancing the normal remineralisation process by preferentially reacting with hydroxyapatite breakdown products to form fluorapatite or a fluoride-enriched apatite.
- inhibiting bacterial metabolism.

Methods of inhibition

The most efficient inhibition of caries occurs through frequent daily contact of low concentrations of fluoride ion with the tooth surface to inhibit demineralisation and enhance remineralisation of that surface. The optimal level necessary to achieve this will vary for each person according to the level of acid ions present in relation to the level of balancing protective agents.

High concentration fluorides store excess fluoride ion as CaF_2 around the apatite crystals. This may lead to heavy remineralisation at the surface of enamel lesions and the fluoride ion may not be able initially to penetrate more deeply into the subsurface body of the lesion. Subsequent acid challenge will progressively ionise this layer to permit free fluoride ions to penetrate more deeply. However, even this additional CaF_2 is quickly lost in the highly acid environment found in the patient with active caries and needs to be replenished more frequently to be effective.

Effect on established lesions

The fluoride ion will not only prevent initial lesions developing, but will also stabilise established lesions. That is, it can:

- contribute to remineralisation of incipient enamel caries
- partly remineralise carious dentine and thus slow down or arrest the caries process in the cavitated coronal lesion
- remineralise root surface lesions to the extent that they may not need restoration.

Topical fluoride is more effective in inhibiting smooth surface caries and in aiding remineralisation of enamel or cementum–dentine. It is less effective in fissure or interproximal caries because of the difficulty of removing stubborn or mature plaque. Daily application of topical fluoride to demineralised root surfaces over a period of 2–4 months will lead to significant hardening of the exposed dentine, indicating that a remineralising balance has been established. Deep and extensive root caries can be hardened within the same period of time but requires the use of higher concentrations of fluoride. The surfaces of such remineralised lesions can become glass-like in texture because of hypermineralisation.

NATURE OF THE ACID ION INTERACTION WITH APATITE AT THE TOOTH SURFACE

To understand the mechanism of the carious process it is necessary to understand the basic nature of the chemical reactions that occur at the tooth surface.

Demineralisation

The mineral component of enamel, dentine and cementum is hydroxyapatite, $Ca_{10}(PO_4)_6(OH)_2$. In a neutral environment, hydroxyapatite is in equilibrium with the local aqueous environment, which is saturated with Ca^{2+} and PO_4^{3-} ions.

Hydroxyapatite is reactive to hydrogen ions at pH 5.5 (the critical pH for hydroxyapatite) and below. H^+ reacts preferentially with the phosphate groups in the aqueous environment immediately adjacent to the crystal surface. The process can be thought of as conversion of PO_4^{3-} to HPO_4^{2-} by the addition of H^+ and the H^+ being buffered at the same time. The HPO_4^{2-} is then not able to contribute to the normal hydroxyapatite equilibrium because it contains PO_4, not HPO_4, and the hydroxyapatite crystal therefore dissolves. This is termed demineralisation.

Remineralisation

The demineralisation process can be reversed if the pH is neutral and there are sufficient Ca^{2+} and PO_4^{3-} ions in the immediate environment. Either the apatite dissolution products can reach neutrality by buffering or the Ca^{2+} and PO_4^{3-} ions in saliva can inhibit the process of dissolution through the common ion effect. This enables rebuilding of partly dissolved apatite crystals and is termed remineralisation.

This interaction can be greatly enhanced by the presence of fluoride ion at the reaction site. The overall reaction, which may be characterised as the 'demineralisation–remineralisation' process, can be symbolised in general terms as shown in **Figure 2.5**.

The chemical basis of the demineralisation–remineralisation process is similar for enamel, dentine and root cementum. However, the different structures and relative quantity of the mineral and organic tissue content of each of these materials causes significant differences in the nature and progress of the carious lesion. These differences will be described later.

Acid reaction with apatite at the tooth surface

Following eruption there is a process of continuing mineralisation of enamel from salivary calcium and phosphate (see Chapter 1). Initially, enamel apatite contains many carbonate and magnesium ions, which are highly soluble in even mild acidic conditions. However, there is a rapid and extensive exchange of hydroxyl and fluoride ions as the magnesium and carbonate are dissolved, leading to a more 'mature' enamel with a greater resistance to acid ion challenge. This level of maturity, or acid resistance, can be greatly enhanced by the presence of fluoride.

When a pulse of acid ions is generated at the tooth surface, regardless of the level of maturity, the general reaction can be symbolised by the diagram in **Figure 2.6**.

As the pH decreases the acid ions react, principally with the phosphates in saliva and plaque (or calculus), until the critical pH for dissociation of hydroxyapatite is reached at approximately pH 5.5–5.2. Further decrease in pH results in progressive interaction of the acid ions with the phosphate groups of hydroxyapatite, causing partial or full dissolution of the surface crystallite. Stored fluoride released in this process reacts with the Ca^{2+} and HPO_4^{2-} ion breakdown products, forming fluorapatite, or fluoride-enriched apatite. If the pH decreases further below 4.5, which is the critical pH for fluorapatite dissolution, even fluorapatite will then dissolve. If acid ions are neutralised, and the Ca^{2+} and HPO_4^{2-} ions are retained in this hypothetical model, the reverse processes of remineralisation are able to occur as shown in Figure 2.6.

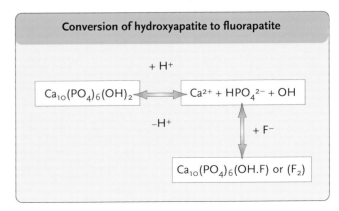

Conversion of hydroxyapatite to fluorapatite

$$Ca_{10}(PO_4)_6(OH)_2 \xrightarrow[-H^+]{+H^+} Ca^{2+} + HPO_4^{2-} + OH$$

$$\xrightarrow{+F^-} Ca_{10}(PO_4)_6(OH.F) \text{ or } (F_2)$$

Fig. 2.5 Conversion of hydroxyapatite to fluorapatite. The chemical reaction taking place at the tooth surface is shown.

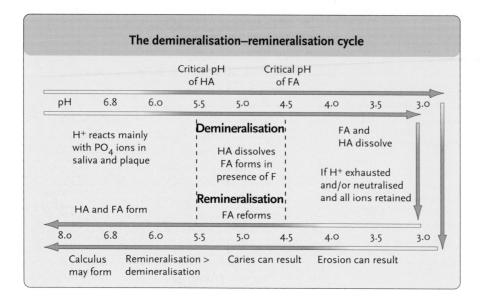

The demineralisation–remineralisation cycle

Critical pH of HA   Critical pH of FA

pH   6.8   6.0   5.5   5.0   4.5   4.0   3.5   3.0

H^+ reacts mainly with PO_4 ions in saliva and plaque

Demineralisation
HA dissolves
FA forms in presence of F

FA and HA dissolve

If H^+ exhausted and/or neutralised and all ions retained

Remineralisation
FA reforms

HA and FA form

8.0   6.8   6.0   5.5   5.0   4.5   4.0   3.5   3.0

Calculus may form   Remineralisation > demineralisation   Caries can result   Erosion can result

Fig. 2.6 The demineralisation–remineralisation cycle. A conceptual chart to demonstrate the levels of pH at which the stages of the demineralisation–remineralisation cycle occur.
F, fluoride; FA, fluorapatite; HA, hydroxyapatite.

In terms of the cycle proposed, in reality, there will be variation in both the level of acid ion production as well as neutralisation under differing situations in the oral cavity. Furthermore, Ca^{2+} and HPO_4^{2-} ions usually diffuse to the tooth surface and may be lost, particularly in the presence of more severe demineralisation. Partial replacement by salivary ions may result in remineralisation occurring in the surface layers, and over time, even in the deeper regions of demineralisation within the lesion (**Fig. 2.7**).

Possible sequelae

It is apparent from the pH cycle diagram that, depending on the strength of the acid that is present, the frequency and duration of its production and the remineralisation potential in each particular situation, any one of the following sequelae can occur:

- the enamel may continue to mature
- chronic caries may develop – slow demineralisation with active remineralisation
- rapid (rampant) caries may arise – rapid demineralisation with inadequate remineralisation
- erosion may occur – very rapid demineralisation with no remineralisation at all.

At every food intake there will be an acid-induced demineralisation in areas of tooth surface beneath mature plaque.

If eating frequency of sugar is low, local fluoride concentration is high and salivary buffering is good, then the mineral loss will be reversible (that is, remineralisation will occur).

If eating frequency is high, local fluoride concentration is low and salivary buffering is poor, then demineralisation outweighs remineralisation. This situation is conducive to dental caries.

It is important for the clinician to identify whether the carious process is chronic or rapidly active as this will determine the degree of urgency and intensity of the control phase. The characteristics of chronic and rampant caries will be discussed.

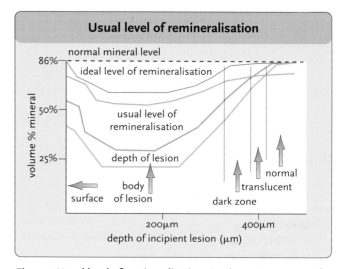

Usual level of remineralisation

86%   normal mineral level
ideal level of remineralisation
50%   usual level of remineralisation
25%   depth of lesion
body of lesion   normal
surface   translucent
dark zone
200μm   400μm
depth of incipient lesion (μm)

volume % mineral

Fig. 2.7 Usual level of remineralisation. A schematic concept of the amount of remineralisation which may take place in enamel following demineralisation. The level will not achieve the theoretical normal but will be adequate to enhance the physical properties of the enamel.

THE PROGRESSING CARIOUS LESION

Early enamel lesion

The initial enamel lesion results when the pH level at the tooth surface exceeds that which can be counterbalanced by remineralisation, but is not low enough to inhibit surface remineralisation. The acid ions penetrate deeply into the prism sheath porosities, leading to subsurface demineralisation. The tooth surface may remain intact through remineralisation, which occurs preferentially at the surface due to increased levels of calcium, phosphate, fluoride ions, and buffering by salivary products (**Fig. 2.8**).

24–37

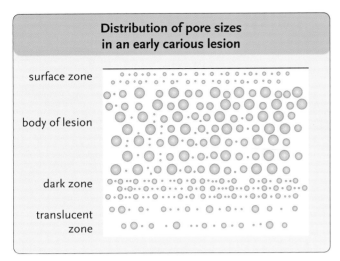

Fig. 2.8 **Distribution of pore sizes in an early carious lesion** (see also Fig. 2.10).

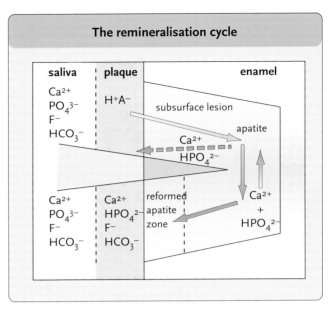

Fig. 2.9 **The remineralisation cycle.** Note that the factors which favour this cycle include increased Ca^{2+}, increased PO_4^{3-}, raised pH and the presence of F^-.

Clinical characteristics
The clinical characteristics of such lesions are:
- loss of normal translucency of enamel with a chalky white appearance, particularly when dehydrated
- a fragile surface layer susceptible to damage from probing, particularly in pits and fissures
- increased porosity, particularly of the subsurface, with increased potential for uptake of stain (**Fig. 2.9**)
- reduced density of the subsurface that may be detectable radiographically or with transillumination
- a potential for remineralisation, with an increased resistance to further acid challenge. The reversed lesion will either regain normal translucency or the chalky appearance may remain and take up stain.

The size of the subsurface lesion may progress until the underlying dentine becomes significantly demineralised. The caries, particularly interproximal lesions, will then become detectable radiographically. Even so, the surface of the tooth may remain intact, and the lesion may still be reversible. This lesion is different from that of erosion, which is described in Chapter 4.

Difficulty of diagnosis
It must be emphasised that assessment of the rate of progress of the lesion at both the incipient and more advanced stages is largely subjective. A wide range of other information relating to past dental history, dietary history and so forth must be investigated to enable the operator to assess the probable demineralisation–remineralisation balance present in each patient's mouth. In reversing incipient enamel lesions, the ideal is to regain the original density of enamel throughout the lesion. In reality, there may be only partial replacement of subsurface density. Even so the partially remineralised incipient lesion of the enamel is more resistant to further acid demineralisation than normal enamel. Hence, it is preferable, where the patient is maintaining good home care, to observe the lesion over time rather than restore the cavity immediately and deny possible remineralisation.

The advancing coronal lesion
If the demineralisation–remineralisation imbalance continues, the surface of the incipient lesion collapses through dissolution of apatite or fracture of the weakened crystallite, resulting in cavitation (**Fig. 2.10**). Plaque can now be retained within the depths of the cavity and the remineralisation phase is rendered more difficult and less effective. The dentine–pulp complex will become involved at this point but there can still be fluctuations in the degree of activity.

Caries into dentine
After bacteria have invaded dentine, the process of demineralisation continues to be driven by dietary substrate. Bacteria will produce acid to dissolve the hydroxyapatite of deeper dentine so there is a front of demineralisation in advance of the bacterial invasion. There may be some pioneer bacteria in, or even beyond, the area of demineralisation, but these are not clinically relevant.

Both the texture and the colour of dentine changes as the lesion advances (**Fig. 2.11**). The texture (hardness) change is caused by demineralisation. The colour will darken because of bacterial products and stains from foods and beverages. In chronic lesions the colour change will be more pronounced and the floor of the cavity will be firmer in texture.

The slowly progressing lesion

If the lesion is left to extend through the dentine the enamel will become progressively undermined and weakened. Collapse of the unsupported enamel may eventually result in a wide open cavity that is relatively self-cleansing and plaque may not be so readily retained. The caries process may then slow down, leading to the development of a hard leathery floor on the cavity which is more or less inactive.

The rampant lesion

In rampant caries the process evolves rapidly. Cavitation in enamel occurs quickly and the dentine floor of the cavity becomes softer to the touch but without significant colour change. The pulp is at risk of irreversible damage because the remineralising and sclerosing process which normally seals the tubules will be unable to keep pace. Rapid protection of the dentine–pulp complex is essential if loss of vitality is to be avoided.

Control of the lesion

It is possible to arrest the progress of dentinal caries at any stage by sealing the cavity and isolating the bacterial flora from its nutrient source, that is, dietary carbohydrate. The remaining bacteria will become dormant and progress in the lesion will cease.

Root surface caries

The early root surface lesion may be very difficult to detect because there is likely to be little or no colour change, only a modification in surface texture (**Fig. 2.12**). The mineral content of dentine is much lower than that of enamel and, when the dentine becomes demineralised, the collagen matrix will rapidly be exposed but it will retain its physical structure so long as it remains well hydrated. The exposed matrix is susceptible to physical damage but appears to be readily remineralised through the repair mechanisms of saliva if the demineralisation–remineralisation balance is stabilised. The surface of advanced root caries lesions may therefore be rehardened through the application of topical fluorides or remineralising solutions and the progression of the lesion may be slowed or arrested.

The advancing lesion will darken over time through bacterial activity and the uptake of dyes from food (**Fig. 2.13**). Identification is then easier but it is always difficult to define the full extent of the lesion. As with all dentine caries there will be an affected zone where the demineralisation is in advance of the bacterial infection. This will be a softened, demineralised, colourless zone of dentine on the floor of the cavity which should not be removed during cavity debridement because it can be sealed from the oral flora and subsequently remineralised. Sealing the surface assists the natural repair mechanisms and leads to reduced challenge to the pulp.

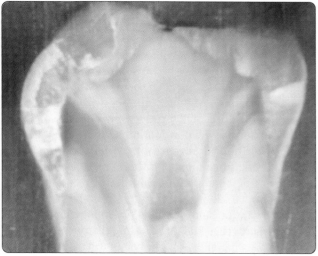

Fig. 2.10 Progress into dentine. The pattern of progress of caries into dentine. The demineralisation follows the dentine tubules downwards and inwards towards the pulp.

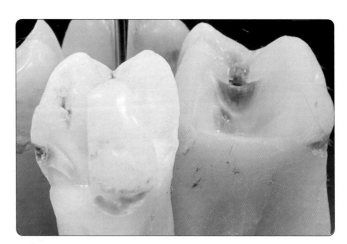

Fig. 2.11 Progress into dentine. Note in the proximal lesion on the left the typical penetration towards the pulp. The occlusal lesion on the right shows penetration to be approximately twice as deep as it is wide.

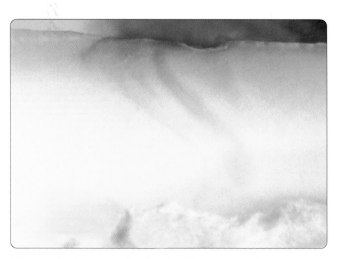

Fig. 2.12 Root caries lesion. Section through an early root caries lesion under transmitted light (x35). Note change in translucency of underlying dentine tubules over a broad area.

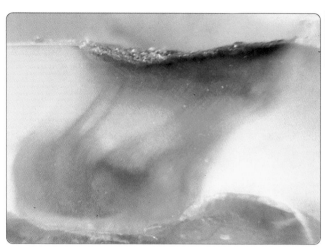

Fig. 2.13 Advanced root caries lesion. The root caries lesion is further advanced, with diffuse distribution on the surface and no clear definition of the margin. Section through a more advanced lesion under polarised light, imbided in quinoline (x100).

FURTHER READING

Featherstone JDB, McIntyre JM, Fu J. Physico-chemical aspects of root caries progression. In: *Dentine and dentine reactions in the oral cavity.* Thylstrup A, Leach SA, Qvist V, eds. Oxford: IRL Press; 1987.

Jensen ME, Wefel JS. Human plaque pH responses to meals and the effect of chewing gum. *Brit Dent J* 1989; **23**: 204–8.

Kidd EA, Jayston-Bechal S. *Essentials of dental caries: the disease and its management.* Dental Practitioners Handbook 31. Bristol: Wright; 1987.

Larsen MJ. Dissolution of enamel. *Scand J Dent Res* 1973; **81**: 518–22.

Newbrun, E. *Cariology.* Chicago: Quintessence Publishing; 1990.

Nikiforuk G. *Understanding Dental caries 1. Aetiology and mechanisms: basic and clinical aspects.* Basel: Karger; 1985.

Silverstone LM, Hicks MJ, Featherstone MJ. *Dynamic factors affecting lesion initiation and progression in human dental enamel II. Surface morphology of sound enamel and caries like lesions of enamel.* Chicago: Quintessence International; 1988.

Silverstone LM, Johnson NW, Hardie JM, Williams RAD. *Dental caries: aetiology, pathology and prevention.* London: Macmillan; 1981.

Ten-Cate JM. 'In vitro' studies on the effects of fluoride on de- and remineralisation. *J Dent Res* 1990; **69**(Special Issue):614–19.

Tenovuo J. Oral defence factors in the elderly. *Endod Dent Traumatol* 1992; **8**:93–8.

Thylstrup A, Fejerskov O. *Textbook of cariology.* Copenhagen: Munksgaard; 1994.

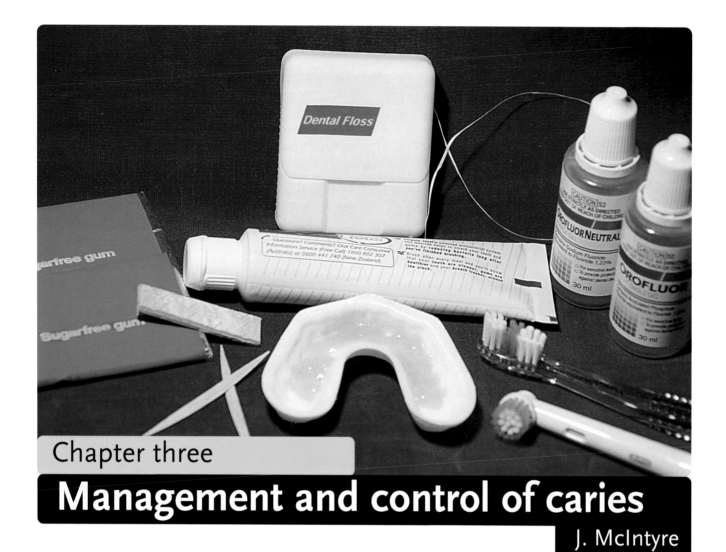

Chapter three

Management and control of caries

J. McIntyre

Using an understanding of the demineralisation–remineralisation cycle discussed in Chapter 2, patients can be advised on strategies to prevent or reverse dental caries.

It is necessary to determine for each patient which is the dominant factor or factors causing the disease. It could be a highly cariogenic diet, poor plaque control or a serious depletion of natural protective factors, causing an otherwise acceptable diet to result in caries.

Irrespective of the cause, it will be necessary first to educate the patient and then to gain control by either reducing the demineralising factors or enhancing the protective factors.

REDUCING THE DEMINERALISING FACTORS

Frequency of fermentable carbohydrate intake

This is the most common and significant cariogenic factor. If acid ions are persistently produced in plaque over sufficient time, they will exhaust the buffering capacity of the saliva, and the remineralising process will no longer be effective.

Where this is the major aetiological factor it will be necessary to work with the patient at recording dietary routines and exploring alternatives to the highly cariogenic component. Continuous monitoring of the effect will be required.

Effective oral hygiene

Notes

Brush teeth before or after eating.

Frequency of sugar intake is the major cause of caries.

First daily clean

The first oral hygiene routine should be carried out in the morning either before or after breakfast. The object is removal of plaque rather than the elimination of food debris so cleaning immediately before eating is just as effective as cleaning after a meal.

Second daily clean

The second oral hygiene routine should be carried out just before retiring for the night. During sleep the salivary flow virtually ceases and any available buffering capacity is lost. Therefore removal of all plaque should be completed with diligence and any prescribed preventive medicines, such as topical fluoride, should be applied at this time. In the absence of plaque, the fluoride will be taken up into the tooth structure more effectively and the subsequent lack of saliva will be of less consequence.

Frequent daily clean

In the presence of rampant caries, oral hygiene routines should be undertaken either before or after each food intake to encourage the patient to recognise the important part played by fermentable carbohydrates in the caries process. Maintenance of the fluoride concentration on the tooth surface is also desirable, so the frequent application of a fluoride-containing tooth paste will help.

ENHANCING THE PROTECTIVE FACTORS

The role of saliva

Saliva is a significant protective factor because it bathes the entire dentition constantly. It is a supersaturated solution of calcium and phosphate ions, contains a low concentration of fluoride ions and has considerable buffering capacity. The flow rate is not necessarily reduced with advancing age but many pharmaceutical products will affect the flow, and these are often prescribed for the ageing patient.

Salivary flow rate

Normal flow rate varies considerably. The unstimulated flow rate is usually 0.3 ml/min. Stimulation by chewing, acidic flavours or conditioned reflex will usually result in an average flow rate of 1.5–2.5 ml/min.

Notes

Xerostomia

A stimulated salivary flow rate below 0.7 ml/min.
• generally the result of pharmaceutical routines
• not necessarily associated with advancing years

Xerostomia is a condition where the stimulated salivary flow rate is reduced to below 0.7 ml/min. Under these circumstances there may be a high caries rate, particularly if other factors have altered at the same time. In the presence of a dry mouth, patients often will seek comfort by eating sweets or drinking sugared drinks more frequently, exceeding the buffering capacity of the saliva.

Effect of drugs

Most mood-altering drugs, such as the tricyclic anti-depressants and antiParkinsonian drugs, will contribute to a reduction in salivary flow (**Fig. 3.1**). Nonprescription psychotrophic agents such as marijuana can produce a similar effect. Where there is severe salivary reduction caused by a particular prescribed drug, it may be possible to try an alternative. However, changing drug routines and

Reduced salivary flow	
drug-induced	antihypertensives anticholinergic antiParkinsonian psychotropic sedatives
anxiety	severe emotional disorders
medical complications	diabetes, malnutrition, glandular infection or obstruction, radiation of head or neck (>70 grays in 6 weeks = total xerostomia) Sjögren's syndrome

Fig. 3.1 Reduced salivary flow. The main causes of xerostomia are shown.

altering the balance of a prescribed series is often a long-term, complex process and should be undertaken only with the cooperation of the other health professionals involved. Even so, modification may be justified if the caries rate is excessive.

Effect of radiation therapy

Radiation therapy in the region of the head and neck may cause xerostomia. The secretory cells of all salivary glands may be irrevocably damaged by large doses of ionising radiation and xerostomia may reach a peak within 6 weeks of commencement of radiation therapy. A slight increase of flow may occur gradually but a severe xerostomia may persist for many years.

Artificial saliva

The discomfort of severe xerostomia can be reduced by the use of artificial salivas, which contain a variety of electrolytes normally present in saliva, and have a similar viscosity. The regular use of sugar-free chewing gum may also provide some relief, as well as reducing caries risk. Great care must be observed in prescribing stimulants to salivary flow because citric acid is often incorporated in commonly used sialogogues and this will lower the intra-oral pH.

The role of fluorides

Theoretically, it should be possible to control all caries, providing there is sufficient fluoride ion in contact with the tooth surface throughout each demineralisation episode. However, when the pH is maintained below 4.5 (the critical pH for fluorapatite) for prolonged periods, the potential for remineralisation will be inhibited. If the normal cariogenic activity from fermenting carbohydrate is taking place, and it is supplemented by periodic contact with highly acid foods or beverages (e.g. cola drinks), then even fluoride ion will be unable to totally inhibit the demineralisation process. In such cases it is essential to assist the patient in controlling the source of strong acids.

The most common fluoride compounds applied topically are: NaF, SnF_2, NH_2F, acidulated phosphate fluoride (APF), and Na_2FPO_3 (sodium monofluorophosphate). The vehicle most commonly used is a dentifrice but there are a variety of other methods of routine application (**Fig. 3.2**). Care must be taken in prescribing because some of them may cause superficial harm. For example, the acidulated gels provide the highest fluoride uptake but at the same time they are likely to remove the glaze from ceramics or roughen the surface of a glass–ionomer or some glass-filled composite resins if applied too often.

Fig. 3.2 Vehicles for topical fluorides.

Vehicles for topical fluorides

Fluoride-containing dentifrices
- Usually as NaF (1.0%), Na_2FPO_3 (0.76%) or SnF_2 (0.4%) = (concentration of fluoride ion by weight).
In general there is approximately 1 mg/g of available fluoride (1000 p.p.m.).
A toothbrush completely covered in paste holds approximately 1.5 mg of fluoride.

Concentrated gels
- APF 1.23% – contains approximately 12.3 mg of fluoride ion/gm or ml of gel or 12 300 p.p.m. fluoride ion at pH 3.5.
- NaF 2% – contains approximately 10 mg of fluoride ion/gm or ml of gel or 10 000 p.p.m. fluoride ion at pH 7.0.
Note that APF gel is more effective than NaF in providing prolonged protection against caries and in counteracting the effects of strong acids. However, it is contraindicated where glass-based restorative materials are present – such as ceramics, glass–ionomers and some glass-filled composite resins.

Concentrated solutions
- SnF_2 20% – dissolved under heat in glycerine for stabilisation, diluted for local topical application as required.

Mouth rinses
- Ranging from 0.02% to 0.2% NaF (0.1–1.0 mg of fluoride per millilitre (100–1000 p.p.m.) of mouth rinse).
- May be acidulated.

Varnishes
- 1.7% NaF in viscous resins/varnishes contains 8 mg of fluoride per millilitre of varnish.
- 5% NaF in viscous varnishes contain 25 mg of fluoride per millilitre.

Note – For patients with a high caries rate, supplemental topical fluoride use should be considered.

Schedules of application

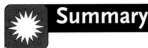

Summary

Factors affecting efficiency of fluoride application:
- oral clearance rate
- concentration applied
- time: overnight best
- duration: 3 minutes minimum
- form: acidulated phosphate fluoride gel offers best uptake

The minimum use of topical fluoride for all patients, irrespective of the apparent caries risk, should be a morning and evening application of fluoride dentifrice as part of the basic daily oral hygiene routine (**Fig. 3.3**).

The following factors should be taken into account:
- Retention rate depends on initial concentration applied. Under normal circumstances, retention rate from a low-concentration mouth rinse is relatively high. The concentrated gels should be used only in the most active cases of caries.
- Time of day for application is important. Application immediately before going to bed will result in prolonged retention because there is a normal decrease in unstimulated salivary flow rate during sleep.
- Duration of application should be at least 3 minutes. Neutral gels work well where there is porous enamel or exposed dentine present on most of the surfaces at risk and the acid environment will aid in fluoride transport into the tooth structure.
- APF gel provides higher uptake as stored fluoride and thus provides a more prolonged period of protection.

If the caries risk is low, use an acidulated gel, professionally applied at 6–12-month intervals.

If the caries rate is high, use the acidulated gel at 6-week intervals. This can be applied at home using a custom made 'pull-down' tray. However, acidulated topical fluoride gels have the potential for etching ceramic or glass-containing restorations if used frequently or for prolonged periods.

Fig. 3.3 Guidelines for additional fluoride therapy.

Guidelines for additional fluoride therapy	
Clinical situation	**Therapy guideline**
To maintain a low rate of caries.	Morning and night fluoride toothpaste plus 12-monthly topical fluoride gel.
Extra protection – orthodontic treatment, partial dentures, pregnancy.	Morning and night fluoride toothpaste plus 0.02% NaF mouthrinse daily.
One to two cavities per year, over 7 years old.	Morning and night fluoride toothpaste plus 0.2% NaF mouthrinse twice per week or 2% NaF gel every 2 weeks.
Three or more new cavities per year, over 7 years old.	Morning and night fluoride toothpaste plus 0.2% NaF mouthrinse daily before bed or 2.0% NaF gel weekly.
Children under 6 years of age with high caries rate.	Supervised brush twice per day with fluoride paste. 1.23% APF gel: very small quantity painted on teeth by parent weekly.
Very dry mouth, scheduled for radiation, surgery or drugs affecting salivary glands.	Morning and night fluoride toothpaste. 0.2% NaF rinse after lunch, and on retiring, or 1.23% APF gel or 2% NaF gel nightly. May use artificial saliva.
Severe erosion – acid reflux, frequent vomiting, excess citrus, wine taster.	1.23% APF gel self-application on retiring during active erosion phase.
Hypersensitive teeth.	Apply fluoride varnish. Paint area with 2% NaF gel twice per day until sensitivity controlled.
Noncompliant home users.	6-weekly visits to the clinic for supervised self-application of 1.23% APF gel.

Fluoride safety factors for adults

Be aware

Fluoride safety for adults

Maximum dose for adults
- 5 mg of fluoride per kilogram of body weight per day

The probable toxic dosage of fluoride ion is 5 mg of fluoride ion per kilogram of body weight per day. For the frail, chronically ill adult, this dosage should be considered high and prescribed doses kept well below this level.

Steps should be taken to minimise ingestion during application. In the office, use adequate suction. During home application, allow the patient to drool liberally over a sink. Have the patient spit out the excess for 1 minute after each application. The amount swallowed will then be well below those levels considered necessary to raise total blood levels to those considered likely to cause chronic toxicity.

The fluoride ion may be retained in the oral cavity for prolonged periods with a relatively slow rate of clearance by ingestion and absorption. It is therefore essential for dentists to prescribe the minimal dose necessary to gain the required result and instruct patients very clearly in the correct means of self-application.

Fluoride safety factors for children

Be aware

Fluoride safety for children

Maximum dose for children
- 5.0 mg of fluoride per kilogram of body weight per day

NOTE – A daily dose greater than 0.07 mg of fluoride per kilogram of body weight per day for children with developing teeth may result in fluorosis. Use topical fluorides with caution

The probable toxic dose of fluoride for children is 5 mg of fluoride ion per kilogram of body weight per day. Containers of fluoride tablets or drops used to supplement systemic fluoride intake should not contain more than 100 mg fluoride ion in total. They should be kept well out of the reach of young children to avoid accidental overdose.

Careful supervision of the amounts of fluoride toothpaste used daily is important because ingestion of more than 1 mg fluoride ion daily may lead to fluorosis. Regular fluoride-containing dentifrice holds up to 0.1% fluoride ion by weight, so a full brush head of paste contains approximately 1.5 mg of fluoride ion.

Particularly for small children, use a 'junior paste' which contains only 0.04% of fluoride ion by weight. Children under 3 years of age are likely to swallow all unused paste unless carefully watched, and those up to 6 years of age may regularly ingest approximately 30% of paste used.

Concentrated gels, and mouth rinses containing 0.2% NaF, should not be prescribed for young children even when infant caries has occurred. Localised application of varnish, or a more concentrated solution, may be undertaken by a dental professional.

Protective sealants

Fissure sealants are a proven protective measure against the development of carious lesions in pits and fissures in children. For the high-risk teenager or young adult patient there is increasing evidence for the benefits of sealing the pits and fissures on the occlusal surfaces of newly erupted teeth using either resin or glass–ionomer cement. Even if the seal is applied subsequent to some degree of demineralisation, the process will be arrested and bacterial activity is likely to become dormant (Chapter 11).

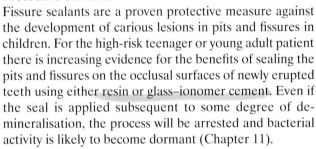

CARIES RISK ASSESSMENT

Caries risk estimation for each patient leads to the development of a thorough picture of the patient's present and future dental health, with an understanding of the need for preventive or surgical intervention. Options for future dental management, and the anticipated cost in time and money of the various options, will be clearer.

The essential components of a proper caries risk-assessment programme include a careful oral examination, a detailed medical and dental history, diagnostic testing of the oral environment and an understanding of the patient's attitude and behaviour.

Examination

A thorough oral examination should assess the extent and location of incipient lesions, cavitated lesions and restorations. It should include an assessment of the activity status of the lesions and the condition of the restorations.

The following evidence should be carefully gathered and recorded:
- Coronal surfaces should be examined for change in colour and translucency and for the presence of cavitation. The use of a fine, sharp explorer is valuable in detecting surface roughness and cavitation within fissures but should be used with caution to avoid damage to a demineralised surface. Bite-wing radiography will reveal the presence of incipient or more advanced lesions under fissures or on proximal surfaces. Occasionally, transillumination may suggest early caries but this should be confirmed by other diagnostic means. Techniques using electronic fissure testing, lasers, ultrasound techniques and fibre-optic probes are being developed to enhance clinical ability to detect the early lesion.
- On the exposed root surface, incipient caries may be

Notes

Examination
- Coronal surface
  colour
  translucency
  cavitation
- Root surface
  texture
  colour
- Radiographs
  cavitation
  pulp
  alveolus
- Transillumination
  possible
- Electronic caries detection
  possible

difficult to detect visually. Demineralised root surfaces are noticeably softer than normal, so gentle exploration using light pressure with a blunt probe (such as a small plastic or periodontal probe) is recommended. Take care to avoid producing cavitation, which may subsequently harbour plaque.

- It is important to be conservative in the interpretation of radiographic evidence of small interproximal lesions, sticky fissures, or white spot lesions. These may have been present for some time and be totally arrested and stable and may not necessarily be evidence of a high caries rate. If these lesions can be remineralised they will be stronger and far less susceptible to further acid challenge than the original tooth surface. Follow-up radiographic examination to assess any change in lesion depth is important.
- For a stable lesion, it is far better to observe progress over time and restore only when essential. Placement of any restoration will weaken remaining tooth structure and no restoration can be regarded as completely permanent.

Patient history

It is necessary to take into account the wider range of historical evidence, including the current status of the major aetiological factors, before deciding if an incipient lesion is able to be arrested or will progress to cavitation. This is particularly so when the initial examination of the teeth suggests a moderate or high rate of caries either now or in the past. The following information should be obtained:

- A thorough history of caries, when restorations were placed, and frequency of repair or replacement.
- An outline of present and past dietary patterns, in particular frequency of refined carbohydrate intake and consumption of acid drinks or foods.

- Past and present fluoride contact, both systemic and topical.
- Medical or social factors that may affect dental health; for example, drugs that may affect salivary flow or that contain high concentrations of sweetening agents.
- Physical or medical problems that may impair a patient's ability to carry out oral hygiene or that exert control over their diet.
- Emotional or other factors resulting in high levels of stress.
- Illnesses or organic problems or medications that result in frequent gastric acid regurgitation.

Diagnostic tests

Summary

Diagnostic tests
- salivary flow: stimulated flow rate ≥ 0.7 ml/min is considered normal
- buffering capacity: low value is a cause for concern
- microbiology: *Streptococcus mutans*, *Lactobacillus* – excessive counts indicate increased risk

Quantity and quality of saliva

This is initially determined by visual observation and questioning. The extremely dry mouth may be identifiable by oral examination. However, depending on cause, this may be periodic in nature, and the patient should be questioned as to whether it is always as dry. Patient experience of dry mouth is very subjective, and is not a reliable indication in itself. Sometimes, the statement that they frequently drink water or other fluids is an indicator of prolonged dryness. Carry out a stimulated salivary flow rate test by asking the patient to chew paraffin wax or gum or use a drop of citric acid on the tongue. Collect the saliva in a small graduated vial over a 2-minute period. Stimulated flow rate of less than 0.7 ml/min should be followed by a further assessment of other risk factors.

Buffering capacity of saliva

It is possible to measure buffering capacity using commercially available kits. However, salivary buffering capacity is usually proportional to flow rate, so the latter is generally considered to be a reasonable indicator.

Microbiological tests

Determination of *Streptococcus mutans* and *Lactobacillus* counts per volume of saliva provides some degree of correlation with risk. *Streptococcus mutans* indicates the potential for caries and will be present when there is active caries in the dentine. However, the correlation is not always reliable, and these results should be considered along with other diagnostic evidence.

Patient attitude and behaviour

An assessment of the patient's interest in altering an obviously caries-active environment is perhaps the most important prediction of future caries risk.

No matter how accurate the determination of natural susceptibility to caries, future risk can only be altered confidently where the patient is committed to altering the home-care factors that are necessary to improve control of the demineralising balance.

The assessment of patient interest does not require more than a basic understanding of behavioural principles. It largely involves applied common sense, some degree of empathy for the patient's situation, and a willingness to communicate well in discussing the nature of the patient's problem. Agreement on preferred professional and home-care management options is required, as well as a reasonable schedule of appointments for immediate treatment, followed up with systematic recalls.

PREVENTIVE MANAGEMENT IN RELATION TO RESTORATIVE MANAGEMENT

Successful management of active caries is dependent on control of the demineralisation–remineralisation balance. The preventive management programme should be instituted before commencing major permanent restorative work. It must be continued while the work is in progress, and be maintained indefinitely following successful completion. The form and intensity of the preventive programme will depend on the changing balance of aetiological factors over time.

Once a favourable balance has been achieved, and restorations are complete, an appropriate recall programme must be instituted. The recall interval will depend on the final risk assessment after completion of the restorations and it may vary from as little as 1 month to as much as 2 years.

FURTHER READING

Anderson MH, Molvar MP, Powell LV. Treating dental caries as an infectious disease. *Oper Dent* 1991; **16**: 21–8.

Axelsson P. The current role of pharmaceuticals in prevention of caries and periodontal disease. *Int Dent J* 1993; **43**:473–82.

Bowen W, Taleak L. *Cariology for the Nineties*. Rochester, NY: University of Rochester Press; 1993.

Edgar WM. Saliva and dental health, clinical implications of saliva: report of a consensus meeting. *Br Dent J* 1990; **169**; 96–8.

Kidd EA, Jayston-Bechal S. *Essentials of dental caries: the disease and its management.* Dental Practitioners Handbook 31. Bristol: Wright; 1987.

Massler M. Changing concepts in the treatment of carious lesions. *Br Dent J* 1967; **123**:547–8.

Massler M. Preventive endodontics: Vital pulp therapy. *Dent Clin North Am* 1967; 663–73.

Newbrun, E. *Cariology*. Chicago: Quintessence Publishing; 1989.

Nikiforuk G. *Understanding dental caries 2. Prevention: Basic and clinical aspects.* Basel: Karger; 1985.

Thylstrup A, Fejerskov O. *Textbook of clinical cariology.*, Munksgaard: Copenhagen; 1994.

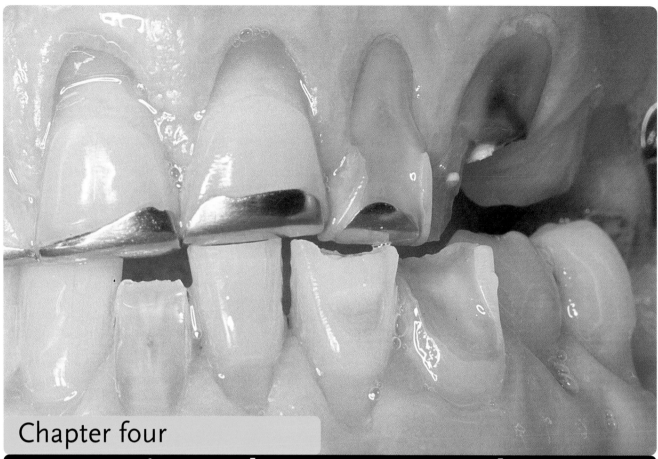

Chapter four

Noncarious changes to tooth crowns

J.A. Kaidonis • L.G. Richards • G.C. Townsend

Apart from dental caries and iatrogenic modification such as cavity preparation by a dentist, the main processes that can change the morphology of a tooth during its lifetime are abrasion, attrition, erosion and fracture. Modern dentistry has evolved into an art and science aimed at restoring the broken-down dentition to its original newly erupted morphology on the assumption that the unworn tooth has the ideal functional form.

A variety of geometric concepts of occlusion have evolved over the years and occlusal reconstruction has tended to follow formal guidelines. This is regardless of the great variability that exists in the architecture of the stomatognathic system within and between populations, as well as in the same individual over time. Fossil records, anthropological research and studies in comparative anatomy, show that the processes responsible for tooth reduction have acted on teeth since prehistoric times. It is therefore reasonable to recognise and accept tooth wear as a normal physiological process, no different from ageing. Changes to masticatory structures as a consequence of wear often represent adaptation and not pathology. Only when the adaptive capabilities of the individual are surpassed will pathology become evident.

This broader concept modifies, to some degree, the philosophy of clinical dentistry. By recognising progressive change in tooth form as a physiologically dynamic process, premature and unnecessary dental intervention may be avoided.

TERMINOLOGY

There is a lack of consistency in the literature in the terminology used to distinguish between and describe the different types of noncarious tooth reduction. The accepted terms abrasion and attrition are often used interchangeably. The term erosion is sometimes considered as tooth wear when in reality it is the result of chemical dissolution of tooth structure, not the rubbing together of surfaces. The confusion has probably arisen because all three forms of tooth loss often occur simultaneously. Fracture is a separate process, also leading to loss of tooth structure.

The term tooth reduction is therefore a useful generic description because it covers all processes that lead to the loss of tooth substance. In this chapter the terms abrasion, attrition, erosion and fracture will each be defined and described because the recognition of the cause of tooth reduction is the principal guide to therapy on those occasions when therapy is indicated.

AETIOLOGY OF TOOTH REDUCTION

Abrasion

Every (1972) described abrasion as 'the wearing of tooth substance that results from friction of exogenous material forced over the surface by incisive, masticatory, and grasping functions.' To this must be added the wear caused by tooth cleaning (**Figs 4.1** and **4.2**).

Within this definition, exogenous material is anything foreign to tooth substance. Included are sand, grit and foreign material found in the food bolus, the natural abrasiveness of some foods, and any solid material held by or forced against the teeth. Abrasion may therefore occur during mastication, when the teeth are being used as tools, or during tooth cleaning.

In general, the action of abrasion is not anatomically selective on the tooth surface. In other words, the abrasive influence of a bolus of food is felt on the whole occlusal surface, affecting the cusp tips, cusp inclines and fissures as well as, to a lesser degree, the occlusal aspects of the buccal and lingual surfaces.

An exception to this lack of specificity may occur when the same two or three teeth are used repeatedly as tools for grasping an object. This may lead to more severe abrasion on these teeth. Examples of this type of abrasion may be related to a broad range of occupations and pursuits, from hunter–gathering to pipe smoking.

An abrasion area, as distinct from an attrition facet, is generally not well defined because abrasion tends to round off or blunt tooth cusps or cutting edges (**Fig. 4.3**). In addition, the tooth surface will have a pitted appearance. Where dentine is exposed it may be 'scooped out' because it is softer than enamel.

Microscopically, an abraded surface generally shows haphazardly oriented scratch marks, numerous pits and various gouge marks (**Fig. 4.4**). Very rarely, abrasive scratches will be almost parallel when the abrasive material is forced in one direction across the tooth surface. The length, depth and width of this microdetail vary depending on the abrasiveness of the food and the pressures applied during mastication.

The distribution and extent of abrasive wear over the dentition is influenced by many variables including type of occlusion, diet, lifestyle, age and oral hygiene.

Occlusion

The type of occlusion is a prime factor in the distribution and pattern of abrasion. As the variability of upper and lower tooth positions is almost limitless, the distribution and pattern of abrasion can also be extremely variable. As a general rule, in an Angle Class I molar relationship, with normal anterior overjet and overbite, abrasive wear will occur on the occluso-buccal aspect of the lower teeth and the occluso-palatal aspect of the upper teeth producing an occlusal slope *ad palatum*. This will normally hold true for the premolars and first permanent molars, but the occlusal slope may be reduced to neutral around the second molars, and finally, may be negative, *ad linguum*, on the third molars

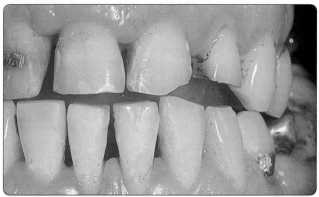

Fig. 4.1 Abrasion on tooth #22. This has been caused by many years of holding a pipe stem in this position.

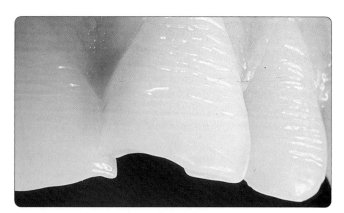

Fig. 4.2 Abrasion on labial of upper anterior teeth. The horizontal, parallel scratch marks were caused by toothbrush abrasion.

(**Fig. 4.5**). The occlusal twist that develops on the occlusal surface of posterior teeth with advanced abrasion is called the helicoidal plane.

Diet and lifestyle

Molnar (1972) described how abrasion is intricately related to diet and culture: 'the varieties of foods consumed by primitive man and the specialised tool function of the teeth have left significant marks in the form of worn occlusal surfaces over the dental arches.' For example, non-industrial populations living in a harsh environment, masticating hard, fibrous foods show more extensive abrasion than those in industrial urban societies consuming soft processed foods.

Age

There is a high correlation between age and tooth wear within all populations. Clearly, newly erupted teeth have less wear than those that have been in function for a longer period. In general, the older the individual the more extensive the abrasion, although there will be individuals who show very little wear indeed.

Oral hygiene techniques

Although routine tooth cleaning is desirable to reduce the risk of periodontal disease and caries, the cleaning process itself may result in the loss of tooth structure through abrasion. The use of an abrasive dentifrice, combined with vigorous brushing with a hard toothbrush, can result in abrasive defects particularly near the gingival margin on the facial surfaces. Such loss of tooth structure can pose a significant problem. When dentine is exposed by abrasion alone the tubules may remain closed by the smear layer. In the presence of acid, the dentinal tubules may be opened through loss of this layer and the pulp may become inflamed and respond to changes in temperature, osmolality and tooth drying. This painful condition is called cervical hypersensitivity. Loss of tooth structure from abrasion may become so severe that the strength of the tooth is threatened.

Although closure of dentinal tubules can overcome cervical hypersensitivity on a temporary basis, for long-term resolution it is necessary to determine the cause of the problem. As will be described below, exposure of the tooth surface to low pH food or drink before brushing may lead to rapid demineralisation, leaving the collagen matrix exposed to damage from a toothbrush. This may exacerbate loss of structure and prevent the natural closure of dentinal tubules by salivary precipitate. Cervical hypersensitivity is discussed further in Chapter 5.

Attrition

The term attrition is used to describe tooth wear caused by tooth-to-tooth contact without the presence of food. It has been defined by Every (1972) as 'wear caused by endogenous material such as microfine particles of enamel prisms caught between two opposing tooth surfaces.' The enamel prisms break off and become caught as the tooth surfaces are forced over one another, producing characteristic parallel striations when viewed microscopically.

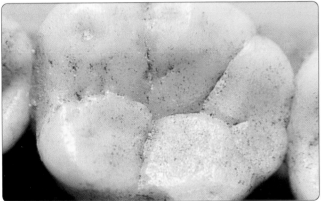

Fig. 4.3 Abrasion on occlusal. An Australian Aboriginal tooth exposed to excessive abrasion. Note the gouge marks and pitting on the occlusal surface.

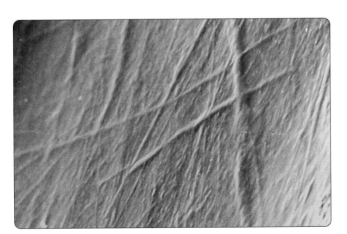

Fig. 4.4 Scanning electron micrograph of abraded surface. Note random pattern of scratch marks on dentine (×100).

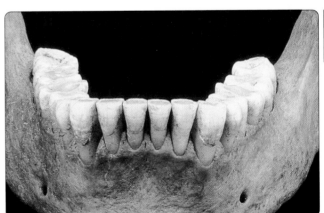

Fig. 4.5 Abrasion pattern on ancient skull specimen. Note the helicoidal wear pattern on posterior teeth emphasising the slope towards the tongue in the third molars.

The characteristic feature is the development of a facet which is a flat surface with a circumscribed and well-defined border (**Figs 4.6** and **4.7**). There will be fine parallel striations in one direction only and within the border of the facet. One facet will match perfectly with another facet on a tooth in the opposite arch and the parallel striations will be lying in the same direction.

The distribution of attrition is influenced by the type of occlusion, the geometry of the stomatognathic system and the characteristic grinding pattern of the individual.

Bruxism and parafunction

Summary

Bruxism

is a universal part of function and should not be regarded as pathological.

Parafunction

is pathological function leading to unusual wear patterns generally associated with, for example
- nail-biting
- pencil-chewing
- occlusal discrepancies

In the past, such terms as bruxism and parafunction have been used synonymously to describe persistent tooth-grinding. This has been described as a pathologic habit leading to temporomandibular joint dysfunction and myofascial pain and it has been suggested that occlusal interference, deflective inclines and stress have all acted, alone or in combination, as trigger mechanisms.

However, it has been noted that the frequency of bruxism in both pre-industrialised and industrialised populations is around 90% in both groups. Children frequently grind their teeth, and even their gums before tooth eruption. These observations suggest that bruxism is a universal behaviour rather than a habit, because habits are learned behaviour patterns. So it is suggested that bruxism should be regarded as a common physiological behaviour of central origin. It is only when stress levels become too high that grinding intensity increases to the point where there is likely to be adaptive changes to the craniofacial structures, including the muscles and joints. When these structures are too slow to adapt, or fail to adapt, then disease may become evident in a variety of forms, for example, craniomandibular disorders.

After all, many other species of mammals grind their teeth. If tooth-grinding were pathological, surely natural selection would have eliminated it by now? Therefore, it is logical to accept that it is a behaviour of central origin, and that only acquired habits such as nail-biting and pencil-chewing should be regarded as parafunction. Occlusal interference cannot be entirely discounted and should be observed and understood in the context of treatment planning. It is not that these latter factors will initiate parafunction but they are likely to provide an environment wherein the direction and intensity of grinding forces may affect teeth, muscles or joints. It seems that tooth wear, caused by tooth-to-tooth contact in the absence of food, may result from a number of distinct behaviours, just as temporomandibular joint pathology and associated muscle pain constitute a number of separate entities under the umbrella of craniomandibular disorders.

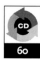

Thegosis

If tooth-grinding is normal physiological behaviour, then it is logical to suggest that there is a reason for such behaviour. The theory of 'thegosis' (Every, 1972) suggests that tooth-grinding is a phylogenic behaviour designed to sharpen

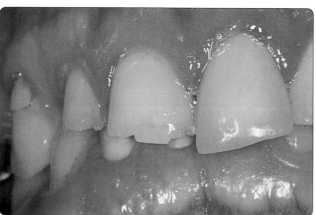

Fig. 4.6 Attrition. Heavy attrition showing on teeth #11 and #12 as well as enamel flaking.

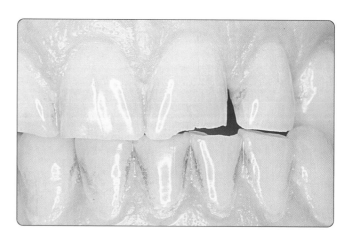

Fig. 4.7 Attrition. Heavy attrition showing on teeth #21 and #22, largely the result of a deflective incline between the second molars on the right side.

teeth both for more efficient mastication, as well as for use as weapons. On the one hand, normal dietary abrasion will make teeth blunt so that they fail to act efficiently as scissor-like blades. On the other hand, empty grinding – bruxing – will reinstate the sharp edges and enhance the blade effect. Certainly many members of the animal kingdom grind their teeth at times of stress, as in the fight-or-flight response or when hungry.

Interproximal attrition

Interproximal attrition occurs on the contacting proximal surfaces of adjacent teeth when they move against one another during occlusal loading, such as mastication or bruxism. Examination of interproximal wear facets in teeth with intact alveolar bone support suggests that the predominant movement is either vertical or near vertical and not buccolingual as has been suggested in the past. The result may be a gradual shortening of the arch length over time, but this is probably not significant in industrialised populations.

Erosion

Erosion of tooth structure is defined as the superficial loss of dental hard tissue due to a chemical process not involving bacteria. The clinical appearance may vary (**Figs 4.8** and **4.9**). In generalised erosion the whole tooth crown may be affected, with a loss of surface definition resulting in a glazed, lifeless appearance with no sharp enamel ridges as these become rounded off. The enamel surface may become relatively concave until the dentine is exposed, whereupon the tooth reduction accelerates because of the comparative softness of the dentine. This causes a scooped-out appearance. Abrasion, attrition, or both, may be superimposed over the erosion process, causing further reduction and possible difficulties in diagnosis.

Any erosive process will be greatly exacerbated if the teeth are brushed while acid is still present in the mouth. This comes about because the demineralisation of the tooth structure leaves the organic matrix of either the dentine or the enamel free and unsupported by the mineral ions. Brushing at this point will remove the organic framework so that remineralisation cannot then take place. If, however, the teeth are not brushed for 2–3 hours after the acid intake, there will have been sufficient remineralisation from the calcium and phosphate ions in the saliva and no permanent loss of tooth structure will occur.

The logical alternative is to advise the patient to brush the teeth before ingestion of acidic food or drink and, possibly, in a chronic situation such as professional wine tasters, use a fluoride mouth wash too. After the acid intake it will be sufficient to merely wash the mouth vigorously with water to remove the acid residue and delay brushing for up to 3 hours. There are, of course, no problems likely to arise from this advice in relation to caries activity because, in the absence of mature plaque, there can be no caries generation, and whether the plaque is removed before or after eating, is not relevant.

Summary

Chemical erosion

There can be a variety of chemical factors involved in erosion. If they do not initiate the erosion they may, at least, exacerbate the problem. The following factors may be involved:

Extrinsic
- acid food
- acid drink – cola drinks, wine
- drugs – hydrochloric acid etc.

Intrinsic
- regurgitation of gastric acid
- gastric reflux
- chronic vomiting

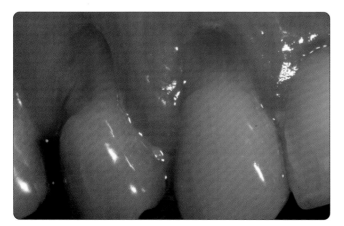

Fig. 4.8 Severe erosion lesions. Teeth #13 and #14 show severe erosion doubtless exacerbated by toothbrush abrasion as well.

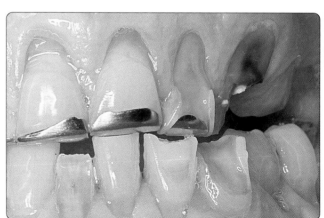

Fig. 4.9 Severe erosion. Another quadrant of teeth showing similar erosion in addition to abrasion.

The acids which cause erosion of the tooth surface may originate from either extrinsic or intrinsic factors.

Extrinsic factors

Acids of extrinsic origin arise from outside the body. Industrial acids can be carried in gaseous form in the air in heavily polluted areas and may cause demineralisation of the labial surfaces of anterior teeth, particularly in a patient who breathes through the mouth. Progress of the erosion may be relatively slow and, therefore, diagnosis is often difficult.

A variety of foods and drinks are acidic and frequent ingestion may cause problems. For example, low-pH cola drinks (including diet colas), cordials and fruit juices may cause erosion. However, individual variations in the method of consumption of these liquids before swallowing may lead to differing patterns.

Certain medications are also acid in nature and the potential for demineralisation must be recognised and the patient counselled. A lack of gastric acid may be compensated for by the oral administration of concentrated hydrochloric acid with advice that it should be taken through a straw or glass tube. However, there is still a tendency to force some of the acid into the oral cavity by the act of swallowing. Erosion on the lingual surfaces of the upper teeth is evidence of this problem and such drugs should preferably be administered in an alternative form.

Intrinsic factors

Gastric acids are the most common intrinsic problem and can often be differentiated from extrinsic acids by observing the distribution of the affected areas. Chronic vomiting will affect the palatal surface of the upper teeth because they are in the path of the gastric contents when emitted, whereas the lower teeth will be protected to a degree by the tongue. However, chronic gastric reflux may erode both upper and lower teeth because the constituents of the reflux are in a gaseous form and may be more widely distributed around the oral cavity.

It should be noted that, in the presence of a reduced salivary flow, the effect of both extrinsic and intrinsic factors will be exacerbated. The buffering capacity of the saliva against acid attack is the best defence against both caries and erosion, but routine use of a fluoride mouth wash, either professionally or applied at home, will assist in reducing the damage.

Abfraction

There is some evidence that excessive buccal or lingual occlusal load may contribute to the erosive process through either compression or tension in the cervical region of the tooth, just above its bony support. This concept, termed abfraction, is currently regarded as theoretical but helps to explain the occurrence of tooth reduction in the cervical region in the form of grooves or notches that cannot otherwise be explained (**Fig. 4.10**). It is suggested that occlusal load causes flexure in the tooth with the point of rotation being at the crest of the alveolar bony support. Under load, the relatively brittle enamel or dentine may disintegrate and release mineral crystals. Subsequent brushing will remove the collagen support for dentine and prevent remineralisation. Differential diagnosis between abfraction and erosion, as discussed below, is difficult.

Tooth fracture

Tooth fracture is a relatively common occurrence, particularly in teeth that have been restored. It may be the result of direct trauma, but other reasons exist, and a careful diagnosis is required rather than just smoothing over the roughened area. The following forms of tooth loss from fracture should be noted.

Enamel flaking

Slivers of enamel of various sizes may fracture from the incisal edges of anterior teeth or from the buccal or lingual edges of posterior teeth, particularly if the occlusal table is flat (**Fig. 4.11**). Occasionally large areas of buccal or lingual enamel plate may split off leaving dentine exposed. It is important to distinguish between chipping from direct trauma and that arising from habits such as biting cotton, biting finger nails or opening hair clips with the teeth. However, enamel flaking is often the result of tooth-grinding and the pattern that results reflects the direction of the mandible during the forceful phase of the grinding stroke.

Observation of the microdetail of wear patterns on facets suggests that they arise from lateral movements of the mandible. There will be lingual to buccal striations on posterior teeth and anterior to lateral striations on the anterior teeth. This means that the condyle on the ipsilateral side acts as a pivot, while the contralateral condyle moves forwards, downwards and medially down the articular eminence. It is the labial incisal edges of the upper incisors and the lingual incisal edges of the lower incisors

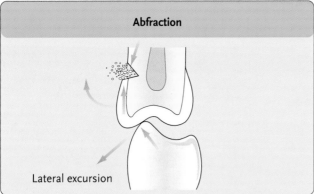

Abfraction

Lateral excursion

Fig. 4.10 Abfraction. This term is used to describe possible flexure of a tooth under heavy lateral load, which may lead to displacement or fracture of enamel rods at the cemento-enamel junction. The lost enamel will expose more dentine, in which dentine tubules may be crushed by the same stresses and more readily demineralised. These factors may account for isolated 'erosion' lesions for which there is no obvious explanation.

that tend to flake, indicating a grinding movement away from the normal intercuspal position.

Occasionally the direction of a forceful grinding stroke is affected by a deflective incline on a posterior tooth, which has become a guiding factor, as a result of a change in the distribution of the posterior teeth. Such guidance may produce a subtle change in wear pattern that is specific for that individual.

Extreme wear patterns

It is possible for the grinding patterns to extend past a normal edge-to-edge position, particularly on canines. It may be a position that the relaxed patient finds uncomfortable or almost impossible to achieve, but it can be shown that the wear facets match entirely (**Fig. 4.12**). The pattern may be more common than thought and it can, on occasion, explain enamel chipping, failure of labial veneers, and even cracks in a porcelain crown or a split in a nonvital root.

Cusp fracture

Fracture may occur from direct physical trauma, as a result of bruxism when the occlusal forces can be very high, during parafunction or, occasionally, during the mastication of food. It is possible for an unrestored tooth to fracture, but it is far more common for this to happen in teeth weakened iatrogenically by the placement of restorations. Cavities designated #2.2 in the new classification (page 138) will double or even triple the length of cusps, substantially increasing the torque at the cusp base and leaving the tooth more prone to fracture. Endodontically treated teeth are also at increased risk because of loss of tooth structure related to access for root canal therapy. Cavities designed to reduce or overcome these problems are described in Chapters 7, 11 and 19.

As a patient ages, teeth develop minor cracks in the enamel that are usually repaired by precipitation of salivary pellicle followed by mineral deposition. However, if the tooth is subject to heavy occlusal load the crack can propagate though to the dentine. Movement of the cusp

during function may then be extremely painful because of hydraulic stimulation of odontoblast sensory nerve receptors. Treatment involves identifying, protecting and strengthening the cusp (see Chapters 7 and 11). The cusps most prone to split and fail are the lingual cusps of lower molars and the buccal or lingual cusps of upper first and second premolars.

Crown fracture

The crowns of anterior teeth are most at risk from extrinsic forces such as direct trauma. The main predisposing factors are the age of the patient and tooth position. From the time of emergence of the permanent anterior teeth to the late teen years there is a combination of immature physical activities with immature facial structures. The teeth tend to protrude beyond both the nose and the chin and are therefore at a higher risk. In the older patient the presence of caries, restorations, erosion, abrasion or attrition may have already weakened the crown structure, and even a minor blow may lead to loss of part or all of a crown. Both crowns and roots are at increased risk of fracture in endodontically treated teeth (see Chapter 19).

ADAPTATION AND PATHOLOGY

The human dentition should remain functional throughout life. Dental caries and the periodontal disease leading to premature tooth loss are modern-day diseases, the incidence of these diseases in prehistoric populations being very low. It is not uncommon to find ancient skeletal material with completely intact dentition and no evidence of caries, only tooth reduction.

The craniofacial skeleton is made up of individual units including the teeth, temporomandibular joints, musculature and the supporting craniofacial skeleton. Any change to one component of the craniofacial anatomy may lead to alterations in associated structures. Because of their physiologic plasticity, the craniofacial structures are in a state of continuous change throughout life, the extent and

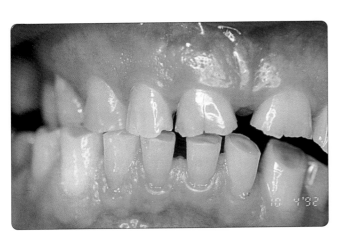

Fig. 4.11 Enamel flaking. Forceful extreme mandibular movement from centric occlusion outwards can cause the enamel flaking on the anteriors.

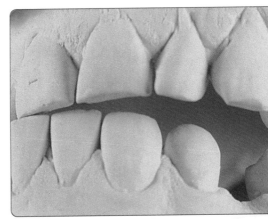

Fig. 4.12 Wear on labial surface. Evidence of extreme mandibular movement during tooth-grinding is shown by the wear facet on the labial incisal edge of the canine.

rate of change being related to a combination of the genetic makeup of the body and the influence of environmental forces. Functional demands imposed upon the system, as well as other factors, can cause change; only when the body cannot adapt or is too slow to adapt to these demands will tissues break down pathologically.

Stability of occlusal vertical dimension

Notes

The vertical dimension is expected to remain essentially unchanged throughout life in spite of wear, abrasion and attrition.

Advanced tooth reduction may also lead to a quantitative change in the craniofacial complex. In the absence of any compensatory or adaptive response from associated structures, a reduction of the occlusal vertical dimension or face height would be expected. However, research suggests that the occlusal vertical dimension is usually maintained by compensatory mechanisms of continual eruption of teeth combined with alveolar bone growth. Further evidence suggests that, if the amount of tooth reduction is small, there may even be an increase in occlusal vertical dimension over time. Face height seems to be dependent on the balance between the rate of occlusal tooth reduction and the adaptive bodily responses of tooth eruption and alveolar bone growth.

Adaptation within the tooth
Progressive tooth reduction also leads to an adaptive change within the tooth with the production of secondary dentine within the pulp chamber. When the rate of loss of tooth substance is slow, secondary dentine will form without damage to the vital pulp, although it may become completely calcified.

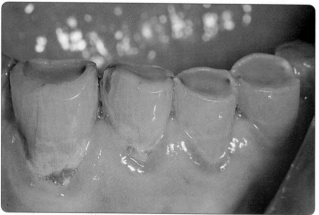

Fig. 4.13 Tooth wear in the ageing patient. The patient is in his 80s and the teeth are well worn but they are still healthy.

However, if the response is not adequate there may be loss of vitality. Furthermore, the gradual loss of cusps causes a wider masticatory stroke which results, in the long term, in anatomical changes to the temporomandibular joint including modification of the articular eminence.

DIAGNOSIS

The causes of tooth reduction have been outlined and it must be noted that more than one process may be acting on teeth simultaneously, with varying intensities and durations. A diagnosis cannot therefore be made using surface appearance alone. Facet borders may not be distinctively sharp, and where surface dissolution is excessive, there may be no facets evident at all. Erosion may remove all fine detail and overwhelm evidence of abrasion. Tooth-grinding, combined with abrasion upon an eroded surface, may remove more tooth substance than normal because of the weakened enamel surface.

This confusion and interplay of forces may complicate clinical diagnosis. However, with a clear understanding of the ways in which tooth reduction may take place, and a thorough medical and dental history, the causes will often become self-evident. Questioning patients about tooth reduction should form a normal part of the history-taking process. The following factors should be taken into account in diagnosis and treatment planning.

Age of the patient
The degree of tooth wear must be related to the age of the patient. An elderly patient may show loss of more than one-half of the clinical crowns, but in the absence of pain and without concern for aesthetics the situation can be considered to be physiological, and the dentition fully functional (**Fig. 4.13**). However, the same degree of wear in a 20-year-old patient could be interpreted as being pathological and the chance of retaining a complete dentition into old age may be remote.

Random loss of teeth
Random loss of posterior teeth will lead to additional load being borne by the remaining teeth; they are then more prone to attrition and abrasion, particularly if the posterior support has fallen below the theoretical minimum (see Chapter 21). The presence of deflective inclines may, in turn, exacerbate this situation, leading bruxing into parafunction, with the development of bizarre wear patterns (**Fig. 4.14**). In the elderly patient the need for treatment may not be so imperative; however, restoration of posterior support to within the minimum, along with restoration of freedom of movement through the absence of deflective inclines, may well prevent further loss of tooth structure and stabilise the situation in a relatively simple fashion.

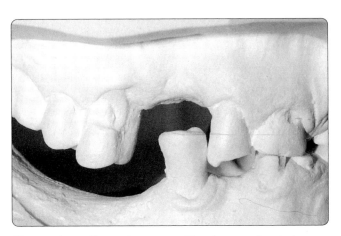

Fig. 4.14 Loss of posterior support. The absence of posterior support leaves all the load on the anteriors, which have worn heavily as a result.

Evidence of active tooth-grinding

A diagnosis of attrition may be difficult to make because of the other factors which may be present concurrently. Observation of the following signs and symptoms may lead to a diagnosis of attrition.

- Shiny facets – well-defined and polished facets indicate active tooth-grinding. The facets should normally be able to be matched between opposing arches but, occasionally, a patient is capable of adopting a bizarre inter-occlusal position during intense concentration or during sleep and will develop a facet in an apparently impossible position such as the labial face of an upper canine. It must be remembered that, in the presence of erosion, the facet may not appear shiny even if the bruxism is active.
- Myofascial pain dysfunction syndrome – myofascial pain dysfunction symptoms may indicate active tooth-grinding and there may be associated pain and tenderness in the temporomandibular joints. Attrition facets may be detectable.
- Stiff jaw – a stiff jaw may result from traumatic injury or infection, but chronic stiffness may indicate active tooth-grinding, particularly if it is apparent upon waking after a night's sleep.
- Use of a night guard for diagnosis – construct a night guard and polish the occlusal surface to a matte finish only. Subsequent tooth-grinding activity will show as highly polished wear facets on the acrylic surface.

Evidence of erosion

Early signs of erosion may be difficult to detect and demonstrate but the following are often indicative of erosion.

- If, in the presence of the usual signs and symptoms of active tooth-grinding, there are no well-defined facets, then there is likely to be active erosion.
- Cervical sensitivity. Gingival recession with exposure of root surfaces or scooped out dentine on the occlusal surfaces is relatively common, but the dentine tubules will normally be burnished closed and, therefore, free of pain. Active erosion will demineralise the dentine surface and may lead to exquisite sensitivity through the open dentine tubules.
- Careful history-taking may be required to confirm the diagnosis because patients are often reluctant to disclose unusual dietary habits. Patient education and counselling may be important if the process is to be arrested.
- Isolated erosion lesions with no apparent cause, where there are adjacent teeth showing no erosion lesions, may well be the result of abfraction.

Evidence of abrasion

As defined above most patients will undergo some degree of abrasion simply through mastication. However, the degree will vary depending on the enthusiasm for chewing displayed by the patient, and the consistency of the food being consumed. The decision as to whether the situation is pathological, and in need of treatment or not, will be taken on the basis of all the above factors. In general, erosion and attrition are the primary aetiological factors and abrasion may be a complicating factor in urban societies.

Diagnosis of active tooth reduction

The best method of making a diagnosis is to study accurate impressions or replicas of teeth under a low-power microscope. This may reveal the microdetail of attrition, abrasion and erosion. Make a shallow scratch with a sharp explorer on a facet or an erosive area before making an impression and compare with further consecutive impressions obtained 1–4 weeks later. The disappearance of the scratch over a reasonably short period of time is good evidence that tooth reduction is active. The decision as to the cause will often be difficult and usually will require careful history-taking and continuing observation.

FURTHER READING

Every RG. *A new terminology for mammalian teeth: founded on the phenomenon of thegosis.* Christchurch: Pegasus Press; 1972:1–64.

Kaidonis JA, Richards LC, Townsend GC. Abrasion: an evolutionary and clinical view. *Aust Prosthodont J* 1992; **6**:9–16.

Kaidonis JA, Richards LC, Townsend GC. Nature and frequency of dental wear facets in an Australian Aboriginal population. *J Oral Rehabil* 1993; **20**:333–40.

Molnar S. Tooth wear and culture: a survey of tooth functions among some prehistoric populations. *Curr Anthropol* 1972; **13**:511–26.

Richards LC. Form and function of the masticatory system. In: Ward GK, ed. *Archaeology at ANZAAS*. Canberra: Australian Institute for Aboriginal Studies; 1984:96–109.

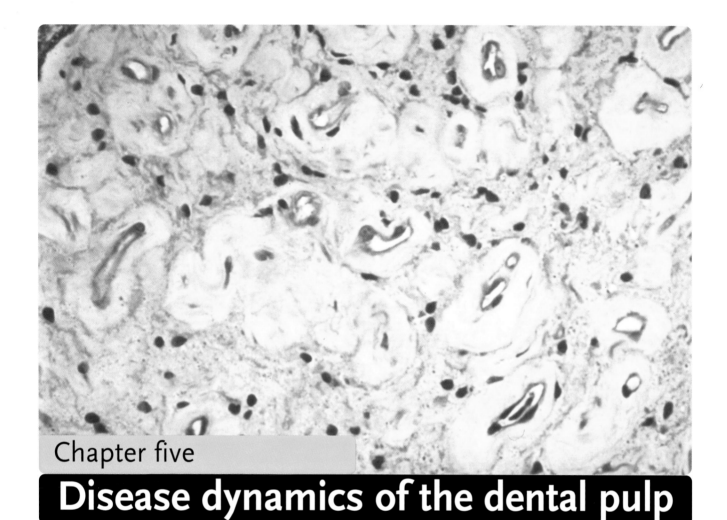

Chapter five

Disease dynamics of the dental pulp

W.R. Hume • W.L.K. Massey

An understanding of the events that occur in the pulp following insult enables the dentist both to protect the tissue and to provide appropriate treatment when it is damaged. Interceptive therapy may make the difference between pulp survival through healing and pulp death. Various therapies may also reduce or eliminate pulpal pain.

In very general terms, the pulp responds to damage in ways similar to other connective tissues; that is, it can undergo various forms of inflammation, it can heal or it can die. However, the pulp is unique among connective tissues in that it is entirely enclosed in dentine and it has processes that extend throughout the dentine; therefore the pulp and the dentine should be regarded as a single entity.

Any trauma or therapy applied to the dentine should be regarded as trauma or therapy applied to the pulp. Insults, such as the carious process or tooth restoration, are unlike those found elsewhere in the body and will challenge the pulp. It is not surprising, therefore, that some aspects of the pulp's response to insult are unique. Some therapies used to treat the dental pulp are also unique.

INSULTS TO THE PULP

The pulp can be damaged or die in one of the three following ways:

Dental caries

Most commonly, the dental pulp can become inflamed and may die as a consequence of the advance of the carious process through dentine. What then occurs is described in detail below. The process can be halted by effective caries treatment or by the application of preventive measures, either alone or in combination with tooth restoration.

Microleakage in restored teeth

Although the restoration of a carious defect in tooth structure is usually in the interests of the patient's health and wellbeing, the action of restoration may not in itself be sufficient to prevent the ultimate death of the pulp, even when carried out in parallel with effective caries preventive measures. The principal reason for pulpal inflammation following restoration is 'microleakage', the existence of a gap between the restorative material and the dentine, into which bacteria can propagate. Evidence for this phenomenon, and the measures that can be taken to minimise it, are described in detail in Chapter 18.

Mechanical, thermal or chemical trauma

Direct mechanical trauma to a tooth can interrupt the blood supply by tearing the fine blood vessels at the root apex, leading to avascular necrosis of the tissue within the tooth. There is little that can be done about this except to encourage those people at high risk of injury (contact sports players) to wear protective mouth guards.

Some pulpal cells, in particular the odontoblasts, can be killed by:

- direct trauma
- heat generated during tooth cutting
- chemicals applied to dentine, particularly when freshly cut
- exposure of pulp tissue during restoration.

It is rare for the entire pulp to be killed in this way and, although these events cause pain, the pulp will usually heal in the weeks after the damage occurs, unless bacteria or their products can reach the damaged tissue.

DEFENCE WITHIN DENTINE

Dentine has a limited capacity for its own defence. Dentinal tubules are a potential pathway for the diffusion of noxious chemicals from the external environment to the pulp and for the inward movement of microorganisms. However, the tubules can be reduced in diameter or totally closed by one or more of the following processes.

Dentinal sclerosis

Dentinal sclerosis is the narrowing of dentinal tubules by the formation of peritubular dentine, dense calcific material laid down through an active, odontoblastic, metabolic process. Sclerosis may progress relatively rapidly in dentine beneath an advancing carious lesion or in dentine that has been exposed to the oral environment through abrasion, attrition or erosion. Sclerosis also occurs more slowly as a natural part of ageing.

Calcium phosphate deposition

Crystals of calcium phosphate may be deposited deep within dentinal tubules as a response to slowly advancing caries by a mechanism that is not understood, but which is presumably mediated by odontoblasts.

Salivary precipitation

Precipitation of salivary calcium and phosphate can occlude dentinal tubules exposed to saliva and effectively desensitise hypersensitive dentine. Remineralisation will not occur in the presence of actively advancing caries or in acid erosion because of the low pH which is integral to these processes. In the presence of active abrasion or attrition there is unlikely to be precipitation, but precipitation will resume if these processes are arrested.

Reparative dentine

Dentine is formed by odontoblasts and, so long as they remain alive, these cells will retain the capacity to make additional dentine in response to injury. There are other cells in the pulp that can form new dentinogenic cells if odontoblasts die, so long as the remainder of the pulp remains vital. The hard tissue which they form has all the constituents of dentine, but may vary in form.

Mild injury

Most odontoblasts beneath the damaged area survive mild injury to dentine, such as damage occurring in attrition or in the preparation of a shallow cavity. Regular reparative dentine, which contains relatively normal tubules, will be laid down at the pulp–dentine interface in the area of damage as a continuation of the main body of dentine.

Moderate to severe injury

If more odontoblasts die because the injury is more severe, in either degree or duration, the pulpal cells will produce reparative hard tissue of widely varying types. The form will depend on the nature and stage of differentiation of the cells that effect the primary calcific repair process. Secondary dentinogenic cells are derived by mitotic activity from the cell-rich subodontoblastic layer. This layer contains a high proportion of both fibroblasts and more primitive mesenchymal cells, either of which may be precursors of the replacement cells. The reparative dentine laid down in this way may be totally atubular, or may be poorly mineralised. In some cases cells in the area of calcification may become entrapped and die, leaving substantial defects in the reparative tissue.

Chronic injury

In the chronically inflamed pulp (see below), diffuse

calcification may occur, presumably because of activation, differentiation and calcific matrix secretion by mesenchymally derived cells. Relatively well-organised dentine may also be laid down within a chronically inflamed pulp to form 'pulp stones'. On rare occasions, pulp stones will form in an otherwise normal pulp for no apparent reason.

PULPAL INFLAMMATION IN RESPONSE TO BACTERIA

Inflammation is a series of events in vascular connective tissue that, ideally, neutralise or eliminate damaging factors and initiate tissue repair. Inflammatory response to bacterial insult in the pulp can be identified by observing degenerative changes in the tissue that are not very different from changes seen in other tissues (**Fig. 5.1**). Early changes include fibrosis and thickening of the basement membrane in associated small vessels. Frustrated repair will often induce calcific foci associated with amorphous, partially mineralised connective tissue matrix with degenerate cells and tissue (**Fig. 5.2**).

Chronic inflammation

Whatever the microbial mix and its pathogenic vectors, it is likely that the first response to caries or microleakage within pulpal tissue will be a low-grade, chronic inflammation, characterised by the presence of greatly increased numbers of T-lymphocytes in the extravascular space. Mild chronic inflammation is usually symptomless because the lymphocytes do not cause release of factors that change the sensitivity of the pulp's sensory nerves.

An infiltrate will form with varying numbers of lymphocytes, monocytes/macrophages and plasma cells within the pulpal connective tissue (**Fig. 5.3**). The capillaries may become engorged and increase in number. Many small vessels in the area may display features resembling high endothelial venules, which are specialised for the exchange of inflammatory and immune cells.

As the inflammation progresses there may be haemorrhagic changes related to extensive leukocyte infiltration (**Fig. 5.4**). There may be extravascular haemorrhage, complete loss of connective tissue architecture and scattered chronic inflammatory infiltrate.

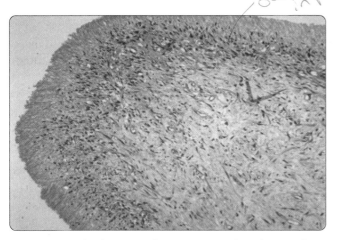

Fig. 5.1 Normal pulp tissue. This represents relatively normal pulp tissue which is a typical loose connective tissue with odontoblasts at the periphery.

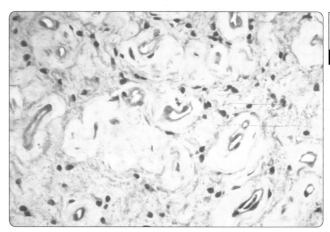

Fig. 5.2 Chronic changes. Calcific foci can generate with an amorphous part-mineralised connective tissue.

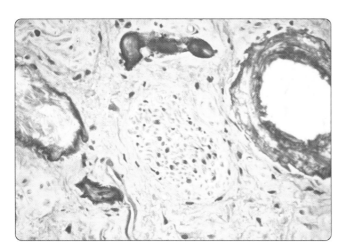

Fig. 5.3 Chronic inflammation. Formation of infiltrate within the pulp with lymphocytes, monocytes/macrophages and plasma cells.

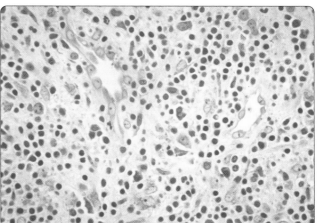

Fig. 5.4 Later stage chronic. Haemorrhagic changes with extensive leukocyte infiltration and loss of connective tissue.

It is likely that the level of response depends to a large degree on the particular bacteria involved. In one individual there may be a small zone of dentinal caries, well removed from the pulp, that evokes a vigorous response because either the lesion contains particularly pathogenic microorganisms or the pulpal response includes a specific immune component related to prior challenge. On the other hand, the microbial mix may be particularly benign in another patient and there may be little or no response until the lesion is large and close to the odontoblast layer. Similarly, a relatively small number of bacteria beneath a leaking restoration may evoke a chronic inflammatory response in one patient but not in another.

Acute inflammation

Foci of acute inflammation can develop within the chronically inflamed tissue if microbially derived toxins damage pulpal cells, bringing about the local synthesis of histamine, bradykinin or prostaglandins. Alternatively, humorally mediated hypersensitivity reactions to microbial components or products themselves may cause tissue damage. If such acute foci develop, the pulpal nerves may become sensitised to normal stimuli and the patient may report sensitivity of short duration to hot or cold food or drink, to cold air, or to osmotic change while eating. The pulp will not necessarily die under these circumstances and the institution of appropriate therapy may well lead to healing.

Reversible pulpitis

The inflammation may resolve if, at the stage of simple chronic inflammation or chronic inflammation with small, acute foci, the aetiological factors are removed by debridement, or denied substrate by the creation of an effective seal. That is to say, the inflammation is reversible. However, it is likely that the pulpal tissue, after such a cycle of inflammation and repair, will be less vascular, less cellular and more fibrous than before, and may therefore be less able to withstand subsequent insults.

Irreversible pulpitis

The tissue changes may become irreversible if the injury is more severe or there is a major immune-mediated response to the microbial challenge. The pulp may then die painlessly over time or, alternatively, total necrosis may take place quite rapidly and cause considerable discomfort. If the level of stimulus remains relatively constant, such as under a leaking but otherwise stable restoration, the ability of the tissue to resist bacterial toxins will decline over time and a reversible inflammatory process may become irreversible. Some form of surgical ablation of the pulp tissue, such as pulpotomy or pulpectomy, will then be required if the tooth is to be retained.

The boundary between reversible and irreversible pulpitis is impossible to define. In a healthy young patient, a pulp in a state of chronic, suppurative inflammation such as occurs with pulp microabscess, may heal after elimination of the causative factor. On the other hand, in older individuals or in teeth which have been subjected to previous episodes of inflammation, a pulp microabscess is more likely to spread because the tissue is less able to repair itself. In such circumstances, toxic products of cell lysis may kill adjacent cells.

Prediction of outcome

Clinically, it is important to develop the ability to discriminate between pulp that will heal following conservative therapy and that which will not. In an adult, irreversible inflammation is characterised by symptoms of severe pain of long duration, in response to hot or cold, or to spontaneous unstimulated pain particularly at night. The patient may not be able to identify accurately which tooth is causing the pain, or whether it is in the maxilla or mandible.

Histological examination of the inflamed tooth will generally reveal at least one pulpal microabscess, often in the area of a pulp horn. A microabscess is an accumulation of polymorphonuclear leukocytes and dead and dying pulp cells in the form of pus. The area of pus formation will be surrounded by fibrous connective tissue infiltrated with polymorphonuclear leukocytes and, slightly further away, chronic inflammatory cells.

A diagnosis can be made on whether the inflammation is reversible or not by removing the infected layer of carious dentine or the leaking restoration and totally sealing the lesion from the oral environment with a glass–ionomer or zinc oxide and eugenol temporary restoration. If the inflammation is reversible, the pain will cease almost immediately and, after a delay of at least 3 weeks to allow healing in the pulp, a definitive restoration can be placed.

Open-form chronic pulpitis

In the presence of a more advanced necrosis of the pulp, tissue drainage may occur from the pulp chamber through the overlying carious dentine (**Fig. 5.5**). The pulpitis is then regarded as ulcerative or open-form, and may not be

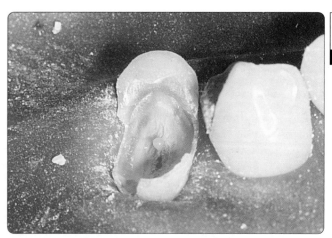

Fig. 5.5 Suppurating pulp. Removal of the last of the affected dentine reveals a bead of pus exuding from the pulp chamber as the result of an irreversible inflammation.

painful. Drainage allows the development of chronic pulpitis, with the inflammatory response being confined to the superficial area. This may persist for a considerable period of time, even years, because of the development of a balance between the injurious agents and tissue resistance. At this point, the elimination of drainage by the placement of a temporary or permanent restoration by a dentist can lead to severe pain, total pulp necrosis and progression to a periapical lesion.

Pulp polyp

In young people with untreated, gross carious lesions that expose the body of the pulp, chronic ulcerative pulpitis may lead to proliferation of hyperplastic granulation tissue into the carious cavity. The hyperplastic tissue, known as a pulp polyp, may have a thin pedicle connecting it to the remainder of the pulp, and may be covered with a well-developed epithelial layer, presumably seeded from desquamated oral epithelial cells carried in the saliva (**Fig. 5.6**).

Diffuse calcification

Chronic pulpal inflammation may also induce the secretion of ectopic dentinal matrix by fibroblasts or undifferentiated mesenchymal cells, causing either diffuse or well-organised calcification, often leading to narrowing or obstruction of the root canal.

Idiopathic resorption

In a small percentage of cases, for reasons that are not fully understood, osteoclasts may proliferate and cause resorption of dentine from the internal surface of the pulp chamber. At the same time as resorption, a disorganised calcification occurs; thus, there is continuing destruction and rebuilding of dentine and progress will be intermittent and irregular. The resorption can commence internally within the pulp tissue or externally at the cemento-enamel junction. It is difficult to recognise in the early stages in both cases.

Internal resorption

Idiopathic internal resorption begins within the pulp tissue, probably at the interface between the pulp and the dentine and, if it is not diagnosed early, can lead to the loss of a tooth. It is generally associated with trauma including cavity preparation or an external blow to a tooth. It will remain asymptomatic and the earliest signs will show radiographically as an ill-defined radiolucency in the pulp chamber (**Fig. 5.7**). Ultimately, it will show as a pink 'blush' through the enamel that, on careful examination, will be revealed as the pulp tissue occupying a large area of the crown. An external lesion may be found at this time at the cemento-enamel junction, often disguised within the gingival crevice. In the early stages, pulpectomy is the only available treatment; however, if it is allowed to progress until it reaches the external surface, the tooth will probably be lost (**Fig. 5.8**).

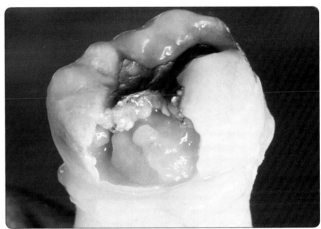

Fig. 5.6 Pulp polyp. A pulp polyp has 'grown out' of the pulp tissue following pulp exposure in a young patient.

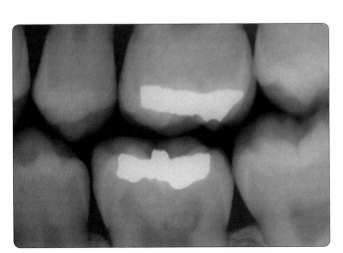

Fig. 5.7 Idiopathic internal resorption. A radiograph shows a bizarre pattern of resorption within the pulp chamber of the lower molar.

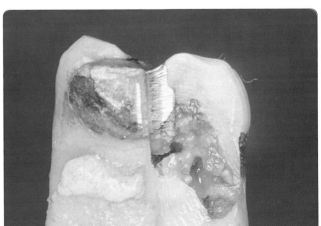

Fig. 5.8 Sectioned tooth. Another molar showing internal resorption, possibly of external origin, following extraction.

External Resorption

The alternative form of resorption commences on the external root surface and is known as idiopathic external resorption (**Fig. 5.9**). It is sometimes associated with trauma or with orthodontic movement of a tooth and generally commences in the region of the cemento-enamel junction. In the early stages it may be successfully treated by careful debridement of the lesion and cauterising with trichloracetic acid followed by placement of a glass–ionomer restoration (**Fig. 5.10**). However, this lesion is very prone to recurrence along the gingival margin; inflammation in the gingival tissue is often observed during recurrence.

INFLAMMATION IN RESPONSE TO MECHANICAL, THERMAL AND CHEMICAL INSULTS

Reversible acute inflammation

Nonbacterial, traumatic stimuli of short duration may kill or damage a few odontoblasts only. The action of cutting dentine or over-heating it during cavity preparation, or the placement directly onto dentine of restorative materials that release toxic chemicals, such as composite resin, may cause a simple, acute inflammatory response. The effect may be direct sensitisation of sensory nerve endings, short-term vasodilatation, a reversible increase in vessel wall permeability, followed by increased local tissue fluid pressure and, possibly, increased lymphatic flow. These effects will be mediated by the release of lysosomal proteins from damaged cells into the extracellular space. Later, there may be release of histamine from mast cells and the synthesis of lysyl-bradykinin from kininogen and of cell membrane fractions following the synthesis of prostaglandins. The sensory nerve effects may include increased responses to otherwise sub-threshold stimuli such as hot or cold foods and represent the body's attempt to remove debris and initiate repair. The pain thus generated may serve no apparent physiological function.

Similarly, a mild, acute inflammatory process may be reversible if the aetiological factors do not persist. The absence of bacteria or their by-products means that the likely course of events may be relatively simple and predictable. The important variables will be the degree of cell damage and the capacity of the host tissues to produce inflammation and repair. Histamine and bradykinin both have a short half-life of about a few minutes only and prostaglandin synthesis ceases when the cell membrane fractions are cleared away by phagocytes, usually within a few days. Repair involves the return to normal tissue fluid dynamics, the redifferentiation of odontoblasts and, subsequently, the deposition of reparative dentine may occur. Although the inflammatory events described above can be regarded as reversible, the pulpal tissue will subsequently be less cellular, less vascular and more fibrous. That is, it will have 'aged', in a manner similar to pulp tissue after chronic inflammation, and will also be less able to withstand subsequent insult in any form.

Acute inflammation leading to pulp death

More severe, nonbacterial insults causing a greater degree of cell damage or death may bring about more marked vaso-dilatation and the movement of substantial amounts of blood fluid and protein into the injured tissues. In the young individual healing may occur through the sequence of events described above, despite the severity of the injury and the initial response. However, in an older patient or in a pulp that has been compromised by previous episodes of inflammation and repair, such damage may lead to the death of the entire pulp. Cell death and disintegration may release lysosomal enzymes into the extracellular environment, causing the death of more cells. The process of cell death almost always ends just short of the root apex. The periapical tissues are more able to resist damage than those of the aged or compromised pulp because they have a rich collateral circulation.

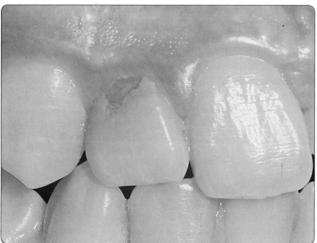

Fig. 5.9 Idiopathic external resorption. The upper right lateral incisor shows the typical 'pink spot' at the gingival margin which is often the first evidence of a resorption lesion.

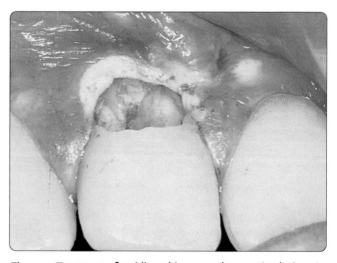

Fig. 5.10 Treatment of an idiopathic external resorption lesion. A lesion similar to that shown in Fig. 5.9 after careful debridement. It will be restored with glass–ionomer cement.

Direct pressure measurements in various areas of normal and inflamed pulps have shown that the tissue behaves as a gel, not a fluid, and that local pressure increases will not spread. The assumption that a pulp is destined to die if it suffers an episode of acute inflammation is therefore not warranted, particularly if bacteria are not involved.

Treatment of the dead pulp

Once blood supply and vitality have been lost, the only predictable therapy that allows long-term tooth retention is the removal of necrotic tissue debris from the pulp space and its replacement with an inert filling material. If this is not done, the tissue debris is likely to become infected at some later time, resulting in periapical infection, inflammation and pain. The anticipated mode of infection consists in anachoresis, the lodgement of bacteria from adjacent tissues, or the blood supply, into the pulp chamber where they can survive and multiply.

PERIAPICAL INFLAMMATION

There is continuity between the pulp and the periodontal ligament through either the apical foramina or the lateral accessory canals. Therefore, inflammatory processes within the pulp tend to affect the periapical or periradicular regions and induce what are generally termed periapical lesions. Most commonly, chronic apical periodontitis develops as a consequence of, and concomitantly with, chronic pulpitis of bacterial origin. Depending on the nature and number of the microorganisms invading the dentine and pulp, this apical response can become well established while all or most of the pulp tissue is still alive.

PULPAL PAIN AND SENSATION

The pulp is richly supplied with sensory nerves, many of which end close to the odontoblastic cell bodies, and will respond to stimuli, such as change of temperature. Application of stimuli may also cause pain via movement of the odontoblast cells through fluid in the dentinal tubules. Finally, cell damage and inflammation within the body of the pulp may stimulate the sensory nerves and also cause pain.

Complete loss of sensibility of the dentine and pulp usually indicates that the entire pulpal tissue is dead. However, there is not an absolute link between sensibility and vitality because patients may report apparently normal sensory responses in teeth that, on histological examination, show no evidence of vital pulp, whereas others have no sensibility in teeth that are otherwise normal.

The periodontal ligament at the root apex is also well innervated. Sensory nerves within the ligament normally provide information to the brainstem nuclei on pressure or mechanical load and tooth displacement. Such sensory information subconsciously contributes to masticatory control and may also be noted consciously as touch,

pressure and pain. Inflammation in the periapical tissues decreases the critical firing threshold of the sensory nerves of the region and allows the initiation of pain by relatively minor tooth movement. Palpation through gentle movement of the tooth with finger pressure, or, alternatively percussion by gently tapping with a solid instrument may well elicit pain under these circumstances.

Tests of pulpal and periapical status

No one test alone can give an accurate picture of the state of the dental pulp or periapex. It is only by the correlation of all available information that the clinician can arrive at a diagnosis. A careful visual examination, using good illumination and magnification, plus a radiographic examination should be used in conjunction with the tests described in **Fig. 5.11**.

Methods for testing pulpal and periapical status	
Heat	Sensibility to heat may be tested by the selective application of hot water from a syringe, heated gutta percha sticks or thermostatically controlled heat applicators.
Cold	Selective application can be carried out using cold water in a syringe, a stick of ice, solid carbon dioxide (dry ice), or ethyl chloride on a cotton pellet.
Percussion	Tap the tooth gently, vertically then laterally, with a suitable solid instrument such as the handle of a mouth mirror. Sharp pain may be elicited, which may persist for a brief time.
Palpation	Digital pressure on the tooth itself, then on the soft tissues adjacent to the root apices may elicit pain or may reveal soft or hard swelling of the tissue.
Electrical	Electric pulp testers may indicate the presence of viable pulp nerves but they do not give a reliable indication of the state of pulpal tissue. They should not be used in individuals with cardiac pacemakers.
Differential anaesthesia	Despite using all of the above tests it may be necessary to use either subperiosteal infiltration or intraligamentary local anaesthesia for individual teeth to help reach a decision on which tooth is causing pain.

Fig. 5.11 Methods for testing pulpal and periapical status.

FURTHER READING

Hilton TJ. Cavity sealers, liners and bases: current philosophies and indications for use. *Oper Dent* 1996; **21**:134–46.

Hume WR, Massey WL. Keeping the pulp alive: the pharmacology and toxicology of agents applied to dentine. *J Aust Dent* 1990; **35**:32–7.

Kim S, Trowbridge H. Pulpal reactions to caries and dentine procedures. In: Cohen S, Burns RC, eds. *Pathways of the pulp, 6th ed.* St Louis: Mosby; 1994.

Smulson MH, Hagen JC, Ellenz SJ. Histopathology and diseases of the dental pulp. In: Weine FS, ed. *Endodontic therapy, 5th ed.* St Louis: Mosby; 1996.

Smulson MH, Hagen JC, Ellenz SJ. Pulpoperiapical pathology and immunological considerations. In: Weine FS, ed. *Endodontic therapy, 5th ed.* St Louis: Mosby; 1996.

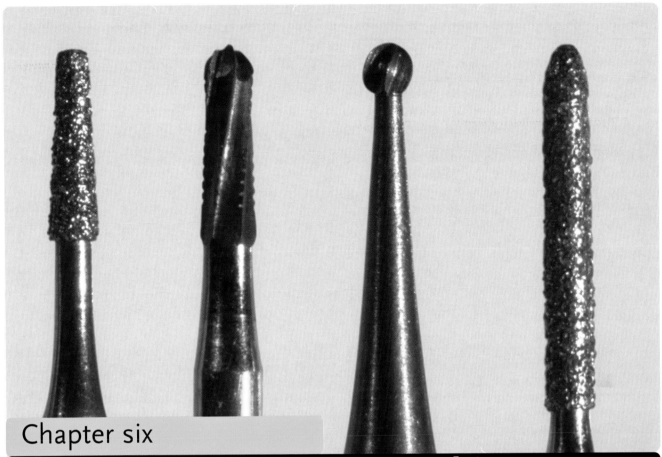

Chapter six

Cutting instruments used in tooth restoration

G.J. Mount

A stage may be reached in the progression of dental caries where preventive therapy and remineralisation techniques will no longer be successful. In the presence of frank cavitation in both enamel and dentine, it will no longer be possible to eliminate plaque. It then becomes necessary to surgically debride the lesion and restore the tooth to its original anatomy, thus preventing further breakdown. It is also sometimes necessary to shape and restore broken teeth, and to remove and replace defective restorations. Each of these actions requires cutting either tooth tissues or hard restorative materials.

Enamel is the hardest material in the body. Some restorative materials are of similar hardness and dentine is only a little softer. Rotating cutting instruments travelling at various speeds are the most effective means of reducing both tooth tissue and restorative material. However, refinement of cavity margins is not always possible with rotary instruments because of difficulties of access and, also, final removal of softened infected dentine may best be carried out using a degree of tactile sense. Under these circumstances, hand instruments remain useful.

ROTARY CUTTING INSTRUMENTS

Classification of burs

There is a vast array of sizes and shapes available in the market and, in an attempt to rationalise the selection, the International Standards Organisation has developed a classification, ISO 6360. The essential dimensions of burs, including the material, shank type, overall length, shape and type of finish of the working head and the size of the head have been ordered numerically (**Fig. 6.1**).

Annoyance factor

The term 'annoyance factor' is used rather loosely to describe the patient's subjective reaction to cavity preparation and is a combination of the pressure applied to the tooth, the vibrations and noise recorded through the bones of the skull, the heat and smell generated at the interface between the tooth and the bur and the time taken to perform a given task (**Fig. 6.2**).

Vibration and noise generation are related closely to the coarseness of the cutting instrument and the speed of rotation. Within limits, the use of higher speeds and smaller instruments reduces vibration, but concentricity is also important and requires maintenance of the handpiece and equipment. The generation of heat and smell are both closely associated with the adequacy of lubrication and the efficiency of the instrument in removing shavings from the tooth.

Surface finish on the cavity

The quality of the surface finish of a completed cavity is clinically significant, particularly if an adhesive restorative material is to be used. Adhesion is best achieved in the presence of smooth surfaces because this will lead to a more intimate adaptation between the two materials and

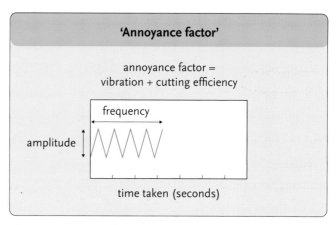

Fig. 6.2 'Annoyance factor'. A diagrammatic representation of the relative discomfort suffered by the patient depending on the selection of bur size, shape and surface as well as the speed of rotation and pressure applied during cutting. These factors are then related to the time taken to complete the task and a factor number can be allocated from 1 to 10.

reduce the possibility of voids at the interface. The surface roughness index (Ra) is designed to define the depth of remaining scratches; it is, therefore, a measure of smoothness. Surface roughness index is usually defined as the arithmetical mean deviation of a profile; it is measured electronically with a machine such as a Surftest-III (Metutoyo, Tokyo, Japan).

VARIETY OF ROTARY CUTTING INSTRUMENTS

Selection of burs

Rotary cutting instruments usually remove tooth structure either by chipping it away or by grinding. Instruments with blades such as steel burs or tungsten carbide burs will lift particles of enamel or dentine depending on the number

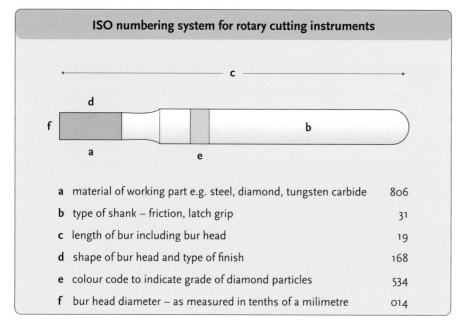

Fig. 6.1 International Standards Organisation (ISO) numbering system for rotary cutting instruments. This is the basic code recommended by ISO to enable a universal numbering system to be developed for recognition of all rotary cutting instruments.

ISO numbering system for rotary cutting instruments

a	material of working part e.g. steel, diamond, tungsten carbide	806
b	type of shank – friction, latch grip	31
c	length of bur including bur head	19
d	shape of bur head and type of finish	168
e	colour code to indicate grade of diamond particles	534
f	bur head diameter – as measured in tenths of a milimetre	014

of blades, the rake angle of the blades and the shavings-removal efficiency of the design of the blades (**Fig. 6.3**). Blades that twist around the shank of the bur will remove debris more readily; even more efficient are those blades with a cross-cut design. Burs with eight or fewer blades are designed for rough or gross cutting; increasing the number of blades on a bur improves the fineness of the surface and the smoothness of the cut. Tungsten carbide burs with 30 or more blades are used for polishing.

Diamond burs will grind away tooth structure: they are available in a range of particle size of about 4–150 μm. Diamonds with a particle size of 150 μm are extremely coarse with a high annoyance factor, so the regular 100 μm particles are usually selected for basic cavity preparation. Finer diamonds with particle sizes ≤ 25 μm are recommended for polishing procedures. The particles are attached to the shank of the bur through either a galvanic metal bond or a sintering process; the quality and efficiency of the bur is dependent upon both the degree of attachment of the particles and the clearance of the shavings.

Steel burs

These were the burs originally used when rotary cutting instruments were first developed, over 100 years ago. They are still valuable for removal of caries and development of retentive elements in dentine. They are designed for slow speeds, under 5000 r.p.m. Each bur usually has eight blades

and some of them have a positive rake angle to ease the cutting of dentine or caries removal. However, this causes steel burs to be fragile and easily chipped along the leading edge; they should not be expected to have a long life in normal practice.

The use of air–water spray during cutting with these burs will increase efficiency, but is not essential. Usually, the shanks are designed for latch-type handpieces but some manufacturers now make burs with friction-grip shanks, which help to maintain concentricity, thereby reducing vibration. Any bur rotating at low speeds will produce a high annoyance factor. A good tactile sense is essential for the operator to avoid over-cutting. Therefore, burs must always be in good condition and visibility must be excellent at all times.

Tungsten carbide burs

After the development of higher speed handpieces, there was a need for stronger steel burs to withstand the heavier stresses and to lengthen their useful life. Tungsten carbide burs are designed almost exclusively for friction-grip handpieces because concentricity is essential and they only cut efficiently at greatly increased speeds. In fact, they do not begin to reach effective cutting capacity until 100 000 r.p.m. and are best used at speeds beyond 300 000 r.p.m. In recent years, one of the main variations in these burs has been to increase the number of blades and to vary the rake angle of the blades (**Fig. 6.4**). The usual bur has six blades and a negative rake angle to provide better support for the cutting edge. For the same reason, many burs have a radial clearance. These burs cut metal and dentine well, but are prone to produce microcracks in enamel, thus weakening the cavosurface margin. However, a tungsten carbide bur with 12 or more blades can be very efficient for polishing enamel margins and dentine surfaces.

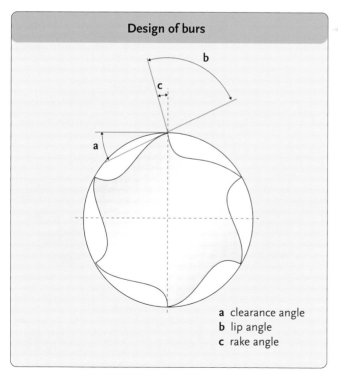

Design of burs

a clearance angle
b lip angle
c rake angle

Fig. 6.3 Design of burs. The design of the blades is predicated on the need to eliminate debris rapidly, at the same time preserving strength in the blades to avoid chipping. Tungsten carbide burs generally have a negative rake angle for additional strength. Many steel burs have a positive rake angle but are prone to chipping.

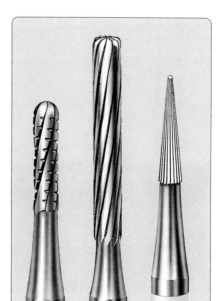

Fig. 6.4 Selection of tungsten carbide burs. These burs show the various blade configurations: cross-cut, plain and multiblade.

It is essential that tungsten carbide burs be used at speeds above 100 000 r.p.m. Air–water spray is mandatory for the removal of debris and for temperature control and burs must be mounted in a friction grip cartridge for concentricity. Probably only a new bur will be truly concentric because any loss of a blade, or even a piece of a blade, will alter the balance, with the result that only every third or fourth blade will contact the tooth and remove material. This means that the clinical life is usually short. The annoyance factor with a new bur at high linear surface speed is very low but a lack of concentricity will be immediately discernible to the patient.

Diamond burs or stones

Diamonds abrade tooth structure rather than cut or chip it and are therefore more efficient over a greater range of speeds; they are also less likely to chip or break, either themselves or the tooth. They are most efficient when used against hard materials such as enamel or porcelain, although very fine diamonds are excellent for reducing dentine to a fine finish. Initially, diamond burs were covered with large diamond particles and were regarded as rather coarse, leaving a finish with a surface roughness index of up to 50 μm. Recently, there have been considerable improvements in the methods of embedding diamond particles into the metal of the bur head; the burs now last longer and there is a much better distribution of particle size. Large particle size ensures rapid removal of porcelain and enamel but leaves a rough surface. Fine particles leave fine scratches and it is possible now to produce a polished surface with particles down to a surface roughness index of 4 μm. There is a variety of grit sizes between 4 μm and 150 μm, to be selected according to the task in hand (Figs 6.5 and 6.6).

Air–water spray is mandatory to enhance clearance and to control heat development, which will be greater as the particle size reduces and clearance is slowed down. Diamond burs will cut efficiently over a wide range of speeds; and, logically, the annoyance factor will be least with the finer grain size if lower speeds are to be utilised.

SIZE AND SHAPE OF ROTARY CUTTING INSTRUMENTS

The original steel burs, designed for low-speed handpieces, were divided into shapes broadly described as follows (**Fig. 6.7**).

- Flat fissure – a parallel sided cylindrical bur of varying length, designed to extend a cavity along a fissure.
- Tapered fissure – similar to a flat fissure but with the sides tapered towards the tip, designed to develop retentive grooves and pin holes.
- Round – spherical burs, designed to remove caries and to develop retentive pinholes.
- Inverted cone – a bur with a flat base and sides tapered towards the shank, designed to develop a flat floor in a cavity as well as undercuts adjacent to the floor for retention of plastic restorative materials.

These shapes have been retained but modified to a considerable extent for increased speed. The original

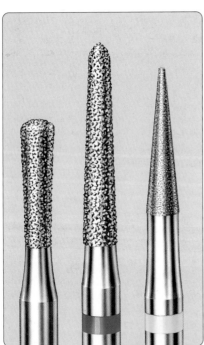

Fig. 6.5 Selection of diamond stones. These show the various grit sizes and distribution.

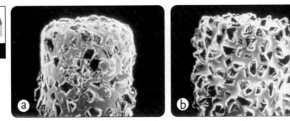

Fig. 6.6 Diamond stones. A comparison of a fine polishing diamond (a) with a coarse diamond (b) showing comparative grit size (×80).

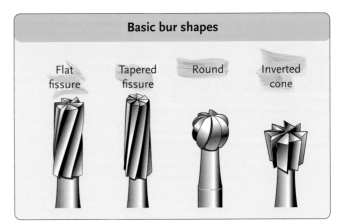

Fig. 6.7 Basic bur shapes. Shown are the four basic shapes in which burs are manufactured. However, the inverted cone is not in common use any longer because the production of undercuts for retention is not required in the presence of adhesion.

subdivision is still valid and burs and their application can still be discussed under those headings, although slightly modified. One complicating factor has been the plethora of rather bizarre bur shapes produced by manufacturers at the whim of individual operators who develop an unusual shape to fulfil one task only in tooth reduction. The result can be a vast array of burs with limited functions that tend to clutter up bur storage and serve very limited purpose. It is recommended that bur shapes and sizes be strictly limited and that the burs of various shapes be used to their full extent.

Elimination of inverted cone

Simplification of bur selection is achieved by eliminating the inverted cone. The original concept behind a bur of this shape was that it should undercut sound enamel and then remove it by being withdrawn vertically through the enamel. This is no longer necessary for cavity preparation and the sharp acute angles which are likely to be produced between the floor and the walls are difficult to restore properly with a plastic restorative material. Retentive features can be developed better with burs of other shapes.

CUTTING EFFICIENCY

Tooth fabric can be removed at different rates depending upon the intended outcome. If it is necessary to remove a large quantity in a short time then, within the constraints of the annoyance factor, a large-diameter coarse-cutting bur rotating at an ultra-high speed with a copious water spray will accomplish this. On the other hand, precise cavity outline form can be achieved with greater accuracy and with conservation of remaining tooth structure at lower speeds with smaller burs and an improved tactile sense.

End cutting or side cutting

It is important to consider whether a bur will cut efficiently at its end or along its side. Entry through intact enamel requires an end cutter; development of cavity outline requires a side cutter. It is possible to combine the two functions in one bur. A logical choice of bur should be made according to the particular task, and the number of burs in a kit should be kept to a minimum.

Linear surface speed

Within limits, the faster the surface of one material passes over the surface of another material, the faster will be the abrasive effect and the greater will be the removal of material. Therefore, the linear surface speed of the rotating bur is significant. The speed can be calculated using the following formula:

$$V = \pi d n$$

where V is the linear surface speed, d is the diameter of the bur and n is revolutions per minute. It must be noted that the linear surface speed of a bur will vary according to the geometry of the bur, which means that the tip of a tapered bur will not travel as fast as the butt. Therefore, cutting efficiency will be different at different positions on the same bur.

In general, higher speeds produce smoother operation; that is, providing the bur is running concentrically, vibration will be reduced as the speed increases. However, there is a limit because centrifugal forces take precedence at ultra-high speeds. For example, a bur with a diameter of 2 mm should not exceed 300 000 r.p.m. or it may bend and break. Also, it is difficult to maintain concentricity in a rotating bur and, at higher speeds, this problem is somewhat 'ironed out': to have only every third or fourth blade working is less significant at ultra-high speeds, and vibration is reduced.

Application of load

As the speed of a bur increases, the load that can be applied without the bur stalling decreases; this is because of torque limitations with air turbines. This means that the tactile sense of the operator also decreases. It is therefore possible to over-cut tooth structure with ultra-high speed burs if visibility is less than excellent. With electric micro-motors, torque can remain high by using an electrical feed-back circuit and tactile sense remains high.

Load before stalling will also be dependent upon the linear surface speed of the bur, the presence or absence of an adequate lubricant and the sharpness of the bur. There is a temptation to extend the life of a bur beyond its useful working life by applying greater load, but in so doing the temperature at the work face will be increased, there will be greater wear and tear on the handpiece bearings and the concentricity of the handpiece will degenerate more rapidly.

The exact amount of load is variable, but usually should be about 60 g and 120 g must be regarded as a maximum. With a given load, the rate of cutting increases with the speed of rotation, but not in direct proportion. At speeds above 100 000 r.p.m. the rate of cutting does not increase greatly; above 400 000 r.p.m. the risks of losing concentricity outweigh the cutting advantages and torque will be substantially reduced.

Lubrication

A coolant applied to the tooth surface and the bur head during cutting reduces the temperature rise and increases the cutting rate by acting as a lubricant. The coolant can be air, water or a combination of the two in the form of a spray. A copious stream of water is the most effective, providing it can directly reach the operative area, but an air–water spray is adequate. It has been shown that cutting dentine with no lubricant may result in a temperature rise at the surface of the tooth in contact with the bur of up to 136°C in only 2 seconds. Air alone will maintain a low temperature but, if used for other than short periods, may dehydrate the tooth and damage the pulp. Using an air–water spray with a water flow rate of 35–50 ml/min, the temperature rise can be limited to 20–30°C. Water alone is even more effective inasmuch as the temperature rise can be limited to 10°C with a flow of only 10 ml/min. However, ensuring that the bur head is adequately bathed with the water is not always easy in the oral cavity and the combined air–water spray is generally regarded as more effective.

Visual contact with the bur head

It is important to maintain visual contact with the working head of the bur during cavity preparation, particularly if the cavity is small and in a confined position. The enamel on the occlusal surface of a molar will be approximately 2–3 mm thick; therefore, if a bur with a head less than 3 mm in length is used to open the fissure, it will disappear from view on reaching the dentine (**Fig. 6.8**). The result can be deep over-cutting and a degree of loss of direction. Penetration into the dentine may be over-extended and the tooth may be unnecessarily weakened.

If the bur head is about 5 mm in length, it will be possible to maintain visual contact at all times and cavity preparation will be more conservative. A diamond cylinder of this dimension is both end-cutting and side-cutting and a fissure can be opened both quickly and efficiently, even when access and visibility is limited. Round or pear-shaped burs are contraindicated for these tasks.

SPEED GROUPINGS

With modern handpieces and the motive power to drive them, rotational speeds from under 1000 r.p.m. to 400 000 r.p.m. are available and, taking into account the above discussions, it is logical to make use of the entire range. However, considering the essential requirements of operative dentistry, it is equally logical to subdivide the stages of cavity preparation and assess the appropriate speed for each activity. Most manufacturers colour-code handpieces (**Fig. 6.9**).

It is usually necessary to enter the lesion through the enamel. The caries can then be removed and the final cavity outline refined to receive the ultimate restoration. Each stage of cavity preparation has its own special requirements in regard to:

- bur selection – diamond, tungsten carbide or steel
- speed of cutting – ultra-high speed, intermediate high speed or low speed
- lubrication – water jet, air alone or combination air–water spray
- visibility – direct or indirect
- reduction of the annoyance factor.

Lubrication with air–water spray is desirable at all speeds for temperature control and removal of cutting debris, but short periods using air alone are acceptable for enhanced visibility.

The speed and efficiency of a rotary cutting instrument will depend to a degree on the engineering and quality of manufacture. It is also necessary to define the optimal size of a bur relative to the linear surface speed and then accurately assess the load to which that bur can be subjected without producing a high annoyance factor (**Fig. 6.10**).

Low speed

- 500–10 000 r.p.m. – green band handpiece
- 1000–25 000 r.p.m. – blue band handpiece

factor = 8

Steel burs are indicated in this speed range and the use of a lubricant is optional. Visibility is better without a lubricant but cutting is faster and cleaner with at least an air spray. Because of the negative rake angle on a modern tungsten carbide bur, they are relatively 'blunt' at this speed. Diamond burs are designed to cut hard tooth material and are not effective in removing soft caries.

The diameter of steel burs can range from 0.5 mm to 3.0 mm; smaller burs have smaller annoyance factors. The size should be selected to fit the particular task. Tasks include removal of caries and development of retentive designs, and placement of pins, grooves and ditches, as well as all stages of polishing to a final finish.

Intermediate high speed

- 20 000–80 000 r.p.m. – red band handpiece
- 20 000–120 000 r.p.m. – orange band handpiece

factor = 3

Diamond burs with a medium to fine grit are the most efficient in this range and use of a lubricant is mandatory. Air alone for very short periods is acceptable because it will enhance visibility, but cutting will be faster under air–water spray.

Tungsten carbide burs tend to 'chatter' at this speed and may cause microcracks in enamel and an increased annoyance factor. Steel burs will not cut at these speeds and the annoyance factor would be far too high. Diameter of the burs to be used in this speed grouping cover a wide range but, logically, the smaller the bur the lower will be

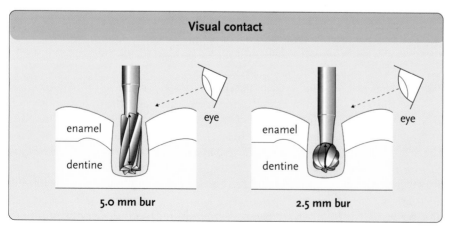

Visual contact

enamel

dentine

eye

5.0 mm bur

enamel

dentine

eye

2.5 mm bur

Fig. 6.8 Visual contact. It is important, wherever possible, to maintain visual contact with the working area of the bur head to minimise depth of penetration and thereby limit the amount of sound tooth fabric removed.

the annoyance factor.

There is a very fine tactile sense available within this speed range and the risk of over-cutting is minimal. Therefore, speeds in this range should be used in the development of small cavities as well as to refine final cavity outline for all restorations. Such speeds are also useful for initial contouring of most restorations, leading to a final polish. This is the correct speed group for refining the occlusions.

Ultra-high speed

- 250 000–400 000 r.p.m. – air turbine only

Tungsten carbide burs are at their most efficient in this range, but diamond burs are also very useful. Lubrication is mandatory with a copious water jet being the most efficient for temperature control.

Tungsten carbide burs cut dentine very smoothly so long as they are not chipped or eccentric. They can also develop a fine margin in enamel, although it must be noted that they cut more smoothly along the margin where the rotating bur enters the cavity; the opposite, exit margin, is likely to chip more readily. Because they are essentially a side-cutting bur, they should not be used to enter through healthy enamel into a new lesion. They cut old metal restorations well.

Diamonds are more versatile and a coarse end-cutting diamond is the preferred bur to enter a new lesion or remove bulk enamel, even though both entry and exit margins will be relatively rough, depending upon the size of the grit being used.

The diameters of burs for this speed group are ≤ 2 mm.

Initial entry to most lesions and the removal of old restorations is achieved best in this speed range. The tactile sense is minimal and over-cutting is possible if visibility is limited at all. Use these speeds only for gross reduction of tooth structure, then reduce to an intermediate high speed when refining the cavity.

Speed grouping	RPM	Handpiece colour	Lubricant
Low speed	500–25 000	Green or blue	Optional
Intermediate high speed	20 000–120 000	Red or orange	Mandatory
Ultra-high speed	250 000–400 000		Mandatory

Fig. 6.9 Colour coding for handpieces. Colour codes used by most manufacturers to indicate the speed at which a handpiece will work best. The variations are achieved by variation in gearing ratios.

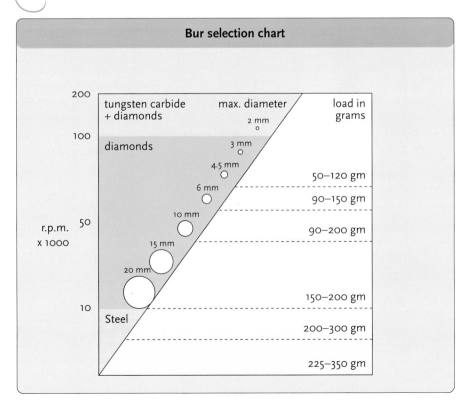

Bur selection chart

Fig. 6.10 Bur selection chart. The chart shows the maximum diameter of a bur relative to the speed available as well as the maximum load which can be applied for optimum efficiency. Note that diamonds have a wide range of speeds available whereas tungsten carbides are efficient only above 100 000 r.p.m. On the other hand, steel burs should only be used below 10 000 r.p.m. Water spray must be used as a lubricant at speeds above 10 000 r.p.m.

HAND INSTRUMENTS

Hand instruments preceded rotary cutting instruments by many years and continued to be used for refining the cavity outline, until the advent of modern high-speed handpieces and adequate lubrication of the cavity. In the beginning, they were the sole means of entering a cavity and GV Black and others developed a wide range of chisels, hatchets and hoes for the efficient removal of enamel and dentine, and spoon excavators for cleaning out remaining caries (**Fig. 6.11**). Now rotary cutting instruments are sophisticated, fast and efficient, the need for hand instruments is greatly reduced. Two instrument types still have a place:

- Gingival margin trimmers for planing the enamel margins in small spaces where access for rotary cutting instruments is limited;
- Spoon excavators for the final removal of softened demineralised infected dentine.

Gingival margin trimmers

According to the classification defined by GV Black, gingival margin trimmers are modified hatchets. The two modifications incorporated in these instruments are, first, that the cutting edge is at an angle to the shaft other than a right angle and, second, that the blade is curved (i.e. it is a double-plane instrument). It is the curve in the blade that makes it a lateral scraping instrument. These are paired instruments, where the blade angle is set for either a left or right function and, in the partner instrument, the

blade angle is set for planing the enamel rods in either a mesial or distal proximal box.

The width of the blade varies from 1.0 mm to 1.5 mm and it is the finer of these two that is recommended for continuing use. Typical numbers in the Black classification are 10.80.7.14 and 10.95.7.14; these are fine enough to trim the cavosurface margins of the average minimal cavity without extending the cavity unduly or damaging the adjacent tooth. It is essential that these instruments be kept very sharp and are used with a light touch otherwise there is a risk of producing microcracks in the enamel walls or of over-extending the cavity outline.

Spoon excavators

The spoon excavator is also a double-plane instrument that can be regarded as a modified hatchet. However, the cutting blade is curved or rounded. It is also designed for lateral scraping and is generally provided with left and right blades at opposite ends of the same shaft. The typical spoon excavator number is 12.90.8.12 for the right side and 12.10.8.12 for the left side; the blades vary in diameter.

It is essential that the blades are maintained in a sharp condition and that they are used with a very light touch so that the demineralised layer on the floor of the average cavity, known as the affected dentine (see Chapters 2 and 18), is maintained rather than removed.

RECOMMENDATIONS FOR INSTRUMENT CHOICE

Selection of burs

It is desirable to maintain only a small selection of burs because a broader selection only leads to confusion and one bur size or shape can perform many functions. The list offered here is brief and is not meant to be exhaustive. The numbers are taken from ISO 6360 and represent only the shape of the bur head and not the size or type of finish; each individual operator is expected to make a choice in those regards, but the burs of the shapes selected will perform all the functions required in general practice, including crowns and bridge preparations (**Fig. 6.12**).

Access through enamel

To gain very conservative access into enamel, such as exploring a fissure before sealing, use a very fine tapered diamond bur (#200Dia) at intermediate high speed under air–water lubrication. The bur should be approximately 0.3 mm at the butt, taper to a fine point and be no more than 5 mm in length. There is a very fine tactile sense under these circumstances and over-extension can be avoided.

To open into a larger carious lesion, use a tapered diamond bur (#168Dia) at ultra-high speed under copious lubricant. The bur should have a diameter of 1.5 mm at the tip and approximately 2.0 mm at the butt. Because the bur will need to be end-cutting, it should have rounded corners at the operative end, with diamond particles

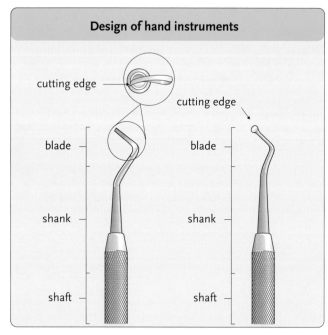

Fig. 6.11 Design of hand instruments. These are typical hand instruments showing the elements in the design. There are infinite variations available in both size and angulation of the blade to the shank as well as the shank to the shaft. Most are double-ended with a left-handed and a right-handed functioning blade on each instrument.

securely attached in that area. The length of the head should not exceed 5 mm. With these dimensions, the bur will attain a high linear surface speed, but have a low annoyance factor.

Extension through enamel for gross cavity outline

A small parallel-sided diamond bur (#156Dia) with similar dimensions to that used for accessing enamel should be used to extend the cavity through the enamel, at ultra-high speed under copious lubricant. To be certain that visual contact with the bur is maintained, the cutting area of the bur must be longer than the thickness of the enamel plus at least 1 mm. Thus, when the cavity has just penetrated into dentine, the butt end of the working head of the bur will remain visible during extension. With care and a concentric bur, a fissure cavity will not require further refinement and over-extension may be avoided. Parallel walls will be sufficiently retentive for both amalgam and composite resin.

At ultra-high speed, vibration will be at a minimum, thus maintaining a low annoyance factor, but tactile sense is low and great care must be exercised to avoid over-cutting.

Refine cavity outline form

The small tapered diamond bur (#168Dia), used for the initial entry, should be used at intermediate high speed. This speed range allows for a fine tactile sense combined with rapid removal of both enamel and dentine and a minimum annoyance factor to the patient. The bur should be approximately 5 mm in length to allow constant visual contact with the butt end, as described in Figure 6.8. Air–water spray is desirable, although short periods with air alone will permit excellent vision for final refinement without undue dehydration of the tooth.

The tapered cylinder diamond bur is both end-cutting and side-cutting and, with medium grit diamonds (15–25 μm), will develop enamel margins that might not require further refining. There will be a need for a light touch, particularly when developing cusp-protection designs (see Chapter 7). Finer polishing diamonds (#223Dia) are

available if there is a need to polish the margin.

The use of tungsten carbide burs in the intermediate high speed range is strictly contraindicated, particularly if the bur has been used previously. When new, these burs will cut both enamel and dentine very cleanly but if there is any eccentricity through chipping of a blade, the bur will contact the tooth on every third or fourth revolution only. The result may be chipping or shattering of the enamel margin leaving it unsuitable, particularly for a cavity being prepared for the placement of an adhesive restorative material.

Removal of caries

Softened demineralised infected dentine is best removed at low speed (about 2000 r.p.m.) with steel burs (#008–016); the use of a lubricant is optional. Steel burs are rather fragile and prone to chipping and should not be expected to last for long, particularly if they come into contact with enamel or an old metal or resin restoration. A good tactile sense is afforded but they may cause considerable vibration if handled carelessly and will add to the annoyance factor. Round burs are side-cutting and will not penetrate easily beyond the softened tooth material. Use the largest bur commensurate with the size of the lesion to enhance the side-cutting effect.

Refine retention form

Retentive grooves and ditches should be cut using a small tapered steel bur (#168MS) at low speed, to retain optimal tactile sense. The bur should be approximately 1 mm in diameter at the tip, to produce a ditch 1 mm wide at the base and up to 1.5 mm wide at the entry. This will facilitate packing the restorative material into the ditch and ensure proper condensation. The ditches should be placed at angles to each other to ensure a retentive design surrounding the central core of the tooth (see Chapter 7).

The placement of pins, either friction-lock or self-threading, is not recommended because of the potential for the development of microcracks in the dentine with subsequent leakage and loss of retention.

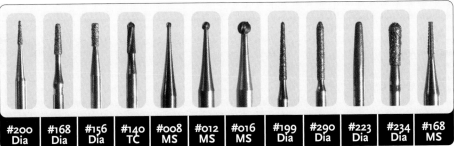

#200 Dia	#168 Dia	#156 Dia	#140 TC	#008 MS	#012 MS	#016 MS	#199 Dia	#290 Dia	#223 Dia	#234 Dia	#168 MS

Fig. 6.12 Standard bur kit. This kit of burs will perform all the standard procedures for cavity preparation as well as preparing extracoronal restorations. There may be occasions where alternatives are useful, but a large range is unnecessary.

PREPARATION FOR RIGID RESTORATION MATERIALS

The burs recommended for cavities for rigid restoration materials can be listed as follows. A relatively coarse parallel-sided diamond cylinder (#290) can be used at ultra high speed for gross reduction of enamel, dentine and old restorative materials. It is too broad to fit safely between adjacent teeth without potential damage so the preparation of mesial and distal surfaces should be carried out with a fine tapered diamond (#199).

Occlusal reduction can be achieved readily with a relatively coarse pear-shaped diamond (#234) and then the entire preparation can be refined and smoothed using a fine sintered diamond (#223). As this bur has a 5° taper the final preparation can also achieve a similar taper. It has a rounded end and will thus produced a champfered margin if that is required.

However development of a gingival shoulder can be achieved using a small fine tapered diamond such as a #168Dia. This same bur will also be used to enhance retentive elements.

The use of hand instruments
As suggested above, the use of hand instruments is very limited in the presence of the extensive range of rotary cutting instruments now available.

Gingival margin trimmer
The use of gingival margin trimmers may be necessary in small cavities where close proximity of the adjacent tooth makes impossible the use of burs without risking damage to adjacent tooth structures. They should be used gently to remove isolated and weakened enamel rods around the cavosurface margin; care must be taken to remove no more than is essential of the remaining enamel. There is a temptation to remove unsupported enamel from the gingival margin simply because it is weak and not supported by sound dentine. However, as it is not subject to occlusal load, it is in no danger of fracture and its retention may keep the margin of the restoration out of the gingival crevice. In many situations, it can be supported and retained by the use of an adhesive glass–ionomer.

Spoon excavator
Spoon excavators are designed for the removal of remaining softened infected dentine at the base of a cavity. However, care must be exercised to avoid producing an unnecessary pulp exposure. The progress of the carious lesion through dentine must be well understood because the deepest layers of softened dentine are merely demineralised and not infected and therefore need not be removed (see Chapter 2, page 15 and Chapter 18, page 213). Certainly, there is no need to remove discoloured dentine. It may be difficult on occasions to define the parameters of affected dentine and a sharp excavator may penetrate deeper than is required for control of the lesion.

FURTHER READING

Benavides R, Herrera V. Rubber dam with washed field evacuation: a new approach. *Oper Dent* 1992; **17**:26–8.

Hartley JL. Comparative evaluation of newer devices and techniques for the removal of tooth structure. *J Prosthet Dent* 1958; **8**:170–82

Hudson DC. Cutting properties of dental burs. National Bureau of Dental Standards, Technical News Bulletin. *J Am Dent Assoc* 1955; **39**:154–6.

Schuchard A, Watkins CE. Thermal and histologic response to high speed and ultra-high speed cutting in tooth structure. *J Am Dent Assoc* 1965; **71**:1451–8.

Schuchard A, Watkins CE. Comparative efficiency of rotary cutting instruments. *J Prosthet Dent* 1965; **15**:908–23.

Thompson EO. Clinical application of the washed field technic in dentistry *J Am Dent Assoc* 1955; **51**:703–13.

Watkins CE. Cutting effectiveness of rotary instruments in a turbine handpiece. *J Prosthet Dent* 1970; **24**:181–5.

Woods RM, Dilts WE. Temperature changes associated with various dental cutting procedures. *J Can Dent Assoc* 1969; **35**:311–4.

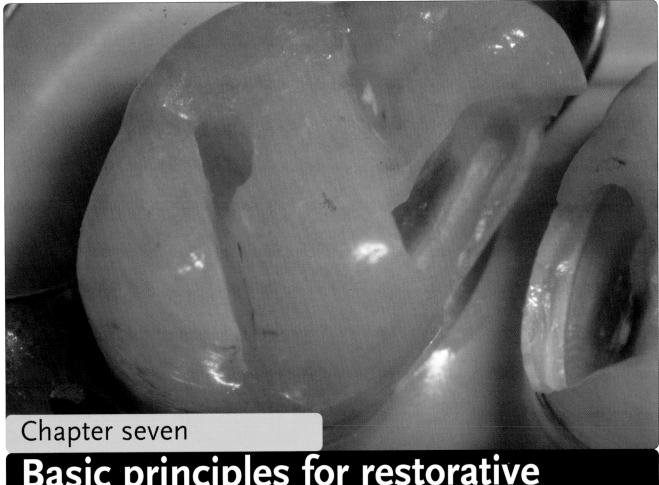

Chapter seven

Basic principles for restorative dentistry

G.J. Mount

When a carious lesion has progressed to the point where it is not possible to remineralise, it is necessary to replace that part which has broken down with a restorative material. If the restoration is to be a success there are a number of factors to be taken into account. This chapter discusses those factors.

No material is universal, and correct selection is important to ensure longevity.

In the following chapters, the commonly used restorative materials will be discussed in sufficient detail to enable the clinician to make a logical selection for each restorative problem.

BASIC PRINCIPLES FOR RESTORATION

When a carious lesion has progressed to a point where it is beyond stabilisation through remineralisation, as discussed in Chapter 2, it is necessary to remove that part of the tooth which is irretrievably broken down and replace it with a restorative material. Selection of the restorative material has a significant effect upon the longevity of the restoration, because the material will help to dictate the longevity of the tooth itself.

Natural tooth structure is a finite commodity and should be preserved and protected as far as possible. There must be a good reason to remove healthy enamel and dentine because it can never be regained. The best restorative material is a poor substitute for the natural material; moreover, rebuilding a tooth to full contour, anatomy and aesthetics is both difficult and expensive. Preparation of a cavity will inevitably weaken remaining tooth structure and each time a restoration is replaced the tooth will become weaker still.

This means that several aspects of each material should be considered before selecting the most appropriate material for a particular task, as shown below.
- Retention of the material within the tooth structure
- Ability to protect remaining tooth structure from further mechanical failure
- Prevention of recurrent caries
- Ability to assist remineralisation of surrounding tooth structure
- Longevity under occlusal load
- Aesthetics.

Principal techniques for placement of restorations
The materials currently in use can be roughly divided into two groups, dictated by the method of clinical placement.

Direct restorative materials
These are classified thus because they are plastic; that is, they are readily deformable when first mixed and are placed into a prepared cavity while still in this condition. After placement, they can be modelled or moulded into the appropriate form before they become rigid and set. They vary in their physical properties, but are expected to achieve a level of strength sufficient to replace effectively missing tooth structure. They can be used to restore a cavity of considerable complexity because of their plasticity, but their physical properties are not always adequate for the tasks imposed.

Indirect restorative materials
These materials are formed on the laboratory bench and the finished restoration is luted into the tooth. Therefore, they require the preparation of a cavity in remaining tooth structure that is completely free of undercuts. An accurate model is made using an impression of the prepared tooth so that the restoration can be fabricated on the model and placed without distortion or stress.

PRINCIPLES OF RETENTION

 Notes

Retention through adhesion is available only with:
- composite resin to enamel (micromechanical)
- glass–ionomer to enamel and dentine (chemical)

A restorative material can be retained on or within a cavity in a tooth either by adhesion or mechanical interlocking. Adhesion can be further subdivided into mechanical interlocking or chemical union through an ion exchange. Either way, successful retention is required both to prevent the restoration from falling out under occlusal load and to prevent microleakage of bacteria into the interface between the restoration and the tooth.

Prevention of microleakage depends largely upon careful manipulation and placement of each of the restorative materials, but retention can be divided into the two categories according to the material used. Composite resin and glass–ionomer are both capable of providing good adhesion and may require no mechanical interlocks. However, amalgam and the rigid restorative materials that are manufactured by indirect techniques rely mainly upon mechanical interlocks, although a degree of adhesion can be developed through the use of luting agents.

Each of the materials will be discussed in relation to their method of retention.

Adhesion with glass–ionomer
Adhesion with glass–ionomer arises entirely through an ion exchange between tooth structure and cement. As the glass powder is mixed with a polyalkenoic acid, calcium and aluminium ions will be released and will form a matrix that will set and hold the particles together. There will also be formation of orthosilicic acid, which will convert to a silica gel as the cement ages and the pH rises, and this will assist further in binding the glass particles together. As the cement is applied to the tooth surface, free polyalkenoic acid will penetrate into both enamel and dentine, displacing calcium and phosphate ions; these will combine with the cement matrix, producing a new ion-enriched material that is firmly bound to both parent materials. The result is a diffusion-based adhesion between the matrix and the glass particles on the one side and the matrix and tooth structure on the other; because the matrix is the weakest material, failure will be cohesive within the cement (**Figs 7.1** and **7.2**).

Although the initial reaction is between the inorganic components of both materials, there is a slow ongoing chemistry that will eventually cause a degree of union with the collagen component of dentine. The cement contains water, and water is a by-product of the chemical reaction, so the presence of further water within the dentine is of little consequence.

In clinical practice, the rather prolonged setting reaction as described in Chapter 8, page 73, must be taken into account. The cement contains a certain amount of bound water, which is essential if the reaction is to occur. There is also some unbound water present which, desirably, should be retained if full physical potential and acceptable translucency are to be achieved in the finally set cement. Hence, it is necessary to maintain the water balance until the set material has reached a degree of maturity.

Also, physical properties are dictated to a degree by the powder content so care must be exercised in both dispensing and mixing. Failure will occur invariably as cohesive failure in the cement, leaving behind an ion-enriched layer firmly attached to the enamel or dentine. This layer is likely to maintain a seal over dentine tubules, thus preventing bacterial microleakage and recurrent caries.

The glass–ionomers adhere in the same manner to both enamel and dentine and the efficiency of adhesion is dictated by:
- use of a high powder:liquid ratio
- placement of the cement onto a clean surface.
- maintenance of the water balance during setting

The technique of placement is relatively simple and straightforward, and longevity is assured following careful application of clinical procedures (see Chapter 8).

Adhesion with composite resin

It is relatively straightforward to develop a mechanical interlock type of adhesion between enamel and composite resin and, in the presence of sound, well supported enamel, this is probably the strongest adhesion available in dentistry. However, adhesion to dentine poses problems because dentine is a very complex material and it is always wet.

Adhesion of composite resin to enamel

Etching with 37% orthophosphoric acid for 15 seconds will cause micropores to appear in the enamel surface, allowing entry of an unfilled low-viscosity resin to a depth of 30–50 μm (**Figs 7.3** and **7.4**). When the resin sets, the strength of the union can be sufficient to withstand a sheer stress of 20 MPa. However, it must be noted that, in setting, the resin contracts and can exert considerable stress upon the union. When bonded to a single surface there may be some flow relaxation during setting, but if placed in a three-dimensional cavity only the outer surface is unbonded and shear stresses of 17–20 MPa are possible. This means that only sound, well-supported enamel should be bonded but, even so, it is possible to overstress weakened cusps in heavily prepared teeth.

CD 102–111

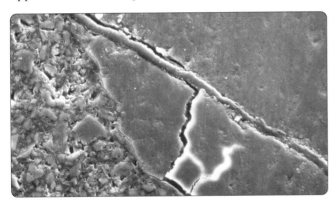

Fig. 7.1 Adhesion of glass–ionomer cement to enamel. A resin-modified glass–ionomer attached to enamel. Note the union with the enamel and some degree of cracking in the enamel (×500).

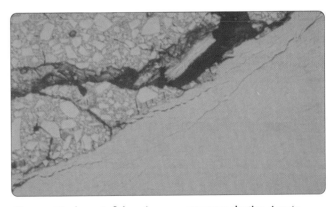

Fig. 7.2 Attachment of glass–ionomer cement to dentine. A resin-modified glass–ionomer cement attached to affected dentine in a simulated ART restoration. Note some cracking in the dentine (× 500).

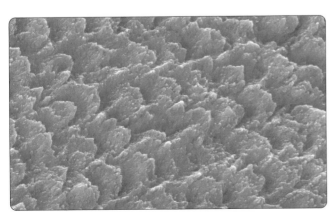

Fig. 7.3 Etched enamel. Enamel surface after 15 seconds of etching with 37% orthophosphoric acid (×2000).

CD 103–111

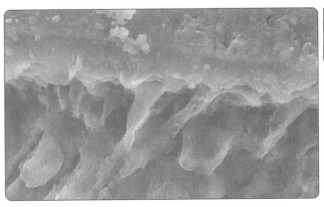

Fig. 7.4 Cross section of composite resin. Composite resin above with resin bond soaked into etched enamel below. Enamel etched away to show penetration (×2000).

Adhesion of composite resin to dentine

Much of the difficulty of bonding composite resin to dentine lies in the complexity of the histological structure and the variable composition of the dentine itself. Dentine is only 45% inorganic, and this component is randomly arranged within an organic matrix that is essentially collagen. Dentine is intimately related to the pulp through the dentine tubules, which are always fluid filled, and each tubule contains an odontoblastic process. There is a constant intrapulpal pressure of 3.3–4.0 kPa, resulting in an outward flow of dentinal fluid. Each tubule is surrounded by a hypermineralised collar of peritubular dentine, with the remaining intertubular dentine being notably less mineralised. The relative area of dentine occupied by tubules decreases as they diverge from the pulp with about 45 000 tubules/mm^2 at the pulp surface, but only 20 000 tubules/mm^2 at the dentino-enamel junction (**Figs 7.5** and **7.6**). In addition, the tubules become narrower as they reach the surface. At the pulp they occupy 22% of the cross-sectional area, whereas near the enamel they occupy only 1%.

The question that must be answered is whether to attempt a chemical adherence to the dentine or whether to develop a micromechanical attachment within the tubules, similar to that achieved so readily with enamel. The former requires a chemical union between a resin, which is essentially hydrophobic, and the dentine which is always wet and contains a complex mix of inorganic and organic material, with greatly varying levels of mineralisation. The latter requires removal of sufficient water for a long enough period to allow penetration of the resin far enough into the tubules to provide an effective mechanical interlock.

A further method involves a micromechanical attachment through development of a so-called hybrid layer. The surface of the intertubular dentine is demineralised and denatured to a depth of approximately 5 μm by the application of an acid, such as 37% orthophosphoric acid (**Fig. 7.7**). Unfilled resin is then led down into the exposed collagen fibres with a hydrophilic leader such as acetone, so that, following activation of the resin, there will be a mechanical interlock with the dentine (**Fig. 7.8**). The composite resin can then be placed into the cavity and

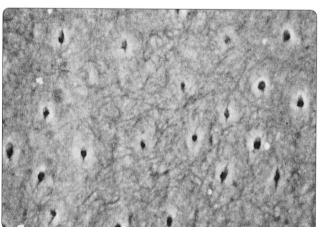

Fig. 7.5 Tubule density. A section close to the dentino-enamel junction shows relatively few small dentine tubules (×1000).

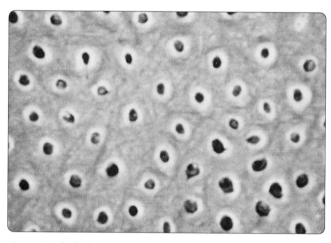

Fig. 7.6 Tubule density. A section close to the pulp chamber. Note size and number of tubules (×1000).

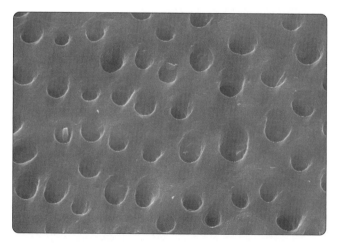

Fig. 7.7 Etched dentine. The surface of dentine after 15 seconds' etch with 37% orthophosphoric acid (×2000).

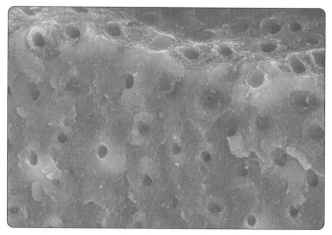

Fig. 7.8 Resin in etched dentine. Resin bond soaked into etched dentine. Note not all tubules are filled with resin (×1000).

united to the adhesive resin layer. Recent in-vitro results suggest high retention strength, but there remain unanswered questions concerning longevity. The long-term effect on collagen is not yet clear and it is possible that demineralising and denaturing the collagen may cause it to be discarded over time. The placement technique is operator sensitive and overall longevity has yet to be tested.

Up to the time of writing, the results of all techniques have been equivocal. Relatively effective adhesion figures can be obtained *in vitro,* but maintaining these figures under the stresses of the oral environment has proved difficult. The main hazards are the dimensional instability during setting and the hydrophobia of the resins, which bind the filler particles together and are the principal constituent of the composite resins. With improvements in these two properties, long-term chemical adhesion to dentine may be developed.

The fillers play no part in adhesion to tooth structure. They are held within the resin matrix either mechanically or through a silane coating which offers some degree of retention to the filler but not to the tooth.

The preferred method of attaching composite resin to dentine is through the use of glass–ionomer cement as the bonding agent, using the lamination technique as discussed in Chapter 8, pages 88–89.

Retention of amalgam

Neither mechanical nor chemical adhesion is available with amalgam, although it is possible to place an adhesive resin or cement layer between amalgam and tooth structure, thus providing a degree of union. At present, in-vitro results appear satisfactory but longevity is unproved. For a small conventional cavity, it is sufficient to provide parallel or slightly convergent walls to retain a section of amalgam, but as the cavity gets larger the problem of retention increases. The major area of strength in remaining tooth structure will lie in the central core of dentine in the gingival one-third of the crown, which suggests that development of retentive elements surrounding that core will offer the best results for extensive restorations. A further consideration is that, often, a large amalgam restoration will subsequently become the foundation for an extracoronal restoration; therefore, maintenance of the central core of dentine is desirable.

Mechanical interlock

Notes

Retention for amalgam should be developed through:
• mechanical interlock
• ditches and grooves
these are safer than:
• self-threading pins, which develop stress in dentine

The best method of developing retention for amalgam within tooth structure is to place ditches and grooves in remaining dentine in such a manner as to engage the central core of dentine (**Figs 7.9–7.11**). Use a small tapered fissure bur at low speed and cut the retentive elements at angles to each other so as to reciprocate from side to side – buccal to lingual or mesial to distal. Individual cusps that are at risk of splitting can be 'tied on', and a tooth showing a mediodistal split can be 'tied together'. Each groove can be made self-retentive by turning the tip of the bur outwards at the end of the groove thus imparting to each retentive element a dovetail shape.

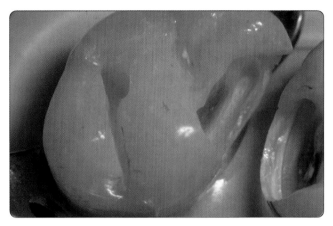

Fig. 7.9 Retentive ditches and grooves. Pronounced groove along the gingival floor of the mesial proximal box provides positive retention.

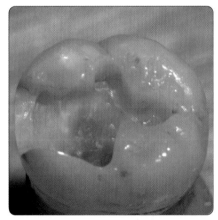

Fig. 7.10 Retentive ditches. Ditches in the floor of the distal proximal box and the end of the buccal groove.

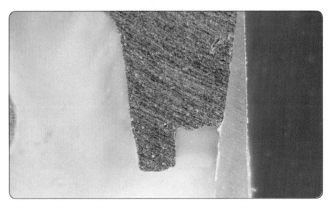

Fig. 7.11 The distal box with a groove approximately 2.0 mm deep.

Use of a tapered fissure bur is recommended because the resultant ditch will be wider at the entry than at the base, and this will facilitate the condensation of amalgam into the groove. Spherical-particle amalgam will flow readily, with the result that it can be fully condensed in a groove up to 3mm deep (**Fig. 7.12**).

Each section of an amalgam restoration should be individually retentive so, as the cavity is extended, ditches and grooves should be incorporated in the design (**Figs 7.13** and **7.14**). An extensive restoration should normally be regarded as a foundation and core for a subsequent extracoronal restoration, which will almost certainly be required as the patient ages. It is essential that it is firmly locked into place (**Figs 7.15** and **7.16**). The amalgam will then become a base, or a dentine replacement, to support the final restoration.

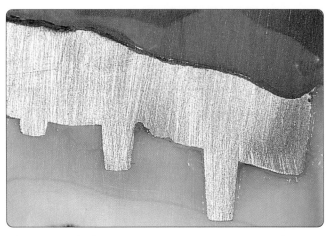

Fig. 7.12 Depth of grooves. Grooves 1.0 mm, 2.0 mm and 3.0 mm in depth, testing amalgam condensation capacity.

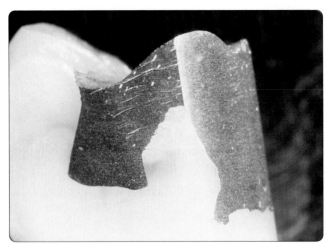

Fig. 7.13 Test cavity with grooves. Cavity prepared in an extracted tooth, restored with amalgam and then cut back to test efficiency of condensation into retentive elements.

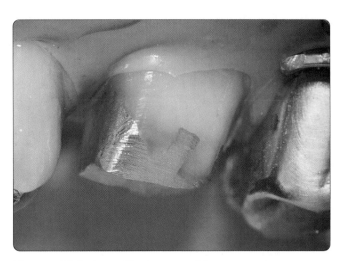

Fig. 7.14 Clinical case. Tooth prepared for a crown shows efficiency of condensation into retentive buccal groove.

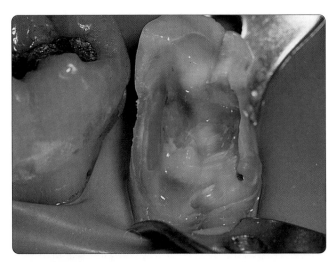

Fig. 7.15 Extensive preparation. Large cavity with grooves and ditches only for retention.

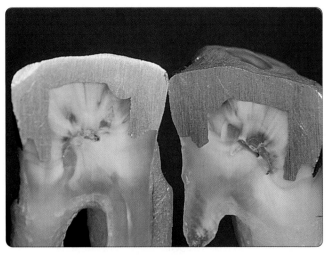

Fig. 7.16 Retention around a central core. The tooth in Figure 7.15 sectioned to demonstrate the central core of dentine embraced by the amalgam.

Supplementary pins

The use of cemented, friction-grip or self-threading pins has been recommended in the past to enhance retention. However, neither cemented nor friction-grip pins offer any mechanical advantage, and self-threading pins place sufficient stress on dentine to lead to subsequent development of microcracks. Their use is not recommended in general, but there may be unusual circumstances where their placement is warranted.

A supplementary pin must be well surrounded by sound tooth structure and will need to lie parallel to both the tooth surface and the pulp chamber. It is worth noting that, at any given point on the root surface, the surface of the root is parallel with the inner surface of the pulp chamber. This means that a periodontal probe placed against the root surface, will give a guide to the direction in which the pulpal wall will be lying. The pin hole should be 2–3 mm in depth; no more than 1 mm of the pin should be left standing in the cavity (**Fig. 7.17**). It is unwise to bend pins after placement because of the risk of propagating cracks in the dentine. If they are properly placed, bending is unnecessary. Shorten a pin using a small diamond stone at ultra-high speed under air–water spray.

Retention of rigid restorations

All rigid restorations will be luted into place with a cement that may have adhesive properties itself. However, any retention offered by the lute will only be as strong as its tensile strength. This may be of some value but the main element of retention will be provided by the design of the cavity preparation (**Fig. 7.18**).

The strength of retention is dictated by three factors:
- it is directly proportional to the area of the vertical walls
- it is affected by the convergence of the walls
- it is only as strong as the weakest link.

In the presence of poor cavity design, the cement should not be relied upon to enhance retention because, generally, with the exception of some resin cements, the tensile strength of a luting cement is not high.

Area of vertical walls

The circumference of the involved tooth will be significant, with the result that a molar tooth will offer more retention than a bicuspid, but the height of the preparation is more significant still. Therefore, it is desirable to rebuild a tooth that is badly broken down to a level similar to its original height before designing the final preparation. If the material with which it is rebuilt is strong and well attached to the underlying tooth, it can be regarded as an integral part of the preparation.

Angle of convergence

The angle of convergence of the walls of the preparation is significant for retention (**Fig. 7.19**). If the angle is less than 5°, it will not be possible to reliably position the restoration all the way on to the preparation. Even the provision of a vent hole in the restoration will not allow elimination of all excess luting cement so the seating will not be complete. On the other hand, if the angle is greater than 10°, retention will be significantly reduced because remaining tooth structure may not provide resistance to rotation of the restoration off the tooth.

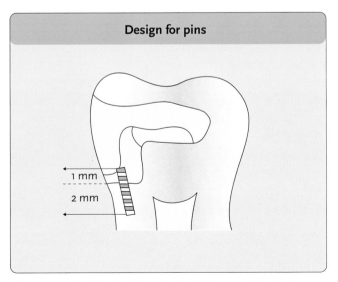

Fig. 7.17 Design for pins. The pin should be parallel with the external surface of the root because it will then be parallel with the wall of the pulp chamber. Leave 1.0 mm in the cavity and 2.0 mm in the dentine. Do not bend the pin after placement.

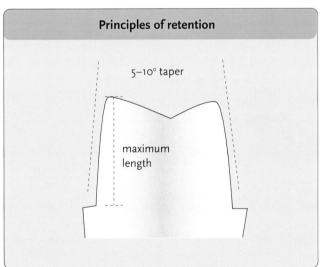

Fig. 7.18 Principles of retention. The basic principle is to provide the largest area possible of vertical wall at a taper of more than 5° and less than 10°. This will often be achieved by rebuilding the crown with a plastic material, such as amalgam, prior to preparation of the final crown design. Logically, a bicuspid crown will not be as retentive as a molar crown because the area of the vertical wall will be less.

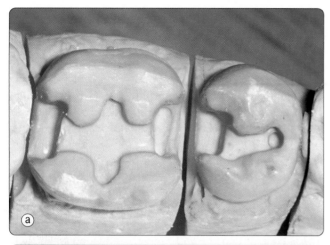

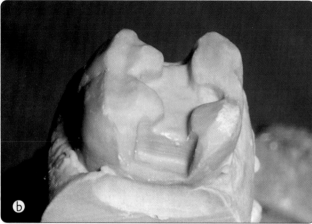

Fig. 7.19a and b Angle of convergence. Preparations for gold inlays showing the fine taper on the walls to allow for a line of withdrawal as well as optimal retention.

Strength of remaining tooth

Strength of remaining tooth structure plays a significant role in retaining a restoration and the weakest link in the chain must be taken into account. An inlay, for example, is retained separately by each of the supporting cusps. If one cusp fails the remaining cusp, or cusps, are at greater risk. The point of rotation of a restoration out of a tooth is at the gingival line angle closest to the point of application of the displacing force. Retention then relies entirely upon the one cusp and the opposite cusp plays no part in supporting the restoration under that particular load.

PROTECTION OF REMAINING TOOTH STRUCTURE

Summary

Protection of tooth structure means using the restoration to protect cuspal inclines.

Preparation of a cavity will compromise the strength of the remaining crown. Preparation of a trench into dentine along a fissure system on the occlusal surface will effectively double the length of a cusp and leave it more susceptible to flexure and fracture. Further preparation of a proximal box in the same tooth will double the length of the cusp again and development of a split at the base becomes more predictable.

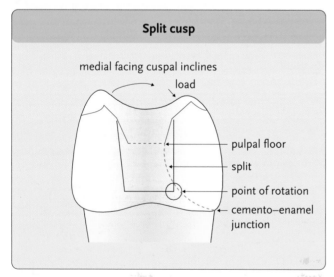

Split cusp

medial facing cuspal inclines
load
pulpal floor
split
point of rotation
cemento–enamel junction

Fig. 7.20 Split cusp. The classic problem leading to a split at the base of a cusp with ultimate cusp failure. The medial facing cusp inclines receive considerable occlusal load so the only way to ensure protection is to cover and protect them. However, an inlay will depend on one cusp only at any one time because the protective bevel will lift off the opposite side. Logically, the larger the cavity, the more prone the tooth will be to developing a split.

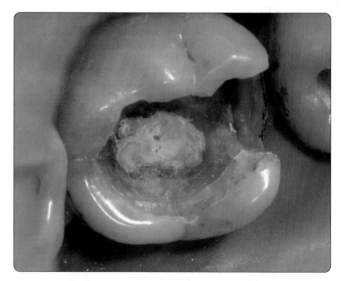

Fig. 7.21 Split cusp. A split shows clearly at the base of the mesiolingual cusp. Best seen when the tooth is completely dry under rubber dam.

Split cusps

Split cusps are frequently encountered in heavily restored teeth and can occur even in unrestored teeth. They are generally the result of frequent loading on sharply angled, medial facing, cusp inclines, often through working side contacts in lateral excursions, and may be difficult to identify (**Figs 7.20** and **7.21**). The patient will report pain on pressure, or possibly, following release of pressure, which will become progressively more consistent over time. The tooth will eventually become temperature sensitive as well. Identification of the failing cusp is difficult in the beginning and testing by the application of pressure to each individual cusp is necessary but not always reliable.

The split generally begins at the level of the pulpal floor of the cavity, at either the buccal or lingual line angle, and progresses on a gentle curve outwards to the cemento-enamel junction (**Fig. 7.22**). When the cusp is lost, the margin will often be just supragingival. However, on occasion, the split will commence more medial to the line angle and may progress through the pulp chamber and out on to the root surface below the epithelial attachment or even the alveolar bone crest. The tooth will then probably lose vitality and restoration may be rather complex or even impossible.

Prevention of splits

Prevention of splits at the base of a cusp, or of their propagation to full fracture, is highly desirable. If a cavity is so extensive that it undermines one or more cusps the cavity should be designed in such a way that the restorative material accepts the occlusal load over the cusp or cusps. Both tooth structure and plastic restorative materials are weak in thin section but are strong in bulk. If the remaining tooth is weak it is necessary to provide bulk in the restoration to protect the tooth from occlusal load. In the conventional #2.2 cavity, there is sufficient strength in both the buccal and lingual walls to support the restoration. The #2.3 category deals with the reverse situation, where it is necessary to rely on the restoration to protect the remaining tooth structure (see Chapter 11, page 142).

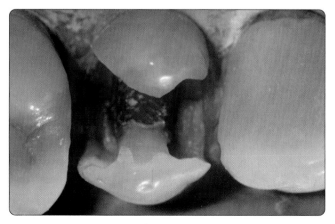

Fig. 7.22 Split at the pulpal floor. The split will normally commence on the pulpal floor and may pass through the pulp chamber.

Restoration of a posterior tooth requires reconstitution of the occlusal anatomy at the correct height with a proper relationship to the opposing tooth. Maintenance of the original cusp height on the tooth to be restored makes it easier to restore the occlusal level, so it is worthwhile trying to retain full cusp length when designing the cavity.

So long as the cavity is simple and at least one marginal ridge remains intact, the risk is not great and the tooth will be strong enough to protect the restoration. Placement of an adhesive restorative material will, in fact, return the tooth to its original strength. However, following removal of the proximal surface as well as trenching the occlusal, it is necessary to consider the need to protect the remaining cusps from undue occlusal load. Further involvement of the central core of dentine will exacerbate the problem and modification to cavity design becomes essential. The stage will be reached where it is necessary to rely upon the restoration itself to accept the occlusal load and this involves both cavity design as well as selection of a restorative material capable of providing strength and protection.

Cavity design for cusp protection

Both tooth structure and most restorative materials, apart from gold, must be regarded as relatively brittle. They are strong enough in bulk to withstand masticatory stress but in thin section will fail rather easily. Therefore modification to cavity design should aim at provision of restorative material in bulk to provide protection for the tooth structure which is now regarded as weak. At the same time it is desirable to retain as much of the gingival one-third of the crown as possible because therein lies strength and retention for the extracoronal restoration which will so often be the final restoration.

It is essential first to remove the weakened tooth structure from undue occlusal load. This can be achieved by eliminating the medially facing inclines from the occlusal end of the cusp and at the same time retaining as much as possible of the original cusp height (**Figs 7.23–7.26**).

Plastic restorative materials

With all plastic restorative materials it is necessary to provide bulk in the restoration. The combined effect can be developed by leaning the facial and lingual walls out from the gingival floor, in a straight line to, or just beyond, the tip of the cusp. A nonworking cusp does not require a great deal of support so it is sufficient to provide approximately 0.5 mm of coverage. However, a working cusp will still be subject to a heavy load and therefore requires up to 2.0 mm of coverage depending on the type of occlusion. By turning the walls outwards in this fashion restorative material can be built over the cusp with a cavosurface margin of close to 90° without compromising the strength of the cusp at the gingival end.

Amalgam is the material of choice for this technique because, properly handled, it has adequate strength. Glass–ionomer is too brittle; composite resin is flexible and the enamel, to which it would (hopefully) gain adhesion, is unsupported and brittle.

Cusp protection

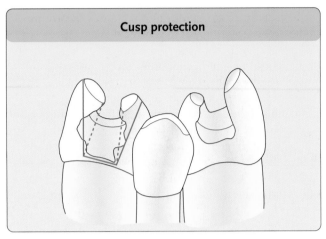

Fig. 7.23 **Cusp protection.** Existing amalgam has been removed and the proposed cavity design superimposed on the original cavity. Note that the medially facing cusp inclines are now protected from occlusal stress.

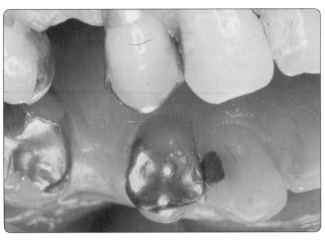

Fig. 7.24 **Protective restoration.** Amalgam *in vivo* showing buccal cusp protected. Note amount of cusp cover required.

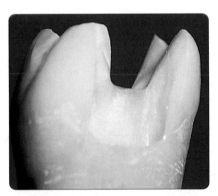

Fig. 7.25 **Cavity outline.** Cavity prepared in extracted tooth showing cavity design.

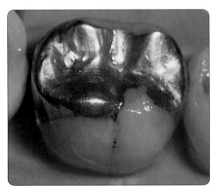

Fig. 7.26 **Working cusp cover.** Amalgam placed in the cavity to show the amount of cover required on a working cusp.

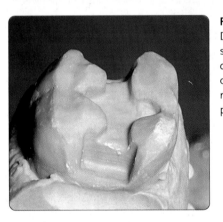

Fig. 7.27 **Gold inlays.** Die for gold inlay showing cavity design and amount of cusp cover required for protection.

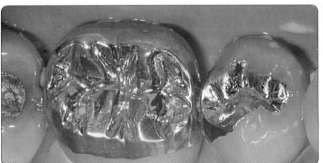

Fig. 7.28 **Inlay *in vivo*.** The inlay in place showing the amount of cover required for the buccal cusps.

Care must be taken not to reduce the cusp height any further than essential because one of the more difficult problems in building a plastic restorative material is to restore the full occlusal height to the tooth. Failure to do so may well compromise the relationship with the opposing tooth and thereby alter the occlusion (see Chapter 21).

Rigid restorative materials

The same principles apply when using a rigid restorative material, such as cast gold, which is indirectly constructed (**Figs 7.27** and **7.28**). It is easier to protect the cusp from load because it can be cast in thin section and the cavity design can be more conservative. However, final success will depend on the strength of both sides of the tooth because, with an intracoronal restoration, the two sides are independently loaded and are not mutually supportive.

Porcelain is a brittle material and must always be used in bulk. A cavity design, such as that proposed for amalgam, may be satisfactory providing both sides of the tooth are sound but thin occlusal sections are not viable.

OTHER SIGNIFICANT FACTORS

Prevention of recurrent caries

Caries will recur in relation to a restoration for one of two reasons:

- microleakage, allowing bacterial ingress between restoration and tooth
- over-contour of restoration, leading to plaque accumulation, particularly at the gingival margin.

Development of correct contour is entirely in the hands of the operator and prevention of microleakage depends also to a degree on the quality of handling and placement techniques. However, there are other aspects which should be considered.

Glass–ionomer

Because of the ion exchange adhesion available there is essentially no microleakage possible in the presence of glass–ionomer. Any failure of adhesion will be cohesive within the cement, leaving a thin layer of ion-enriched cement behind and maintaining a seal over dentine.

The continuing fluoride release will also discourage the formation of bacterial plaque as well as encouraging a degree of remineralisation of surrounding tooth structure, particularly areas already moderately demineralised.

Composite resin

The micromechanical adhesion available between enamel and composite resin will prevent ingress of bacterial contamination but the union with dentine is regarded as less durable. The present recommendation is that a glass–ionomer base be placed first to provide adhesion with dentine, and a composite resin then being laminated over this, thus providing adhesion to both enamel and dentine.

Attempts have been made to develop a composite resin which will release a reliable flow of fluoride at a similar level to that attained from glass–ionomer. There are a few materials capable of fluoride release but at a level substantially below the amount required to have any effect on the development of recurrent caries.

Amalgam

Amalgam shows no adhesion to tooth structure but it does corrode reasonably rapidly in the oral environment. A fortunate side effect from this is that it has a tendency to seal the interface between the restoration and the tooth with corrosion by-products which in turn will prevent microleakage. The development of the sealing effect can be controlled to a degree by painting the cavity surface with one or two layers of copal varnish before placing the restoration. The varnish is soluble in the oral environment so it will slowly wash out of the interface. As it dissolves, the corrosion will occur and the by-products – largely tin ions – will seal the margin.

An alternative currently being explored is to apply a resin or glass–ionomer bond to the tooth surface and then pack the amalgam directly into the cavity while the bond is curing. In-vitro testing suggests acceptable levels of retention but the strength will only be as great as the weakest link and the bonding material is likely to be the first to give. There may be an advantage to be gained from the release of fluoride by glass–ionomer, but such bonding agents should not be relied upon to hold amalgam in place or to reinforce the tooth structure in the presence of poor cavity design.

Amalgam has no in-built resistance to plaque accumulation and attempts to incorporate fluoride have not been successful.

Longevity under occlusal load

All the restorative materials are capable of withstanding normal occlusal loads although it must be accepted that there is a wide variation within the bounds of normal. The actual physical properties will be discussed in the following chapters. The development of these properties to their full extent in the oral cavity is in the hands of the operator.

Aesthetics

Aesthetics must be regarded as a matter of opinion and warrants full discussion with the patient. Nothing can be regarded as permanent and stable inasmuch as natural tooth structure is constantly maturing and changing colour, with the result that a good colour match initially may not remain so. It is unwise to select a material entirely on the grounds of aesthetics. Longevity is by far the more important property because every time a restoration is replaced there will be further loss of tooth structure, resulting in progressive weakening of that which remains.

THE FINAL SELECTION

The following factors should be taken into account when deciding the final treatment plan both from the point of view of selection of material to be used and the other factors discussed above.

Advantages of direct plastic restorative materials:

- possible to conserve remaining tooth structure
- relatively simple to place, to repair and to replace
- relatively economical in time and material
- some materials offer acceptable aesthetics
- some materials allow mechanical adhesion to enamel and some allow chemical adhesion to both enamel and dentine
- some materials release small amounts of fluoride and therefore discourage formation of further caries.

Factors in favour

Keeping these factors in mind, a direct plastic restorative material is the obvious choice for the small initial lesion where removal of natural tooth structure can be kept to a minimum. Removing enamel and dentine to make room for the restorative material is highly undesirable and the use of modern adhesive materials obviates this to a large extent.

The fact that these restorations can be readily, and relatively inexpensively, added to, modified, repaired or replaced makes them the logical choice in the young patient where caries activity is difficult to monitor or is unpredictable. Also for the older patient who presents with an apparent acute attack of active caries, it is probably wise, in the first instance, to restore with these materials until such time as the caries rate is again stabilised.

Factors against

Because the operator is working in a very confined space, with limited access and only one direction of approach, there are limitations to the ability to rebuild a tooth crown to its original anatomy. This means there is a constant risk to both the occlusal and proximal contours of a tooth with the ever present risk of leading to a continuance of dental disease rather than its elimination. These problems will be addressed further in Chapters 16, 20 and 21.

Indirect rigid restorative materials

- Restorations are constructed indirectly on the laboratory bench.
- Accurate reproduction is possible for occlusal anatomy in relation to opposing teeth and proximal anatomy in relation to adjacent teeth and gingival tissues.
- Some materials can be used in thin section to protect remaining tooth structure from occlusal load.
- Some materials are ideal for the long-term reproduction of aesthetics.

Factors in favour

The ability to reproduce the original anatomy of the crown of a tooth is of great value to ensure the longevity of a restoration. Undesirable alterations to occlusal anatomy can lead to bruxing, clenching and grinding of teeth and may result in further splitting of remaining tooth crowns. Maintenance of correct emergence profile and contact areas is essential for the health of periodontal tissues and the avoidance of recurrent caries.

Ceramic restorations provide the best aesthetic results available and can only be constructed indirectly.

Factors against

It is necessary to develop a cavity with divergent walls to make it possible to obtain an accurate model of the tooth and to provide a path of insertion of the restoration without stress. This requires further destruction of sound tooth structure. It is possible, when using gold, to protect a remaining cusp with the metal in very thin section but there is still undue tooth reduction necessary to develop a suitable line of withdrawal.

There are many stages required for the completion of the restoration and each stage is open to error. Excellence in the end-result demands excellence at each stage and this inevitably leads to additional cost. This means that indirect restorations are relatively costly and time consuming. However, the cost factors must be balanced against the potential longevity before a final decision is made.

Further discussion

The next four chapters will deal with direct plastic materials, ending with cavity preparation procedures and placement techniques. A new cavity classification will be presented in Chapter 11 which will take into account the present ability to develop reliable adhesion in the oral environment as discussed above.

Discussion will begin with glass–ionomer cement, composite resin and amalgam, because these are the materials used most commonly in general dental practice. The nature and use of the rigid restorative materials will then be described in the two chapters following the classification.

The purpose of these chapters is to provide information that will enable the dental student and practising dentist to achieve optimum clinical results by understanding better the reasons for material selection, and the manipulative requirements for clinical success. To achieve this, three closely linked aspects of each material are discussed.

- Composition, setting mechanisms and structure relevant to material selection and clinical performance.
- Properties and clinical characteristics likely to influence success and failure.
- Clinical considerations which are relevant to the development of an optimum end result under the limitations imposed by either placing the materials direct into the oral cavity or constructing them indirectly on the laboratory bench.

THE USE OF RUBBER DAM

There have been arguments offered both for and against the use of rubber dam as a routine during cavity preparation and restoration and there are many substitutes available designed to maintain access and saliva control. None are as effective and simple to place and maintain as dam and its use is strongly encouraged.

Use lightweight or medium weight dam and the minimum of instruments for placement. It should be regarded as a four-handed operation with a well trained chairside assistant although it can be done single handed. Wingless clamps are recommended because they are less bulky and ligatures are seldom required.

As a general routine it is best to expose a full quadrant on every occasion even when restoring a single tooth. This means going at least to the midline and, for preference, extend to the next tooth beyond. Where possible place the clamp at least one tooth distal to the one to be restored although a matrix can be positioned to replace the clamp when the restorative material is to be inserted.

The major advantages are as follows:
- Enhanced visibility for both operator and chairside assistant.
- High degree of cleanliness available for operator and patient.

- Complete sterility can be achieved.
- Operator has both hands free to concentrate on the task in hand.
- Patient can relax the tongue and cheeks knowing that they cannot interfere with access for the operator.

With practised teamwork it should be possible to place a dam in even the most difficult situation within 2 minutes.

Some degree of training and discussion may be required for a patient with a high gag reflex but there is no doubt they will be more comfortable and secure once the dam is placed. If necessary cut a small hole high up in the dam to make it easier for the patient to breath through, although mostly they will breathe around it.

FURTHER READING

Davis SP, Summitt JB, Mayhew RB, Hawley RJ. Self-threading pins and amalgapins compared in resistance form for complex amalgam restorations. *Oper Dent* 1983; **8**:88–93.

Durkowski JS, Pelleu JB, Harris RK, Harper RH. Effect of diameter of self-threading pins and channel location on enamel crazing. *Oper Dent* 1982; **7**:86–91.

Evans JR, Wetz JH. The pinned amalgam restoration. Part 1. A review. *J Prosthet Dent* 1977; **37**:37–41.

Garman TA, Outhwaite WC, Hawkins IK, Smith CD. A clinical comparison of dentinal slot retention with metallic pin retention. *J Am Dent Assoc* 1983; **107**:762–3.

Glantz PO. Adhesion to teeth. *Int Dent J* 1977; **27**:324–31.

Proceedings of the International Symposium on Adhesives in Dentistry. Barkmeier WW, Garnnett AJ, Reticf H (eds). *Oper Dent* 1991; **(Suppl 5)**.

Khera SC, Rittman BRJ. Dentinal crazing and inter-pin distance. *J Prosthet Dent* 1978; **40**:538–43.

McMaster DR, House RC, Anderson MH, Pelleu GB. The effect of slot preparation length on the transverse strength of slot retained restorations. *J Prosthet Dent* 1992; **67**:472–7.

Mount GJ. The use of amalgam to protect remaining tooth structure. *N Z Dent J* 1977; **73**:15–20.

Mount GJ. The three stages of the amalgam restoration. *Aust Dent J* 1978; **23**:75–80.

Mount GJ. Adhesion of glass–ionomer cement in the clinical environment. *Oper Dent* 1991; **16**:141–8.

Oilo G. Bond strength testing – what does it mean? *Int Dent J* 1993; **43**:492–8.

Outhwaite WC, Garman TA, Pashley DH. Pin vs slot retention in extensive amalgam restorations. *J Prosthet Dent* 1979; **41**:396.

Papa J, Wilson PR, Tyas MJ. Pins for direct restorations. *J Dent* 1995; **21**:259–64.

Phillips RW. Structure of matter: Adhesion. In: *Skinner's science of dental materials, 9th ed.* Philadelphia: WB Saunders; 1991:11–28.

Plasmans PJJM, Willi PR, Vrijhoef MMA. The tensile resistance of extensive amalgam restorations with auxiliary retention. *Quintessence Int* 1986; **17**:411–4.

Plasmans PJJM, Kusters ST, de Jonge BA, van't Hof MA, Vrihoef MMA. *In vitro* resistance of extensive amalgam restorations using various retention methods. *J Prosthet Dent* 1987; **57**:16–20.

Starr CB. Amalgam crown restorations for posterior pulpless teeth. *J Prosthet Dent* 1990; **63**:614–9.

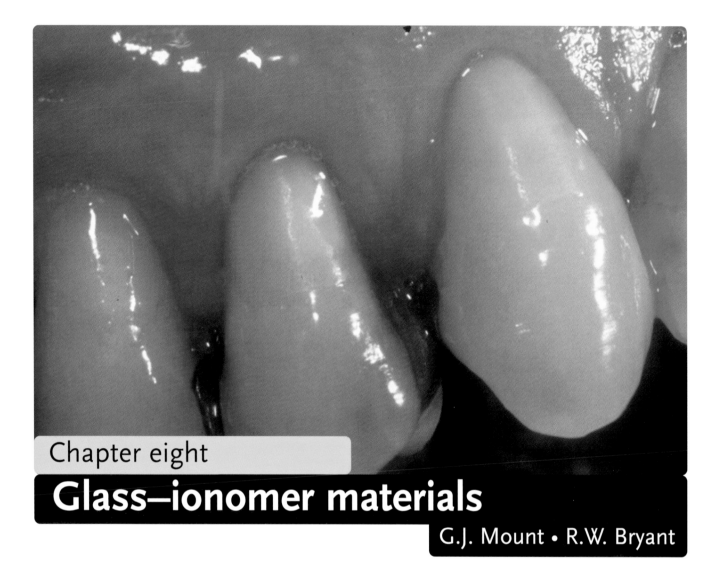

Chapter eight

Glass–ionomer materials

G.J. Mount • R.W. Bryant

Glass–ionomer was developed in England and first reported by Wilson and Kent in 1972. At that time glass–ionomer was recommended for the restoration of class V abrasion lesions, but the early versions lacked aesthetic appeal and translucency. Subsequent development and research by the manufacturers has produced a number of very useful materials in this class that can be used for a variety of functions in restorative dentistry, including luting rigid restorative materials and lining and basing cavities before placement of other restorative materials, as well as making aesthetic translucent restorations in their own right.

Since their development, glass–ionomers have increasingly become an essential part of the dentist's armamentarium for providing treatment that conserves tooth structure and assists in its remineralisation while maintaining aesthetic appeal.

Of glass–ionomer's numerous attractive characteristics, the most significant are the ability to bond chemically to dentine and enamel through an ion-exchange mechanism, long-term fluoride release without high solubility and the ability to reabsorb fluoride ions and therefore act as a fluoride reservoir. The principal negative feature, at this point, is susceptibility to brittle fracture – the material is unable to withstand undue occlusal–incisal loading.

DEFINITIONS AND TERMINOLOGY

A glass–ionomer cement is formed from the reaction of an ion-leachable calcium aluminosilicate glass powder containing fluoride and a polyalkenoic acid. The official ISO terminology for glass–ionomer cements, 'glass poly-alkenoate cements', indicates the principal components.

Developments in the glass–ionomer type of materials in recent years have resulted in the availability of a range of materials extending from the traditional glass–ionomer cement at one end to a modified composite resin at the other. In between is a variety of blends, using different proportions of acid–base and free-radical reactions to bring about setting or 'curing'.

The following terminology is consistent with current understanding of the chemistry and the properties of the materials and has received general endorsement (McLean *et al.*, 1994).

Glass–ionomer

This refers to a material in which an acid–base reaction contributes to a setting process which takes place within a clinically acceptable time (that is, a few minutes). There are two types of glass–ionomers.

Glass–ionomer cement

This term is reserved exclusively for a material consisting of an acid-decomposable glass and a water soluble acid that sets by neutralisation reaction. There are, to date, two subgroups and others are likely to be developed.
- Glass polyalkenoates
- Glass polyphosphonates.

Resin-modified glass–ionomer materials

> ## ! Be aware
>
> There is a significant difference between resin-modified glass–ionomer and polyacid-modified composite resin.

These materials consist of the components of a glass–ionomer, as described above, modified by the inclusion of a small quantity of additional resin – mostly HEMA (hydroxyethyl methacrylate). They set partly by an acid–base reaction and partly by a photochemical polymerisation. In addition, in some materials, the polymerisation of the resin component may involve a chemical initiator mechanism.

General description

Glass–ionomer materials contain water, both bound in and free, the system therefore being regarded as water based. In the early stages of setting, the material can take up extra water and, as the newly forming calcium polyacrylate chains will be highly soluble, it is possible that they may wash out and be lost. Also, during the setting period, if the material is left exposed to air, water may be lost rapidly and physical properties will be downgraded. However, these problems can be minimised during the manufacturing process by the removal of excess calcium ions from the surface of the glass particles, thus speeding the setting process. The result is a material that is water stable in the early stages of setting but, in this fast-setting form, lacks translucency.

'Dual-cure' and 'tri-cure'

> ## ✦ Summary
>
> **Types of cure**
> - autocure: chemical cure acid–base reaction
> - dual-cure: light initiation followed by acid–base reaction
> - tri-cure: auto cure resin reaction in remaining uncured resin

A modification to the setting process is to include a light activation mechanism using HEMA, photo-initiators and traces of other resins and reactive chemicals. The first stages of the chemistry, the acid–base reaction between the glass and the polyalkenoic acid, will still take place as described above; however, at the moment that light activation is undertaken, water contamination will be eliminated. The polyacrylate chain formation will continue in the same fashion but at a slower rate under a protective umbrella of set resins. In the long term, any cement not set by light activation will set by autocure and achieve the same physical properties. Finally, in the presence of an incorporated 'oxidation–reduction' reaction, remaining unset resins will also autocure, ensuring that the total restoration is cured throughout.

Development of aesthetics

Two possible solutions exist for a translucent restoration. When using an autocure material, it is necessary to maintain the restoration in complete isolation from the oral environment for at least 1 hour after placement by the application of a completely waterproof sealant. Alternatively, with the use of the dual-cure or resin-modified materials, there is no need to seal.

Polyacid-modified composite resin (compomers)

There is a further group of materials that contain either or both of the essential components of a glass–ionomer material, but at levels insufficient to promote the acid–base setting reaction in the dark; that is, they will not set without light activation. They do not belong in the glass–ionomer category and are best regarded as being a polyacid-modified composite resin. Commonly called 'compomers' they can be quite useful materials as long as their limitations are recognised. It is not possible for a compomer to bond to tooth structure through an ion-exchange mechanism because the acid–base reaction does not occur for some time after placement. For the same reason, the fluoride-reservoir effect of the glass–ionomers is not available, although there is a small degree of fluoride release beginning after some months.

The critical difference which distinguishes glass–ionomers from polyacid-modified compomers is the ability to set in the dark in a clinically acceptable time through the ongoing acid–base reaction.

Notes

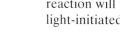

Test the difference between resin-modified glass–ionomer and polyacid-modified composite resin.

Clinical test to distinguish resin-modified glass–ionomer from polyacid-modified composite resin

For the clinician to differentiate between the resin-modified glass–ionomers (dual-cured or tri-cured) and a polyacid-modified composite resin, mix a sample and place a small quantity on to a glass slab for testing. Immediately after mixing, place the sample under a lightproof cover and test it at brief intervals to check the degree of set. The true dual-cure material will be reasonably hard to touch within 10–15 minutes. The other materials will not set at all, although a few may achieve a rubbery consistency within 15 minutes. However, they will not set beyond this point without being subjected to light activation (**Figs 8.1** and **8.2**).

The remainder of this chapter describes and discusses two types of glass–ionomers, one of which sets by an acid–base neutralisation reaction alone; the other sets by a dual-cure or a tri-cure reaction as a result of the inclusion of a small quantity of additional resin – principally HEMA. In both these materials, the acid–base reaction will take place but, in the latter, there is also a light-initiated setting reaction caused by the additional

resins incorporated in the formula. This group is termed resin-modified glass–ionomers and the continuing dominance of the acid–base reaction distinguishes it from the polyacid-modified composite resins (compomers).

COMPOSITION

The composition and chemistry of all the members of this group of materials remains essentially the same and therefore the following discussion can be regarded as universal. They are supplied as a powder and a liquid, as a powder that is mixed with water, or in an encapsulated form. When the polyalkenoic acid is dehydrated and incorporated in the powder, the liquid is usually water or tartaric acid diluted with water. For both practical and patent reasons, there is a considerable difference between the powders and liquids produced by different manufacturers. Therefore, components of various products must not be interchanged under any circumstances.

Glass powder

The approximate composition of the calcium fluoroalumino-silicate glass that forms the basis of the powder component in glass–ionomer cements, is shown in **Figure 8.3**.

The mixture is fused, quenched, ground and sieved to obtain a particle size of 4–50 μm, depending upon the proposed clinical application for each material. Generally, finer particles are used for luting cements and for some lining cements; coarser particles are used for restorative materials because these are likely to provide better translucency. The range and particle size distribution will have a bearing on the working properties and final physical properties of each material. The glass powder can be modified in many ways and research will continue with the aim of improving physical properties and therapeutic potential. One manufacturer has incorporated lanthanum to improve radiopacity and another has entirely replaced the calcium with strontium for the same reason. As calcium and strontium are closely related on the periodic table they behave in a similar fashion and it is even possible to develop a strontium apatite in tooth structure.

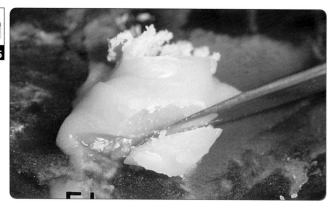

Fig. 8.1 Setting time – true dual-cure. A resin-modified glass–ionomer sets 7 minutes after the start of mix.

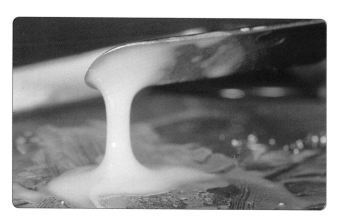

Fig. 8.2 Setting time – polyacid-modified composite resin. After 20 minutes, there is no sign of the cement setting.

Reactivity
The reactivity of the glass is controlled by the fusion temperature and the heat history. Materials formed with higher temperature glasses, set more quickly and reactivity can be varied by modifying the annealing process.

Radiopacity
Radiopacity can be achieved by the incorporation of barium, strontium or lanthanum, by fusing metal to the glass particles (as in cermet powders) or by mixing with dental amalgam alloy or zinc oxide.

Resin-modified powder
In some of the resin-modified materials in which the setting mechanism is initiated by light, incorporated in the powder is part of the light-activated catalyst, thus making the powder susceptible to ambient light. Always follow the manufacturer's instructions; do not dispense either the powder or liquid until immediately before mixing.

of powder part of glass ionomer

Composition of calcium fluoroaluminosilicate glass	
Component	**Weight %**
SiO_2 (quartz)	29.0
Al_2O_3 (alumina)	16.6
CaF_2 (fluorite)	34.2
Na_3AlF_6 (cryolite)	5.0
AlF_3	5.3
$AlPO_4$	9.9

Fig. 8.3 Composition of calcium fluoroaluminosilicate glass. Adapted from Prosser *et al.*1982.

Cermets
Cermet (ceramic–metal) powder particles are formed by sintering a metal such as silver or gold to the glass particles. Up to 5% (by weight) of titanium oxide may then be added to the powder to restore the material to a clinically acceptable colour.

The alternative of adding metal flakes or spheres, such as amalgam alloy, to the powder may improve the abrasion resistance but does not appear to improve other physical properties to any great extent. The physical properties of the basic material seems to be of greater importance than the inclusion of metals (**Figs 8.4** and **8.5**).

Fluoride content
Fluoride is an essential component because of its effect on the temperature of glass fusion, working characteristics and ultimate physical properties. Its presence promotes remineralisation in surrounding tooth structure. The fluoride content of the glass can be varied and a moderate fluoride reduction will enhance translucency without unduly reducing the remineralisation potential. It also has some inhibitory effect on plaque formation in the vicinity of a restoration, although it is becoming apparent that other metal ions, such as zinc, may be as effective, or more so, in this regard.

Poly(alkenoic acid) liquid
A typical liquid for a glass–ionomer contains a 40–55% solution of 2 : 1 acrylic-acid–itaconic-acid copolymer in water or, alternatively, a copolymer of maleic acid and acrylic acid. The use of copolymers improves storage compared with the aqueous solution of polyacrylic acid used in the original glass–ionomers, which tended to become more viscous relatively quickly. It is also possible to incorporate variations in the liquid.

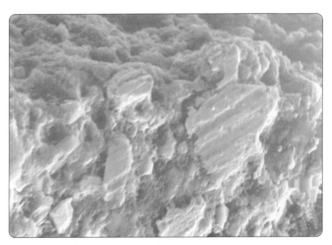

Fig. 8.4 Cermet. A scanning electron micrograph of a specimen of a true cermet. There is a very fine layer of microfine silver powder sintered to the surface of the glass particles.

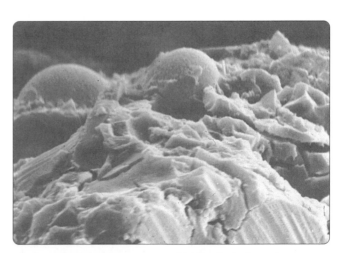

Fig. 8.5 Glass–ionomer cement with alloy inclusions. A glass–ionomer cement with spherical amalgam alloy inclusions designed to increase abrasion resistance.

Tartaric acid

To control the setting reaction, small quantities (5–15%) of the optically active isomers of tartaric acid are added to the liquid. This assists the extraction of ions from the glass powder, retains the working time and sharpens the setting time. It also allows the use of lower fluoride-containing glasses, which are more translucent, thereby improving the aesthetic characteristics of the set cement.

Anhydrous cement

Summary

'Anhydrous' means that the acid has been freeze-dried and included in the powder.

The liquid is now water.

The term 'anhydrous' is a misnomer, inasmuch as the glass–ionomers are water-based cements and water is an essential component of all types. However, the polyacrylic acid can be vacuum dried and incorporated with the glass powder, the liquid then used being either water or a dilute aqueous solution of tartaric acid. On mixing, these cements have a relatively low viscosity and are particularly suitable for luting or lining purposes. Also, a polyacrylic acid of higher molecular weight can be used under these circumstances resulting in moderately improved strength.

Liquid for resin-modified systems

In resin-modified systems the liquid contains a 15–25% resin component in the form of HEMA together with <1% polymerisable groups and a photoinitiator. After initial light-activation of the resin, the usual acid–base chemical reaction continues with the final maturation being achieved over approximately the same time span as for the autocure materials. Depending upon the powder : liquid ratio used in the mix, there will be a residual HEMA content in the set cement ranging from 4.5% where there is a high powder content, to possibly 15% in a thinly mixed lining cement. Because HEMA is hydrophilic, there is potential for water uptake and subsequent degradation with release of HEMA into the surrounding dentine. Some manufacturers incorporate further trace chemicals into the liquid, to create an oxidation–reduction reaction thereby enhancing the set in any remaining unset resins and reducing the susceptibility to water uptake.

SETTING REACTIONS

Be aware

The autocure cement has a three-stage setting reaction.

The setting mechanism involves the dissolution of the surface of the glass particles with the release of calcium and aluminium ions, which then combine with the polyacrylic acid to form calcium and aluminium polyacrylate chains. The calcium chains form first, producing an early set, but are fragile and highly soluble in water. The aluminium chains form thereafter; these are strong and insoluble and provide the major physical properties of the set restoration.

The essential setting mechanism is an acid–base reaction between the poly(alkenoic acid) liquid and the glass, which leads to a diffusion-based adhesion between the glass particles and the matrix. Calcium and aluminium ions are released by proton attack on the surface of the glass particles; these ions ultimately cross-link the polyacid chains into a network that remains porous, thus allowing free passage of both hydroxyl and fluoride ions out of and back into the cement matrix. Three stages have been described in this setting reaction, which is regarded as a long-term reaction continuing for at least 1 month after placement and, probably, much longer (**Fig. 8.6**).

Stage 1 – dissolution

The surface layer of the glass particles is attacked by the polyacid to produce a diffusion-based adhesion between the glass particles and the matrix. Approximately 20–30% of the glass is decomposed and ions (including calcium, aluminium and fluoride ions) are released, leading to formation of a cement sol.

Stage 2 – precipitation of salts; gelation and hardening

During this stage, calcium and aluminium ions bind to polyanions via the carboxylate groups. The initial clinical set is achieved by cross-linking of the more readily available calcium ions. This reaction is relatively rapid, usually forming a clinically 'hard' surface within 4–10 minutes from the start of mixing. Maturation occurs over the next 24 hours as the less mobile aluminium ions become bound within the cement matrix, leading to more rigid cross-linking between the poly(alkenoic acid) chains. Fluoride and phosphate ions form insoluble salts and complexes. Sodium ions contribute to the formation of an orthosilicic acid on the surface of the particles and, as the pH rises, this converts to a silica gel which assists in binding the powder to the matrix.

Stage 3 – hydration of salts

Associated with the maturation phase is a progressive hydration of the matrix salts, leading to a sharp improvement in the physical properties.

Rate of setting

The rate of setting depends on a number of manufacturer-controlled variables, such as glass composition, glass fusion temperature, powder particle size, tartaric acid concentration, liquid composition and the possible inclusion of a resin component and photoinitiators. The setting rate is also dependent on several operator-controlled factors.

- Mixing temperature. Storage of the mixing slab and the

bottle of powder in a refrigerator increases the working time by up to 25%. The liquid should not be refrigerated because it is likely to become gelatinous.

- Powder : liquid ratio. Although a higher powder content will yield improved physical properties, sufficient liquid must be present to wet the surface of all the powder particles. Inadequate liquid results in a decline in translucency as well as a decline in physical properties.
- Variations in the ratio of powder to liquid will alter clinical handling characteristics. A luting cement, for example, will be mixed with a lower powder content because it needs to be able to flow sufficiently to allow a fine film thickness between the restoration and the tooth. However, physical properties will be reduced.

Setting reaction of the resin-modified glass–ionomers

In theory, two distinct types of curing/setting reactions occur in this type of glass–ionomer (**Fig. 8.7**).

- Acid–base neutralisation reaction.
- Free-radical methacrylate cure.

The relationship between these two reactions may take one of two forms.

- Formation of two separate matrices – an ionomer salt hydrogel and a poly-HEMA matrix. This system may cause complete inhibition of the acid–base reaction.
- Multiple cross-linking – pendant methacrylate groups may replace a small fraction only of the carboxylate groups of the polyalkenoic acid, thus preventing the separation of the two potential matrices.

Cross-linking of the polymer chains may then take place

through one or more of the following reactions.

- Acid–base reaction.
- Light-cure mechanism (in the presence of a photo-initiator such as camphorquinone.
- Oxidation–reduction reaction (resin autocure mechanism).

Following mixing and placement of the material, application of the activator light will result in rapid hardening to the depth of penetration of the light. There will be photo-cross-linking, both of the HEMA and of the methacrylate groups of the polymer, and the restoration can be regarded as clinically set. However, full physical properties will not be achieved for some days while the acid–base reaction continues (in the same way as for the autocure materials, although probably at a reduced rate).

Effect of powder : liquid ratio

Variations in the powder : liquid ratio will cause the physical properties to vary. Strength will increase with increased powder content, up to the point where there is insufficient liquid to completely wet the powder particles.

Structure of the set glass–ionomer

The set material contains particles of unreacted glass, surrounded and supported by a siliceous hydrogel, embedded in a polysalt matrix of cross-linked polyalkenoic acid molecules rich in calcium (or strontium) and aluminium ions. This framework can be regarded as porous to the extent that ions with small dimensions (such as hydroxyl and fluoride ions) are free to move through the material.

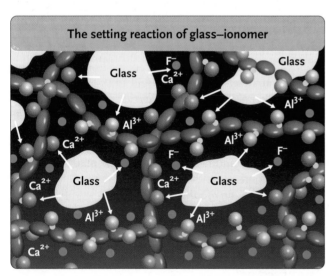

Fig. 8.6 The setting reaction of glass–ionomer. The calcium polyacrylate chains form first, followed by the aluminium polyacrylate chains. Note that fluoride ions are released from the glass, but lie free within the matrix and are therefore able to move out of the set cement and return back to the matrix. Also note that only the surface of the glass particles is involved and a silica gel forms in relation to the glass surfaces.

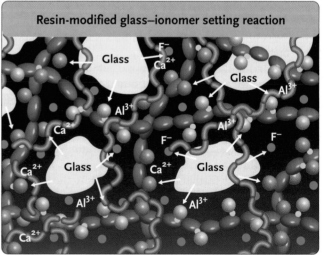

Fig. 8.7 Resin-modified glass–ionomer setting reaction. Note that the same acid–base reaction as discussed in Figure 8.6 still occurs but the resin included in the formula, which is principally HEMA (hydroxyethyl methacrylate), will set following light initiation and will provide protection to the autocure system from immediate water uptake. The HEMA is represented in this diagram by the additional chains superimposed over the acid–base reaction pictorially demonstrated in Figure 8.6.

The set cement contains water, both bound in and free, so it is regarded as a water-based cement. In the early stages immediately following mixing, the calcium polyacrylate chains can take up further water and be washed out and lost. On the other hand, if the cement is exposed to air it may lose some of the unbound water and dehydrate, losing both physical integrity and strength. These problems can be modified at the time of manufacture by washing off some of the excess calcium ions from the surface of the glass powder, thus producing a fast-set cement. However, this in turn will lower the translucency of the set material, with the result that fast-set cements are not aesthetic.

Classification for glass–ionomer cements

The following is the accepted classification for glass–ionomer cements

Type I – Luting
Use – cementation of crowns, bridges, inlays, orthodontic appliances
Setting rate – fast set
Powder : liquid ratio – 1.5 : 1
Radiopaque – generally
Film thickness – ≤20 μm

Type II – Restorative

Type II.1 Restorative aesthetic
Use – aesthetic restorations
Setting rate:
autocure – slow resistance to water uptake and loss
resin-modified – fast set, immediate resistance to water uptake
Powder : liquid ratio – 3 : 1 or greater
Radiopaque – most materials

Type II.2 Restorative reinforced
Use – where increased physical properties are required but aesthetics not important
Setting rate – fast set
Powder : liquid ratio – 3 : 1 or greater
Radiopaque – always

Type III – Lining or Base

Lining
Use – in thin section as thermal barrier under metal restorations
Setting rate – fast set
Powder : liquid ratio – 1.5 : 1

Base – dentine substitute
Use – in combination with composite resin in lamination technique
Setting rate – fast set
Powder : liquid ratio – 3 : 1 or greater
Radiopaque – always

The resin-modified materials are presumed to have either a multiple cross-linked matrix or a matrix containing two separate phases (polysalt matrix and poly-HEMA matrix). Either or both of these will inhibit water exchange in the early stages, but, in the long term, will not prevent further development and maturation via the acid–base reaction.

DISPENSING AND MIXING

Glass–ionomers are available commercially in two forms.
• Encapsulated, for mechanical mixing.
• Powder and liquid supplied separately, for hand-mixing.

Capsules
There are several types of capsule available and use of such a system provides a consistent and satisfactory powder : liquid ratio. This results in standardised mixing and setting times, and ensures optimum physical properties. A further advantage lies in the fact that the capsule also acts as a syringe for placement of the mixed material into the cavity. Quality control in the manufacture of the capsules is generally very high, but care must be taken in activating a capsule to ensure the full release of the liquid into the chamber containing the powder. Also pay attention to the manufacturer's directions on machine mixing. The time of mixing will vary from one manufacturer to another and there may be variations in the consistency of the energy provision of different mixing machines.

Loss of gloss/slump test

Notes

Test the efficiency of the mixing machine.

Learn to recognise a properly mixed capsulated specimen by carrying out a loss of gloss/slump test. Make a trial mix and express the cement on to a glass slab. Lift the top of the pile of cement with a small instrument until the cement breaks and slumps back on to the slab. There will come a point where the cement breaks but does not slump. Measure that time and subtract 30 seconds to determine the working time. Normally, this should be between 60 and 90 seconds but for the resin-modified glass–ionomers it will be nearer to 3–3.5 minutes (**Fig. 8.8**).

Hand mixing

Be aware

Note the significance of the powder : liquid ratio when hand mixing.

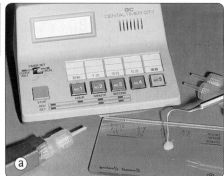
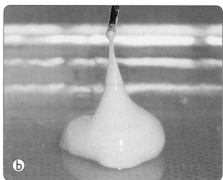
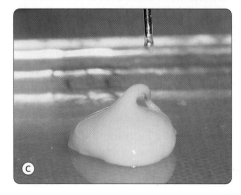
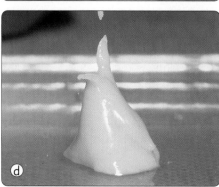

Fig. 8.8 Loss of gloss/slump test. (a) Mix capsule contents for the required time and express the resultant mix on to a glass slab. Start timing. **(b)** Lift the mixed cement with a small instrument until it strings out and breaks off. **(c)** Initially the cement will slump back into the original pile . It will still be soft and glossy and will slump readily. **(d)** At a given point the cement will break off and remain strung out and stiff and the surface will lose its gloss. The exact time is difficult to determine, so take off 30 seconds from the estimated time and that will be the working time for that particular mixer.

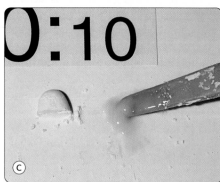
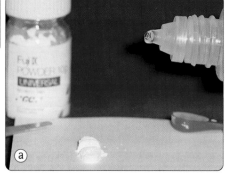
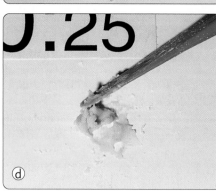
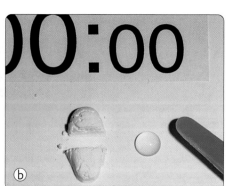

Fig. 8.9 Hand mixing routine.
(a) Dispense both powder and liquid carefully. Turn the liquid bottle to the horizontal briefly to allow liquid to flow into the tip before turning it to the vertical and squeezing out a single drop. **(b)** Divide the powder into two equal parts and prepare to mix. **(c)** Incorporate the first half of the powder within 10 seconds, rolling the powder into the liquid without spreading the mix over the slab. Do not spatulate too much. **(d)** Complete the mixing within 25–30 seconds. For preference, place into a disposable syringe for transfer to the cavity.

Hand mixing of all types of cements is possible, although great care is required when dispensing the powder to avoid under-dispensing or over-dispensing. Physical properties are heavily dependent upon the powder content; for optimum results, full measure is imperative. It is not possible to vary reliably the size of a drop of liquid, and it is difficult to dispense accurately by hand a spoon of powder; therefore, it is unwise to attempt to dispense a partial mix.

The principal objective in mixing these materials is to wet the surface of each glass particle, without dissolving the powder completely in the liquid. The strength of the set cement lies in the remaining glass particles rather than in the matrix. Therefore, the mix should be undertaken quickly on a cool dry glass slab without spreading the mix around or spatulating heavily. The powder should be dispensed onto the slab, then divided in half and mixed in two parts. The first part should be incorporated by gently but rapidly rolling the powder into the liquid within 10 seconds. Now, include the second part entirely, leaving no residue, and finish the mixing within a further 15 seconds. The finished mixed material should be 'glossy wet' on the surface and the working time should now be between 60–90 seconds. For convenience, it should be transferred to a disposable syringe for accurate and positive placement into the cavity (**Fig. 8.9**).

WATER BALANCE

Successful management of the water balance of the glass–ionomer material is probably the most significant factor in ensuring long-term success with the autocure cements. Approximately 24% of the set glass–ionomer is water; susceptibility to water uptake and loss is summarised in **Figure 8.10**. The cement is most susceptible to moisture contamination during stage 2 of the setting process, before the calcium ions have been locked in to the resistant gel matrix.

Slow-set autocure cements

This initial setting stage is prolonged for type II.1 autocure aesthetic materials and early water contamination will result in loss of calcium polyacrylate chains, absorption of water, loss of translucency and loss of physical properties, which leave the cement susceptible to erosion (**Fig. 8.11**). On the other hand, dehydration will result in loss of water and will lead to cracking and fissuring of the cement, softening of the surface and loss of the matrix-forming ions.

Therefore, care must be taken to seal the restoration, immediately it has achieved its initial set, to isolate it from the oral environment and ensure water stability for the next 24 hours. This can best be achieved using a single-component, very low viscosity, light-activated resin–enamel bonding agent, containing a polyalkenoic acid such as maleic acid. A generous layer should be flowed over the cement, just as the matrix is removed. The cement can be trimmed through the unset resin sealant, only if essential, and then the sealant can be light-activated to provide a waterproof seal. At the same time, any surface porosity will be filled, resulting in further improvement in aesthetics and resistance to stain uptake. Final contouring should be delayed for at least 24 hours and must always be carried out under air–water spray to avoid dehydration.

Fast-set autocure cements

Except for the slow-set materials, all types of autocure cements are modified during manufacture to remove some of the excess calcium ions. This reduces their susceptibility to water to ensure that they are fast setting, and therefore, resistant to water uptake at about 4 minutes after mixing. The main limitation is that they lack translucency, although they may have superior physical properties. It must be noted that they remain susceptible to water loss, and therefore cracking, for about 2 weeks after placement. If, in that period, the cement is likely to be exposed to air for more than 5 minutes it should be sealed with a resin–enamel bonding agent as discussed above.

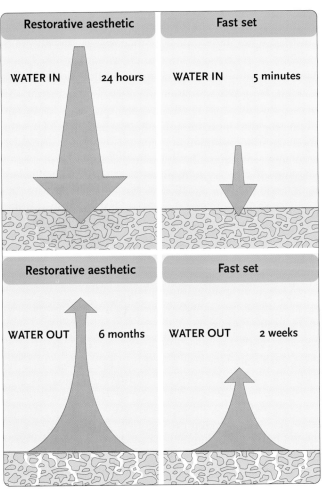

Fig. 8.10 Water balance. The autocure glass–ionomer cements are susceptible to water uptake and water loss during the early setting stages. The restorative aesthetic cements, in particular, need to be protected because water uptake will severely reduce the degree of translucency of the set cement as well as reduce physical properties.

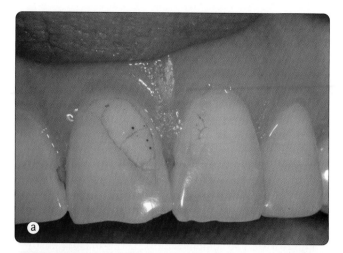

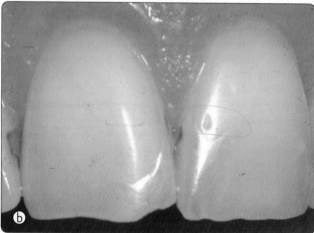

Fig. 8.11 Effect of contamination. (a) The glass–ionomers on the labial of these two upper central incisors were subjected to both early hydration and subsequent dehydration the first time they were placed. Subsequently they were replaced and properly protected with a resin sealant. (b) 8 years after replacement

Resin-modified glass–ionomers

Modifications to allow for light initiation of the glass–ionomers mean that these cements can then be regarded as a fast-setting with immediate resistance to water uptake and some protection against water loss. The addition of 5–15% HEMA, as well as light-activation catalysts, offers protection to the calcium polyacrylate chains against dissolution in water while the usual acid–base reaction continues. However, glass–ionomers seem to perform like mild hydrogels with a rapid water uptake over the next 5–7 days, which can lead to swelling and some possible stain uptake. After adequate light activation, the material can immediately be contoured under air–water spray at an intermediate high speed without interfering with the setting reaction. However, it should be noted that it is still possible to dehydrate the restoration any time over the next 2 weeks. Also, it is logical to seal the surface of the newly placed and contoured restoration with a low-viscosity resin sealant because this will fill any exposed porosity and scratches and leave a smoother surface for patient comfort and aesthetics.

ADHESION TO TOOTH STRUCTURE

Bond to mineralised tissue

One of the most important characteristics of glass–ionomer materials is their ability to adhere chemically to mineralised tissues. The probable mechanism of adhesion is based upon both diffusion and adsorption phenomena. Adhesion is initiated by the polyalkenoic acid when freshly mixed material contacts the tooth surface. Phosphate ions are displaced from apatite by carboxyl groups, each phosphate ion taking a calcium ion with it to retain electrical neutrality (**Fig. 8.12**). The setting of the material and dissolution of the enamel or dentine surface result in buffering of the polyacid, a rise in local pH and reprecipitation of minerals at the cement–tooth interface. Therefore, it appears that chemical bonding is achieved by a calcium phosphate–polyalkenoate crystalline structure acting as an interface between enamel or dentine and the set material. This can be described as a 'diffusion-based adhesion'.

Further evidence of the presence of such a highly mineralised interface is shown in **Fig. 8.13**. A glass–ionomer restoration has been sectioned, polished and lightly etched for 10 seconds with 37% orthophosphoric acid. When viewed under a scanning electron microscope (SEM) with a cryo-vac stage, in which the water content of both the tooth and the cement is stabilised, it is seen that the intermediate layer is more resistant to etching and is revealed as a rather prominent ridge between the two. The specimen in **Fig. 8.14** was examined on a standard SEM, for which the specimen had to be completely dehydrated. This resulted in cracking of the cement and separation from the tooth structure, leaving behind the ion-enriched layer still adherent to the tooth.

The significance of this method of bonding lies in the fact that there cannot be adhesive failure between the two materials, tooth structure and glass–ionomer, but, if a restoration is to be lost, there will need to be cohesive failure in one or the other. As the tensile strength of glass–ionomer is notably lower than that of tooth structure the ion-exchange layer will generally be found still attached to the dentine or enamel. There may, of course, be occasions where there are already micro-cracks in the enamel, resulting in failure in tooth structure.

Bond to collagen

Adhesion to the organic component of the dentine may also occur through either hydrogen bonding or metallic ion bridging between the carboxyl groups on the polyacid and the collagen molecules of the dentine.

The strength of the union has not yet been measured because failure, under normal circumstances, is cohesive in the cement. The ion-exchange layer described above is

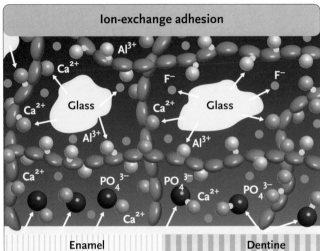

Fig. 8.12 **Ion-exchange adhesion between glass ionomer and tooth structure.** Polyalkenoic acid attacks the dentine and enamel and displaces phosphate and calcium (or strontium) ions. These migrate into the cement and develop an ion enriched layer firmly attached to the tooth structure. Failure will be cohesive within the cement and not at the interface. Dentinal tubules will remain sealed and microleakage can only occur into the cement.

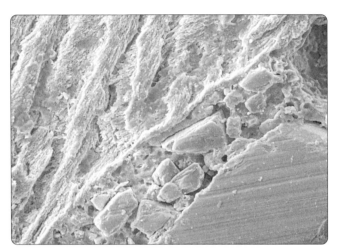

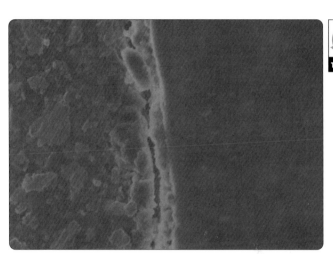

Fig. 8.13 **Ion-exchange adhesion.** The ion-enriched layer is shown clearly in this SEM taken on a cryo-vac stage. The surface has been lightly etched and the new material shows greater resistance to etching than either the enamel or the glass–ionomer.

Fig. 8.14 **Ion-exchange layer.** The ion-exchange layer attached to the dentine with cohesive failure in cement.

always present, so tests purporting to reveal the strength of adhesion will reveal the tensile strength of the relevant cement rather than the adhesion.

Conditioning the tooth surface

Notes

Always 'condition' the tooth surface for glass–ionomers.

Never 'etch': etching is reserved for composite resin only.

Logically, adhesion will take place best in a clean environment. Various agents have been proposed to remove some or all of the smear layer and possibly pre-activate the enamel or dentine. Low molecular weight acids such as citric acid or hydrogen peroxide were recommended initially, but the most desirable material has proved to be a low-concentration polyacrylic acid applied for a brief period and then washed thoroughly from the tooth surface (**Figs 8.15** and **8.16**). Polyacrylic acid is a part of the glass–ionomer system; therefore, any remaining residue will not interfere with the setting reaction. Both glass–ionomer and the tooth structure have a high surface energy and application of the polyacrylic acid will lower the surface energy of the tooth and thus increase the wettability of the surface and encourage the adaptation

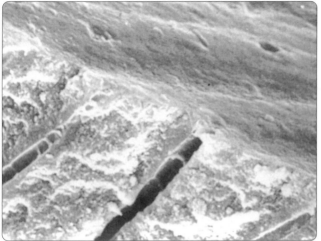

Fig. 8.15 Smear layer. A cross-section of dentine showing intact smear layer covering the dentinal tubules.

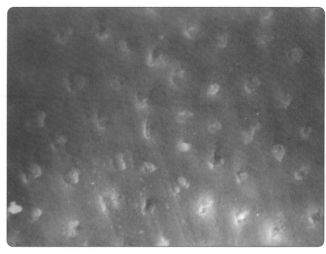

Fig. 8.16 Conditioned dentine. Smear layer removed by 10-second application of 10% polyacrylic acid.

of the material to the tooth. Polyacrylic acid is a mild acid with a high molecular weight and will not demineralise the tooth surface unduly or penetrate the dentine tubules. After an application time of 10 seconds, plugs will still be present in the dentine tubules, discouraging dentine fluid flow and helping to keep the cavity dry until the restoration is in place.

An alternative to removal of the smear layer is to apply a mineralising solution to the tooth surface, such as ITS solution (see Causten and Johnson, 1982) or 25% tannic acid, and leave it in place for 1–2 minutes before washing thoroughly. The smear layer will now be included in the ion-exchange layer and will not interfere with the adhesion.

When using these cements for luting full crowns, it is more logical to apply a mineralising solution, as suggested above, or a dentine bonding agent containing a poly(alkenoic acid). Either of these will seal the dentine tubules, thus avoiding the risk of opening the tubules and allowing the hydraulic pressure of cementation to permit permeation of polyacrylic acid towards the pulp.

Placement routine

The following routine is recommended for the placement of any glass–ionomer material.

- Prepare the cavity surface as smooth as possible.
- Clean the tooth surface, where access permits, using a slurry of plain pumice and water.
- Apply a liberal coat of 10% polyacrylic acid for 10 seconds.
- Wash vigorously with air–water spray for 10 seconds.
- Dry lightly but do not dehydrate the surface.

The glass–ionomer is now immediately syringed into place and supported positively with a matrix to assist adaptation between the glass–ionomer and the dentine and enamel.

PROPERTIES
Biocompatibility
Resistance to plaque

It has been shown that bacterial plaque fails to thrive on the surface of glass–ionomer; this, in turn, means that there is a high level of tolerance in surrounding soft tissue. *Streptococcus mutans* is the major pathogen found in dental plaque, and it is thought that it is unable to thrive in the presence of fluoride. Thus, the response of all soft tissues to glass–ionomer restorations is favourable (**Figs 8.17** and **8.18**).

Pulp response to glass–ionomer

The pulpal response to glass–ionomer materials is favourable. The freshly mixed material is very acid with the pH ranging between 0.9 and 1.6. However, dentine is an excellent buffer and even thin layers of dentine remaining between the restoration and the pulp are sufficient to prevent a reduction of pH within the pulp tissue. A mild inflammatory response has been noted by several authors but, as the pH rises again within the first hour, the inflammation will resolve within 10–20 days. It is therefore probably unnecessary to place a sublining, such as calcium hydroxide, under a glass–ionomer because it will serve no purpose. To a certain extent, the relatively mild pulpal irritation may be accounted for by the high buffering capacity of the hydroxyapatite itself. Also, the low mobility and chelating capacity of the large polyalkenoic acid molecules may be significant factors (**Fig. 8.19**).

Recent work suggests that glass–ionomer can be used to cover and protect a mechanical or traumatic exposure of an otherwise healthy pulp, because formation of a dentine bridge can occur in spite of the lowered pH. This supports the previously held concept that it is only bacteria or their

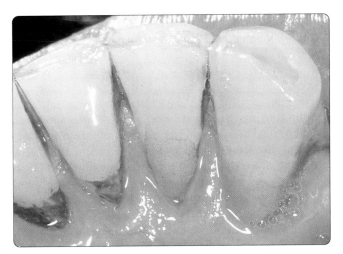

Fig. 8.17 Resistance to plaque. Two glass–ionomer restorations at the cervical of the lateral incisor and canine. Note the lack of plaque build-up relative to the two adjacent central incisors.

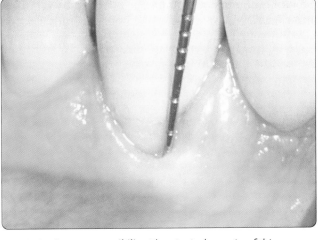

Fig. 8.18 Tissue compatibility. The gingival margin of this glass–ionomer cement restoration is 2 mm beneath the gingiva. Note the excellent tissue response to its presence.

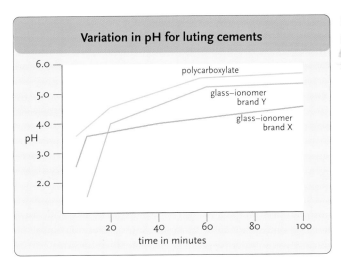

Variation in pH for luting cements

polycarboxylate
glass–ionomer brand Y
glass–ionomer brand X

pH: 6.0, 5.0, 4.0, 3.0, 2.0

time in minutes: 20, 40, 60, 80, 100

Fig. 8.19 Variation in pH for luting cements. Although the glass–ionomers show a very low pH when first mixed, the pH will rise quite rapidly within the first 20 minutes. It would seem that the early pH is not a cause of postinsertion sensitivity.

toxins that cause a continuing pulpal inflammation and not a restorative material in itself. However, if there is any doubt, particularly concerning the possibility of bacterial infection, a small quantity of calcium hydroxide over the actual exposure will have a predictable result (see Chapter 17).

Sensitivity to luting materials

Summary

> Postinsertion sensitivity is the same for glass–ionomers and zinc phosphate.

It has been suggested that glass–ionomer can be the cause of postinsertion sensitivity when used as a luting agent under full crowns. However, it has been shown that the results are the same when using zinc phosphate cement, so there are likely to be other causes. In a tooth which requires

a crown, it is likely that the pulp has already become inflamed as a result of its original condition and the following preparation procedures. It is therefore desirable to treat it with considerable care. Do not remove the smear layer by conditioning or scrubbing the dentine in an attempt to develop adhesion. For preference, seal the dentine tubules by applying a mineralising solution or a resin–dentine bond at the time of cavity preparation and before recording the impression. Then, at the time of cementation, mix the cement at the correct powder : liquid ratio, taking care not to dehydrate the dentine before placement.

Because the tensile strength of a luting cement is not high, it is unwise to expect it to add significantly to retention; therefore, no cement should be used to compensate for a poor cavity design. The reasons for selecting a glass–ionomer for cementation of indirect restorations include:
- thixotropic flow properties
- excellent ultimate film thickness
- fluoride release
- low solubility.

Solubility and disintegration

In a clinically relevant organic acid solution, such as lactic acid, the solubility of glass–ionomer is low compared with zinc phosphate and zinc polycarboxylate cements. Solubility in water is less than that of silicate cements, but slightly greater than that of several other cements, including resin materials.

However, the surface of glass–ionomer can be damaged in the presence of a low pH, such as occurs during the application of some topical fluoride solutions. Acid phosphate fluoride solution has a pH of 3.0, whereas neutral sodium fluoride is about pH 6.5. Therefore, it is possible for roughening of the cement surface to occur if a phosphate–fluoride solution is applied regularly. Caution should be exercised when using these solutions near glass–ionomers, particularly in hostile environments such as those found in patients with xerostomia. In conditions of severe xerostomia, such as found in Sjogren's syndrome, autocure glass–ionomers will often only last for a year or so before disintegrating, unless they are laminated with composite resin.

Resin-modified glass–ionomers appear to be more resistant to solubility and disintegration than the autocure glass–ionomers, but it is still probably wise to use topical fluorides with a higher pH.

Fluoride release

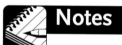

Notes

Fluoride ions are released and returned throughout the life of the restoration.

The prolonged and substantial release of fluoride ions from all glass–ionomer materials is of major clinical significance. It is likely that a further release is available from the glass particles themselves because they can be regarded as being porous to ions such as these. The large release of fluoride ions during the first few days after placement declines rapidly during the first week and stabilises after 2–3 months. The long-term rate of release, although substantially lower, appears to be sufficient to ensure protection from caries for the surrounding tooth structure as well as adjacent teeth. There is evidence to indicate a continuing release for at least 8 years after placement of a restoration and almost certainly longer.

The fluoride ions arise initially from the surface of the glass powder and are held in the siliceous hydrogel matrix. The fluoride ion is not a structural part of the matrix and is of approximately the same size and mobility as the hydroxyl ion. This means that a continuing exchange of fluoride ions can occur, depending on the gradient of fluoride available in the mouth at any given time. Fluoride release normally takes place from the matrix into the adjacent environment but, in the presence of a high fluoride concentration in the mouth (such as during a professional application of fluoride as a preventive measure), fluoride ions can be taken up into the cement again. Glass–ionomer materials can, therefore, be regarded as a fluoride reservoir (**Figs 8.20** and **8.21**).

It is suggested that, for the fluoride concentration to be effective in initiating remineralisation, the concentration in saliva should be at least 10 p.p.m. It is this level that is available from glass–ionomer materials; any concentration below this level will be of little clinical significance.

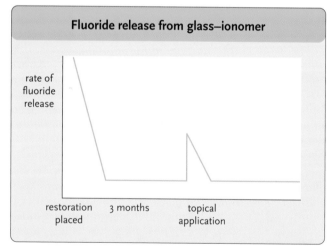

Fig. 8.20 Fluoride release from glass–ionomer. The initial release is high but declines rapidly over the first 3 months. It will then continue at that level for many years – probably for the life of the restoration. A topical application of fluoride will increase the release for the short term, so a glass–ionomer restoration can be regarded as a fluoride reservoir.

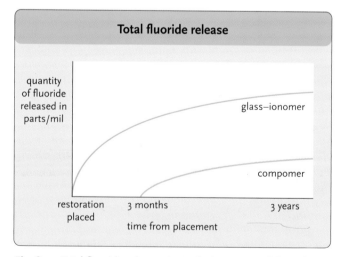

Fig. 8.21 Total fluoride release. A graph showing total fluoride release over time for the average glass–ionomer compared with a compomer which does not begin to release fluoride for the first 3 months after placement. The amount released thereafter is insignificant, and remains so.

Dimensional change

A free-standing specimen of a glass–ionomer material will, if correctly manipulated and protected from early exposure to moisture, show a volumetric setting contraction of approximately 3%, which develops slowly through the setting process. In the presence of adhesion, through ion exchange with tooth structure, the shrinkage is controlled and, in view of the time taken for the setting reaction, there is a degree of stress relaxation leading to a reduced marginal discrepancy.

For the slower setting cements, such as type II.1 restorative aesthetic autocure cements, early exposure to water will result in dissolution of the calcium polyacrylate chains as well as excess water uptake. This may minimise shrinkage, but will reduce physical properties. Protection can be provided by the application of a light-activated resin bonding agent or a varnish.

The resin-modified glass–ionomer restorative materials contain <5% of additional resin and show a very small initial shrinkage of the resin component at the time of light activation. Subsequent shrinkage from the continuing acid–base reaction will develop rather slowly and is controlled to a degree by adhesion. In contrast, light-activated composite resins show immediate shrinkage, with development of considerable stress at the tooth–resin interface.

Resistance to fracture

One of the major limitations of glass–ionomers is their susceptibility to brittle fracture. Compared with hybrid composite resins and dental amalgams, glass–ionomer materials are weak and lack rigidity. Clinical use should avoid situations that subject the restoration to heavy occlusal load or bending. There is a difference in strength among various glass–ionomers, with a substantial difference between the original autocure glass–ionomers and composite resins or amalgams. The resin-modified glass–ionomers are stronger, with the best of them showing more than double the fracture resistance: they are nearly as resistant as the microfill composite resins. Recent research is leading to improvement in the physical properties of the autocure materials and there are a number now being sold with strengths comparable to, or slightly above, those of the resin-modified materials, and very close to those of the microfilled resins. Further improvements are expected. Typical 7-day strengths are shown in **Figure 8.22**.

It should be noted that the presence of silver does not impart additional fracture toughness to silver cermets although it does improve abrasion resistance. Cermets are not indicated where occlusal loading precludes the use of other glass–ionomer materials.

The modulus of elasticity, which measures rigidity, ranges from 7 GPa to 13 GPa and the silver cermets tend to have a relatively low elastic modulus.

Abrasion resistance

Immediately after placement, glass–ionomers are less resistant to abrasion than composite resins, but their resistance improves considerably as they mature. So long as the material is well supported and protected with remaining tooth structure, abrasion resistance is satisfactory. Because abrasion results in loss of matrix, there will be an increase in surface roughness over time with exposure of internal porosities.

The silver cermet materials, where the silver particles are incorporated in the glass, have more resistance to abrasion because, under loading, the silver is smeared across the surface of the set cement during finishing and under occlusal load. The result is a so-called Beilby layer of burnished metal, such as is found following polishing of most soft metals. However, the inclusion of amalgam alloy or silver particles may not be quite as effective in providing resistance to abrasion (**Figs 8.23** and **8.24**).

Thermal diffusivity

This property governs the insulating efficiency of a material under transient conditions. Representative values for several materials are listed in **Figure 8.25**.

Strengths (after 7 days) of glass–ionomer cements				
Type of glass–ionomer	Compressive strength (MPa)	Diametral tensile strength (MPa)	Flexural strength (MPa)	Shear punch (MPa)
Type II.1 aesthetic	70–220	12–20	8–40	30–40
Type II.2 reinforced	140–220	13–16	22–30	35–45
Type I luting	70–150	6–15	4–18	20–25
Resin modified	110–220	15–16		60–70
Type II.2 new version				70–80

Fig. 8.22 Strengths (after 7 days) of glass–ionomer cements. Differences among commercial products and in experimental conditions account for the large variations.

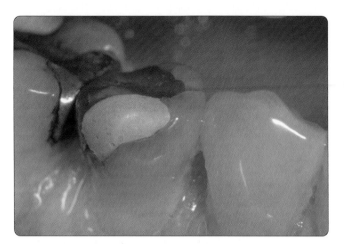

Fig. 8.23 Abrasion resistance. The cermet repair on the buccal cusp of the bicuspid has been in place for 6 years and appears stable.

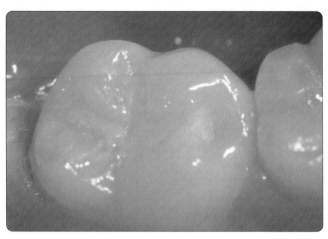

Fig. 8.24 Abrasion of autocure. There is a site 1, size 1 (#1.1) autocure restoration on the molar that is 8 years old. It shows little sign of wear.

Thermal expansion and diffusivity		
Type of material	Linear coefficient of thermal expansion (K x 10⁻⁶)	Thermal diffusivity x 10⁻⁶/°C (mm²/sec)
Casting gold	15.0	90.0
Dental amalgam	22–28	9.40
Composite resin	20–60	0.25
Glass–ionomer materials	10–11	
Type I. luting		0.15
Type II.1 aesthetic restorative		0.19
Type II.2 silver – cermet		0.19
Type III base/lining – autocure		0.35
Type III lining – dual-cure		0.19
Tooth	11.4	
Dentine		0.18
Enamel		0.47
Water		0.14

Fig. 8.25 Thermal expansion and diffusivity. The figure shows the relative thermal expansion and thermal diffusivity of various materials compared with tooth structure. The glass–ionomers are very similar in both properties to tooth structure.

Thermal diffusivity increases with increased powder : liquid ratio; therefore, type III lining cements show a higher value than type II restorative cements. Despite its silver content, the silver cermet behaves as a cement rather than as a metallic material and has a diffusivity lower than that of polycarboxylate cements.

Colour and translucency

The type II.1 restorative aesthetic materials, both autocure and resin modified, provide adequate colour matching and translucency, although translucency will take several days to develop in the autocure cements. The greatest problem with the autocure type is that it may be seriously affected by early exposure to water; therefore, careful sealing immediately after placement is essential. If colour selection is correct, careful clinical placement, with final contouring undertaken at least 24 hours later, can lead to entirely satisfactory results. If the colour match or translucency is not satisfactory after maturation over 1 week, the restoration may be laminated with composite resin (**Figs 8.26** and **8.27**).

On the other hand, resin-modified glass–ionomers show excellent translucency immediately after light activation. Over the following day or two, the actual measure of translucency will decline, although this is not detectable clinically. Within the first week, the restoration will have

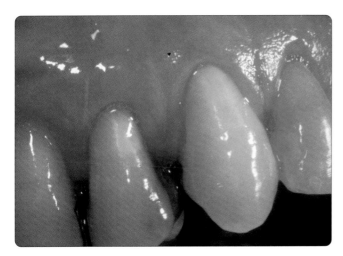

Fig. 8.26 Autocure aesthetics. There are three site 3, size 1 (#3.1) restorations in these three teeth 7 years after placement. The aesthetic result is entirely satisfactory.

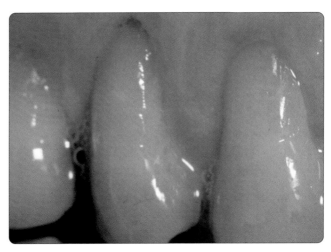

Fig. 8.27 Resin-modified aesthetics. The two site 3, size 1 (#3.1) restorations are now 18 months old and still aesthetically satisfactory.

recovered completely and may in fact have surpassed the original degree of translucency. The ultimate restoration compares favourably with composite resin and lamination is normally not justified.

Radiopacity

Most of the glass–ionomers are more radiopaque than dentine and several exceed the radiopacity of enamel. Some of the autocure type II.1 restorative aesthetic cements are entirely radiolucent, because the incorporation of a radiopacifier may alter their translucency. The silver cermet has a radiopacity approaching that of dental amalgam.

CLINICAL CONSIDERATIONS

Taking into account the factors above, it is suggested that during clinical placement of each of the types, consideration should be given to the following factors.

Type I – Luting
Reasons for use
The following are the main reasons for regarding glass–ionomer as useful for luting indirect restorations.
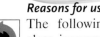
- Fine ultimate film thickness, easily obtained because of good flow properties.
- Low solubility in oral environment.
- Tensile strength and abrasion resistance equivalent to zinc phosphate.
- Presence of continuing fluoride release.
- High tissue tolerance of both pulp and gingival tissue.

Strength of retention
Strength of retention with an indirectly fabricated restoration is directly proportional to the area of the vertical walls of the preparation and the accuracy of fit. It

is unwise to expect to enhance the retention with a luting agent because the tensile strength of the cement is only about 2–4 MPa. Therefore, glass–ionomer cement should not be used for its retention properties and conditioning of the tooth structure before cementation to enhance adhesion is undesirable. Removal of the smear layer will open the dentine tubules and this may allow acid to be forced into the dentine, or even the pulp chamber, under the high hydraulic pressure that develops during placement of a full crown. It is better that the dentine is sealed and protected with a mineralising solution or a resin-bonding agent at the time of preparation of the cavity or, alternatively, immediately before cementation.

Fast setting
The luting cements are fast setting with early resistance to water uptake, so it is unnecessary to seal the cement immediately after placement. Subgingival margins will not be available for sealing anyway. Leave the excess cement, which has extruded out from around the gingival margin, until the cement is fully set. External contamination of the excess will not matter. As soon as the excess is hard, break it off and any cement exposed at the margin will, by then, be resistant to water uptake.

Thixotropic flow
The freshly mixed cement shows properties of thixotropic flow, so it is unnecessary to maintain pressure on the newly placed restoration after it is fully seated. For preparations with long, parallel sides it may still be wise to vent the crown to encourage full seating.

Small particle size
The powder in the luting cement should contain particles of sizes $\leq 10\,\mu m$ to allow for optimal film thickness.

Correct powder:liquid ratio

The prescribed powder:liquid ratio is usually 1.5:1.0, and it is important to achieve this during mixing. Capsulation is the preferred method of dispensing and mixing. Too little powder will leave an excess of liquid, with an increased risk of postinsertion sensitivity and increased solubility. An excess of powder will reduce the ability to achieve complete seating of the restoration, thus altering the fit and the occlusion.

Type II.1 – Restorative aesthetic

Reasons for use

The following are the main reasons for using these materials as restoratives in their own right.

- Adequate aesthetics and translucency are available in both the autocure and the resin-modified materials.
- Physical properties are sufficient so long as the restoration is fully supported by surrounding tooth structure and it is not subject to undue occlusal load.
- Adhesion can be achieved with underlying tooth structure through the ion-exchange mechanism, thus completely eliminating microleakage. Conditioning with 10% polyacrylic acid for 10 seconds is sufficient to remove the smear layer following cavity preparation to achieve the ion exchange.
- The material acts as a fluoride reservoir. The continuing release of fluoride inhibits plaque formation on the restoration, thereby enhancing tissue tolerance as well as providing a source of fluoride for remineralisation of any adjacent demineralised tooth structure.

Dispensing and placement

The prescribed powder:liquid ratio is 3:1 or greater and, for optimum physical properties, the powder content should not be reduced. Capsulation is the preferred technique for dispensing and mixing because it is always reliable.

If the cement is to be hand mixed, it is desirable to transfer it, after mixing, to a disposable syringe for placement into the cavity because this will enhance the placement and minimise the inclusion of air bubbles and voids.

Adaptation of the material to the original crown form through the use of a matrix is desirable to improve adaptation to the cavity floor. This also minimises the subsequent need to contour and polish the restoration, as well as reducing the possibility of voids on the surface.

Water balance

Maintenance of the water balance of the autocure cements in this category is essential. Some manufacturers claim to provide a cement that is resistant to water uptake within 15 minutes of mixing, but all these materials develop superior translucency if they are protected with a waterproof sealant for at least the first hour. The result is better still if the seal remains intact for 24 hours.

Light activation

Manufacturers recommend 20–40 seconds of light activation for the resin-modified materials. However, as it is not possible to light-activate excessively, it is recommended that the light is applied for at least 20 seconds in each of several directions to ensure the material is fully cured. Incremental build-up is desirable for any restoration which is more than 2–3 mm in depth (**Fig. 8.28**).

Contour and polish

Initial contouring is best carried out using fine diamonds at an intermediate high speed under air–water spray. Take care not to dehydrate the cement in the first 6 months after placement. Because the material must be mixed, the cement will always contain some porosity so it is not possible to achieve a fine surface sheen. However, an adequate surface finish can be obtained with both autocure and dual-cure materials by using very fine diamonds and progressing finally to graded aluminium oxide discs under air–water spray. Application of a low-viscosity resin sealant will impart a gloss, at least in the short term, and will fill the surface porosities and scratches.

Type II.2 – Restorative reinforced

Reasons for use

In situations where a fast-setting material is desirable with increased physical properties, but where the colour match of the restoration with the tooth is not important.

Physical properties

The physical properties of this group, particularly the tensile strength, ultimate compressive strength and the fracture resistance, are not yet comparable with amalgam and will never be as good as those of gold. However, considerable progress is being made in improving these properties, so their uses will expand. There are now materials, both with and without metal inclusions, with strength values (assessed by a shear punch test) close to those of microfilled composite resins.

Core build-up

The term 'core build-up', although widely used in relation to these materials, is really a misnomer. Although they can be used to a limited degree for rebuilding a badly broken down tooth in preparation for the placement of a full crown, their physical properties are such that they cannot be relied upon to accept any undue occlusal or lateral load. It is essential that there is still adequate remaining natural tooth structure strong enough to withstand the stresses to which the crown is likely to be subjected (see Chapter 19, page 222). There should be at least one-half of the original crown bulk present, with a cuff of at least 3 mm of natural dentine around the gingival margin involved in the preparation. In the absence of the dentine, reinforcement with pins and posts will not be sufficient on its own (**Figs 8.29** and **8.30**).

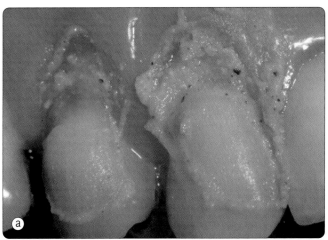

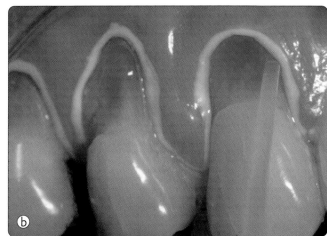

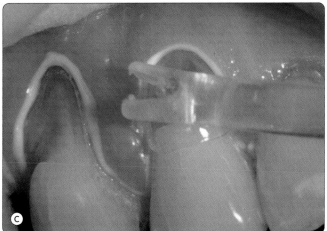

Fig. 8.28 Placement of a resin-modified glass–ionomer. (a) Clean an erosion lesion with pumice and water. **(b)** Condition with 10% polyacrylic acid for 10 seconds. For this patient, the gingival tissue has been treated with trichloroacetic acid to overcome minor haemorrhage and gingival seepage. **(c)** Test a translucent matrix and use it to apply positive pressure to the cement during placement to minimise porosity and ensure good wetting of the tooth. **(d)** Immediately following light activation a dual-cure cement can be trimmed and contoured under air–water spray. Finally, seal with a light activated resin sealant to improve the surface finish.

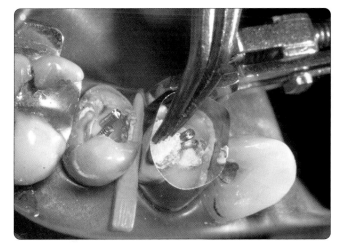

Fig. 8.29 Cermet placement. Using a standard matrix, syringe the cermet into place and tamp it in with a dry plastic sponge.

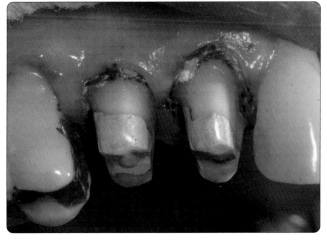

Fig. 8.30 Developing a core. Allow about 10 minutes to set and trim and contour under air–water spray. Note that the gingival one-third of the core is natural tooth structure.

Inclusion of metals

The presence of the metal inclusions, such as silver particles or amalgam alloys, will not, by themselves, improve physical properties. There may, in fact, be a reduction in both the strength of the adhesion and the fluoride release. However, abrasion resistance will be mildly enhanced and there are other methods of improving physical properties available.

Modifications to chemistry

Further modifications to the chemistry of this group are being researched and already the resin-modified materials have physical properties approximately 100% better than those of the autocure materials. There is a trend back to the original autocure chemistry, particularly in situations not requiring translucency. It is difficult to include translucency as well as increased strength, but physical properties are already close to the microfilled composite resins, and further strengthening is anticipated. It is reasonable to expect significant changes in the near future, such that the applications for this group of materials will be extended, although it is likely they will always be rather more brittle than desirable. They will probably not become a universal restorative material, but will remain a very valuable adjunct.

Type III – Lining and base cements
Reasons for use

There are two different applications for this group depending on the powder : liquid ratio used.

- Low powder content (ratio 1.5 : 1.0). Used only as a lining under another restoration to prevent thermal change irritating the pulp and to seal dentinal tubules, preventing dentinal fluid flow into any space under the restoration.
- High powder content (ratio 3.0 : 1.0 or greater). Used as a base or dentine substitute.

Lining cements

Lining cements have relatively low physical properties and are designed to be entirely covered by another restorative material. They should be used in thin section to fill voids in cavity design and act as a thermal insulator to prevent pulpal insult. Because of their physical properties, they should not be expected to act as a bonding agent for the overlying restorative material. Under no circumstances should they be left exposed to the oral environment (Figs 8.31 and 8.32).

Dentine substitute

When the cement is mixed with a high powder content, it can be regarded as a dentine substitute and a significant part of a total restoration. Always use the strongest material available with the highest possible powder content and completely restore the cavity with glass–ionomer. It can then be cut back to make room for a stronger material, such as amalgam or composite resin, to be laminated over it. This will improve both the ultimate physical properties and the adhesion to dentine of the combined restoration.

The lamination or 'sandwich' technique

The concept of using two different materials to form one final restoration is new to dentistry and leads to some confusion. The rationale behind the technique is to make the most of the physical and aesthetic properties of each material and, in the presence of adhesion, to achieve as close as possible a single monolithic reconstruction of a tooth. It has been shown that a tooth can be restored to its original physical strength by this method with no compromise in aesthetics.

225+

As long as there remains doubt about the longevity of bonding resin to dentine, this must be the preferred system for the placement of a composite resin restoration in any cavity where at least one margin is located on dentine. Also, where a cavity extends deeply interproximally and the

213, 214

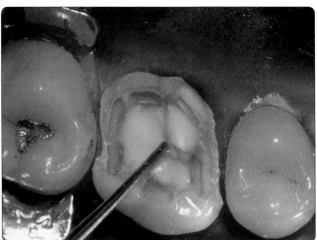

Fig. 8.31 Glass–ionomer cement as a lining. The cement should be mixed at a ratio of 1.5 : 1.0 so that it is thin and will flow readily.

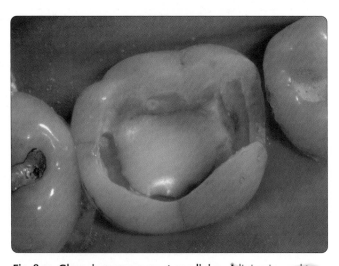

Fig. 8.32 Glass–ionomer cement as a lining. A lining is used to protect the pulp from temperature change so the lining needs to be only 0.5 mm thick overall.

ultimate restoration is to be amalgam, then it is simpler to place a glass–ionomer base in the gingival half of the proximal box and laminate over that.

The result will be that, with either composite resin or amalgam, the section of the restoration that is likely to be subgingival will have an ion-exchange adhesion to the dentine, will release fluoride and will show a resistance to plaque formation. In both situations, the physical limitations of the glass–ionomer will be compensated for by having the stronger material laminated over the glass–ionomer.

There are further practical advantages to be gained from placing the glass–ionomer as a dentine substitute.

- Less composite resin to be placed, thus minimising the ultimate shrinkage of the composite resin, which will occur during light activation.
- Minimisation of the number of increments of composite resin to be placed and light-activated, thus saving time.

Principles of lamination

To obtain the maximum benefits from the technique the following principles must be observed (**Figs 8.33–8.36**).

- Use the strongest glass–ionomer available; place it in quantity; and regard it as a dentine substitute.
- Avoid the placement of a sub-base such as calcium hydroxide, if possible, because it will reduce the area of adhesion of the glass–ionomer to the dentine.
- Condition the cavity as usual to develop full ion-exchange adhesion with the underlying tooth structure.
- Place the glass–ionomer and allow it to set fully, either chemically or by light initiation, before proceeding.
- Once set, cut the glass–ionomer back to expose all the enamel margins, because the composite resin union to sound enamel is the strongest available.
- Allow sufficient space for a reasonable thickness of composite resin, taking into account its relative flexibility under load.

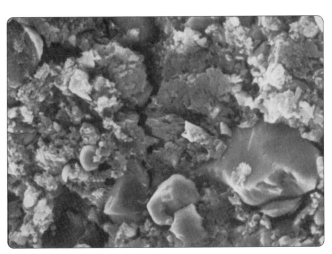

Fig. 8.33 Glass–ionomer cement as a base. The entire cavity should be filled with glass–ionomer cement; then cut back to expose sound enamel margins.

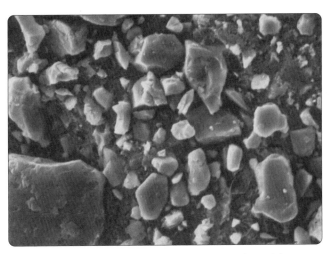

Fig. 8.34 Cross-section. A cross-section of the tooth in Figure 8.33 showing the extent of the glass–ionomer cement base. Any sound enamel can be etched to bond directly to composite.

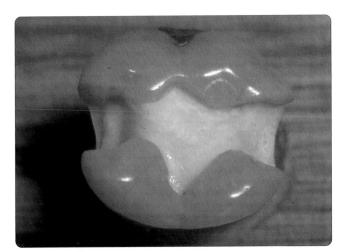

Fig. 8.35 Unetched glass–ionomer cement. Scanning electron micrograph of a glass–ionomer cement before etching. Note the matrix covering the cement.

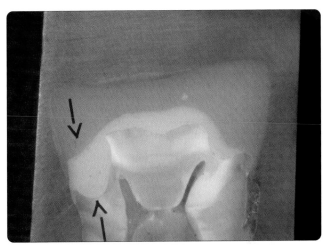

Fig. 8.36 Etched glass–ionomer cement. The surface of the glass–ionomer cement following 15 seconds etching with orthophosphoric acid.

- Build the contact area in composite resin rather than glass–ionomer.
- Develop a union between the glass–ionomer and the composite resin so as to obtain optimum advantage from the 'monolithic reconstruction' concept.
- Always use a radiopaque glass–ionomer.

Lamination over autocure glass–ionomer

It is possible to develop a mechanical interlock between an autocure glass–ionomer and composite resin similar to the union between composite resin and enamel. As soon as the material is set, apply a standard etchant to both the glass–ionomer and enamel and leave for 15 seconds only. Wash thoroughly and dry lightly, but do not dehydrate the glass–ionomer. Apply a thin layer of a low-viscosity enamel-bonding resin. There is no need to use a complex dentine-bonding routine because there is no dentine still exposed. Finally, place the composite resin using a standard incremental build-up technique.

Lamination over resin-modified glass–ionomer

It is unnecessary to etch a resin-modified glass–ionomer when laminating it with composite resin, because there appears to be sufficient bonding capacity in the HEMA, incorporated in the cement, to ensure an adequate chemical bond between the two materials. If etchant does flow over the cement, however, it will do no harm.

Follow the same routine as described above, but etch the enamel only. Apply a thin coat of an enamel-bonding resin and blow off the excess. Light-activate the bonding resin and build the composite resin incrementally as usual.

Lamination with amalgam

This combination is likely to be used in restoration of a molar tooth that is expected to withstand a relatively heavy occlusal load. Use the strongest glass–ionomer available as the base, either autocured or resin-modified, and develop the full ion-exchange adhesion to tooth structure. Ensure the material is fully set, then cut back generously to allow sufficient space to compensate for the relatively brittle nature of the amalgam. Expose all the enamel margins and develop a mechanical interlock design in both the glass–ionomer and the remaining tooth structure so that the amalgam is firmly locked into position in the usual style (**Figs 8.37** and **8.38**).

It is possible to develop a degree of chemical union between the glass–ionomer and the amalgam by wiping a small quantity of 45% polyacrylic acid over the set cement just before packing the amalgam. Wipe off any excess but leave a fine layer of acid on the cement only. The freshly packed amalgam will now unite with the glass–ionomer to some degree, although the value of such union is questionable.

SUMMARY

It is apparent that the glass–ionomers can play a useful part in restorative dentistry. No one material is universal and it is unlikely that such an ideal will ever be achieved. All current materials have limitations but, each one, used to its full potential, has a place. There have been 20 years of close clinical observation of the glass–ionomers and their main advantages, as listed above, make them a valuable adjunct to restorative dentistry.

The ion-exchange adhesion is unique and particularly valuable in view of the fact that micro-leakage is such a problem with all other restorative materials. Whilst the micro-mechanical attachment of composite resin is arguably the strongest union in dentistry it is dependent upon the strength and condition of the enamel around the entire margin. An effective long-term union between composite resin and dentine has still to be perfected. As

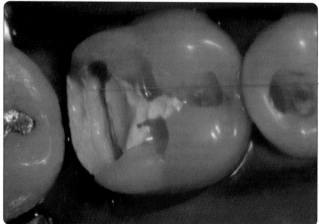

Fig. 8.37 Lamination over amalgam. A very deep proximal box is restored first with a type II.2 glass–ionomer; amalgam is then placed over.

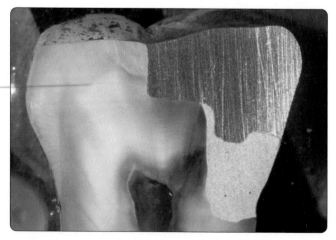

Fig. 8.38 Cross-section. A cross-section of a similar cavity in an extracted tooth. Note the mechanical interlock developed to enhance the union between the two materials.

compomers require the use of a resin bonding agent they must be placed within the composite resin category when discussing adhesion.

It has been shown that glass–ionomers will act reliably as a fluoride reservoir, probably for the life of the restoration. The compomers show a low fluoride release in the early stages following water uptake but it has not yet been shown to be sustained. The potential for antibacterial activity and stimulation of remineralisation has been proven for glass–ionomer and other advantages such as biocompatibility and usefulness in minimal cavity design stem from these properties.

FURTHER READING

Akinmade AO. Adhesion of glass–polyalkenoate cement to collagen. *J Dent Res* [Special Issue] 1994; Abstr. 633:181.

Akinmade AO, Nicholson JW. Glass–ionomer cements as adhesives. Part 1. Fundamental aspects and their clinical relevance [Review]. *J Material Sci Med* 1993; 4:95–101.

Causten BE, Johnson NW. Improvement of polycarboxylate adhesion to dentine by the use of a new calcifying solution. *Br Dent J* 1982; **152**:9–11.

Cox CF, Suzuki S. Re-evaluating pulp protection: Calcium hydroxide liners v. cohesive hybridization. *J Amer Dent Assoc* 1994; **125**:823–31.

Doray P. Color stability of direct esthetic restorative materials. In: Hunt P, ed. *Proceedings of the second symposium on glass–ionomers*. Philadelphia; 1994:199–209.

Earl MSA, Mount GJ, Hume WR. The effect of varnishes and other surface treatments on water movement across the surface of a glass–ionomer cement: II. *Aust Dent J* 1989; **34**:326–9.

Ellis J, Braybook JH. A new glass–ionomer cement based on polyvinyl phosphonic acid. *J Dent* 1990; **18**:77–81.

Forsten L. *Fluoride release and uptake by five year old glass–ionomer specimens*. 2nd NOF/CED Joint Meeting, Kolding, Denmark.1993; Abstr. 005,

Forsten L. Fluoride release of glass–ionomers. In: Hunt P, ed. *Proceedings of the second symposium on glass–ionomers*. Philadelphia; 1994:241–9.

Hume WR. Pulpal responses to glass–ionomers.In: Hunt P, ed. *Proceedings of the second symposium on glass–ionomers*. Philadelphia; 1994:143–150.

Hunt P. *Glass–ionomers: the next generation*. Philadelphia: 1994.

Matis BA, Cochran M, Carlson T. Longevity of glass–ionomer restorative materials; results of a 10 year evaluation. *Quintessence International* 1996; **27**:373–82

McLean JW. Dentinal bonding agents versus glass–ionomer cements. *Quintessence Intl* 1996; **25**:659–67.

McLean JW, Nicholson JW, Wilson AD. Proposed nomenclature for glass–ionomer dental cements and related materials [Guest editorial]. *Quintessence Int* 1994; **25**:587–589.

Meiers JC, Miller GA. Antibacterial activity of dentin bonding systems, resin-modified glass–ionomers and poly-acid modified composite resins. *Oper Dent* 1997; **21**:257–67.

Mount GJ. Clinical requirements for a successful "sandwich" – dentine to glass–ionomer cement to composite resin. *Aust Dent J* 1989; **34**:159–265.

Mount GJ. Adhesion of glass–ionomer cement in the clinical environment. *Oper Dent* 1991; **16**:141–8.

Mount GJ. Clinical placement of modern glass ionomer cements. *Quintessence Int* 1993; **24**:107–11.

Mount GJ. *An atlas of glass–ionomer cement: a clinician's guide,* 2nd ed. London: Martin Dunitz; 1994.

Mount GJ. Longevity in glass–ionomer restorations: review of a successful technique. *Quintessence Int* 1997; **28**:643–50.

Mount GJ, Makinson OF, Peters MCRB. The strength of auto-cured and light-cured materials. The shear punch test. *Aust Dent J* 1996; **41**:118–23.

Ngo H, Mount GJ, Peters MCRB. A study of glass–ionomer cement and its interface with the enamel and dentin using a low-temperature, high resolution scanning electron microscope technique. *Quintessence Int* 1997; **28**:63–9.

Nicholson JW, Anstice M. The development of modified glass–ionomer cements for dentistry. *Trends Polymer Sci* 1994; **2**:272–6.

Nicholson JW, Anstice HM, McLean JW. A preliminary report on the effect of storage in water on the properties of commercial light cured glass–ionomer cements. *Br Dent J* 1992; **173**:98–101.

Nicholson JW, Czarnecka B, Limanowska-Shaw H. Effect of glass–ionomer and related dental cements on the pH of lactic acid storage solutions. *J Dent Res* [in press].

Palenik CJ, Bhnen MJ, Setcos JC, Miller CH. Inhibition of microbial adherents and growth by various glass–ionomers in vitro. *Dent Mater* 1992; 16–20.

Peutzfeldt A. Compomers and glass–ionomers: bond strength to dentine and mechanical properties. *Am J Dent* 1996; **9**: 159–263.

Prosser *et al*. *J Biomed Material Res* 1982; **16**:431.

Serra MC, Cury JA. The in vitro effect of glass–ionomer cement restoration on enamel subjected to demineralisation and remineralisation model. *Quintessence Int* 1992; **23**:143–7.

Sidhu SK, Watson TF. Resin-modified glass–ionomer materials– a status report for the American Journal of Dentistry. *Am J Dent* 1995; **8**:59–67.

Svanberg M, Krasse B, Omerfeldt H-O. Mutans Streptococci in interproximal plaque from amalgam and glass–ionomer restorations. *Caries Res* 1990; **24**:133–6.

Tam LE, Chan G P-l, Yim D. In vitro caries inhibition effects by conventional and resin modified glass–ionomer restorations. *Oper Dent* 1997; **22**:4–14.

Ten-Cate, JM, van Duinen RNB. Hypermineralisation of dentinal lesions adjacent to glass–ionomer cement restorations. *J Dent Res* 1995; **74**:1266–71.

Tyas MJ. Cario-static effect of glass–ionomer cement: a five year clinical study. *Aust Dent J* 1991; **36**:236–39.

Watson TW, Banerjee A. Effectiveness of glass–ionomer surface protection treatments: a scanning optical microscope study. *J Prosthodont Restorat Dent* 1993; **2**:85–90.

Watson TF, Billington RW, Williams JA. The interfacial region of the tooth/glass–ionomer restoration: a confocal microscope study. *Am J Dent* 1991; **3**:303–10.

Wilson AD, Kent BE. A new translucent cement for dentistry: the glass–ionomer cement. *Br Dent J* 1972; **132**:133–5.

Wilson AD, McLean JW. *Glass–ionomer cement.* London: Quintessence; 1989.

Wilson AD, Nicholson JW. *Acid–base cements: their biomedical and industrial applications.* Cambridge: Cambridge University Press; 1993.

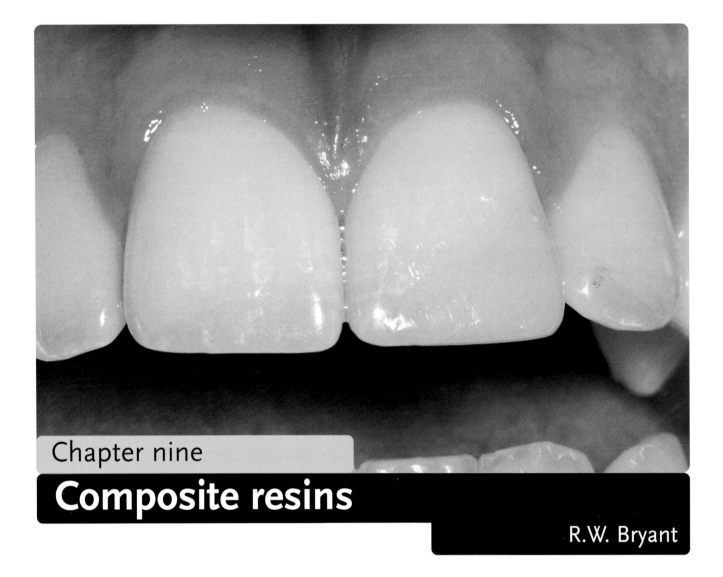

Chapter nine

Composite resins

R.W. Bryant

Dental composite resins were introduced commercially in the mid-1960s. The addition of inorganic fillers to synthetic resins created composite (or 'filled') resins with substantially better strength, stiffness and colour and considerably less shrinkage than unfilled resins.

Mechanical bonding of resins to enamel by acid-etching had already been developed in the 1950s and became common usage by the mid-1970s. Activation of the polymerisation by intense visible light, developed in the late 1970s, increased the range of clinical uses of these materials.

Chemically activated (autocure) materials are still available and dual-activated composites, (activated both chemically and by light) are available for luting purposes.

The principal use of composite resin is for direct placement into a prepared cavity or for lamination over the outside of a tooth to improve aesthetics. However, it can also be used indirectly, using a technique where a composite resin inlay is indirectly fabricated and then luted into a prepared cavity with a resin-luting agent.

COMPONENTS OF A COMPOSITE RESIN

Dental composite resins are complex materials and contain:
- an organic resin component that forms the matrix
- inorganic filler
- coupling (interfacial) agent, to unite the resin with the filler
- initiator system, to activate the setting mechanism
- stabilisers (inhibitors)
- pigments.

Resin component

> ## Notes
>
> **Composite resin consists of**
> - resins
> - inorganic fillers
> - silane coupling agent

Composite resins vary in their resin component but all the variations are diacrylates. Most systems contain the high-viscosity aromatic monomer, bis-GMA (bisphenol-A diglycidyl dimethacrylate), which was synthesised by Bowen in the USA in the 1960s. The lengthy diacrylate chains of this monomer minimise the polymerisation contraction. Some systems contain oligomeric compounds based on urethane dimethacrylate to replace bis-GMA either partially or completely.

Low-viscosity monomers are also incorporated, such as TEGDMA (triethylene glycol dimethacrylate), EGDMA (ethylene glycol dimethacrylate), and HEMA (hydroxy-ethyl methacrylate), to facilitate clinical handling. There must be carbon–carbon double bonds at each end of the monomer chain to allow polymerisation and cross-linking.

Inorganic fillers

The term 'filler loading' is used to refer to the percentage of inorganic filler present in the cured composite resin. Filler loading may range from 52% (by weight) for a micro-filled composite resin to 88% (by weight) for a 'heavily' filled hybrid composite.

Commercially, the filler loading is usually expressed as 'weight per cent'. However, the 'volume per cent' is more relevant to the ultimate physical properties and clinical performance. As a guide, the volume per cent is usually 11–16% less than the weight per cent for commercial composite resins.

Macrofillers

Macrofiller particles are prepared from some form of glass, quartz or ceramic by crushing, grinding and sieving to achieve splinter-shaped particles. The average size of the particles in traditional formulations is 5–30 μm. In the hybrid materials, the average size is 0.5–8 μm. Barium (Ba), strontium (Sr) or lanthanum (La) glasses are usually included to provide radiopacity.

Microfillers

Microfiller particles are amorphous silica (SiO_2) of average **diameter** 0.04 μm prepared by hydrolysis and precipitation; they are radiolucent.

Coupling agent

The filler particles are treated with a silane coupling agent to produce a bond between the particles and the resin matrix. The usual coupling agent is γ-methacryloxypropyl trimethoxysilane. The quality of the silane coupling affects the durability of the composite resin inasmuch as loss of the coupling releases particles and leads to surface breakdown.

TYPES OF COMPOSITE RESINS

There are a number of classifications of composite resins available but the one described by Lutz and Phillips (1983), based on the filler particle size and distribution, is simple and logical (**Fig. 9.1**). In addition to the composite resins described in the following two classifications, polyacid-modified composite resins (compomers), with a fluoride-release mechanism similar to glass–ionomers, are briefly discussed below.

Lutz and Phillips classification

Type 1. Macrofilled composite resin

This type contains only macrofiller particles and is usually referred to as 'conventional' or 'traditional'. Largely because of the particle size, this type exhibits a pattern of unacceptable wear, both of itself and of the opposing tooth.

Type 2. Microfilled composite resin

The fillers in these composites are amorphous silica particles of 0.04 μm average diameter. Four different particle groupings have been developed to maximise the filler loading while retaining acceptable clinical handling.
- Homogeneous – consists of directly admixed microfiller particles.
- Splintered prepolymerised particles. Microfilled resin with optimal filler loading is polymerised and then ground to form 'filler blocks' up to 80 μm in size. These 'filler blocks' or 'prepolymerised particles' are then incorporated into fresh resin containing additional microfiller particles, ready for curing after placement into a cavity. The results of this technique are improved filler loading and reduced polymerisation contraction.
- Spherical prepolymerised particles. Particles of selected size allow optimal packing together.
- Agglomerated microfiller complexes. The $SiO2$ micro-filler particles are sintered to a porous mass and then ground to form coarse particles of agglomerated $SiO2$ up to 25 μm in size. These are incorporated, with additional microfiller particles, into uncured resin.

Using a combination of splintered prepolymerised particles in combination with agglomerated microfiller complexes, inorganic filler contents of up to 75% by weight can be achieved. Incorporation of ytterbium or zirconium can provide radiopacity but most microfilled composites are radiolucent.

Type 3. Hybrid composite resin
These are also often known as 'small-particle composites'. They contain a combination of macrofiller particles with a proportion of microfiller particles and are probably the most commonly used composite resins. The main variation is in the proportion and distribution of the various particles of different sizes because this will control the ability to 'fill' the resin and increase the percentage loading.

Willems classification
The classification scheme developed by Willems *et al.* (1992) is far more complex, but provides more information on mean particle size, filler distribution, filler content, Young's modulus, surface roughness, compressive strength, surface hardness and filler morphology. Thus, it links the composition with a number of important clinical characteristics and physical properties. This classification is shown in **Figure 9.2**.

POLYMERISATION AND STRUCTURE

Initiator systems
Visible-light-activated systems
Single-paste, visible-light-activated composite resin systems contain a two-component initiator system, comprising a di-ketone and a tertiary amine. The photosensitive di-ketone, usually 0.2–0.7% camphorquinone, absorbs the radiant energy of wavelength approximately 470 nm (blue light). At the appropriate stage of excitation, the di-ketone combines with the amine to form a complex that breaks down to release free radicals which then initiate polymerisation of the resin.

When placing light-activated composite resin, care must be taken to avoid premature initiation of the light-activation mechanism by ambient light levels, such as dental operating lights. These have peak light levels of 17–22 klx, whereas the activator light will show approximately 200 klx at the tip of the instrument. Some composite resins, particularly those with high inorganic filler contents, may allow less than 60 seconds of working time when exposed to 20 klx illumination. This means that the operating light beam may need to be moved away from the restoration site while placing a new increment of resin to extend the working time.

Chemically activated systems
These materials are marketed as two-paste or powder–liquid systems. One part will contain an initiator, benzoyl peroxide, and the other part a tertiary aromatic amine accelerator; combination of the two parts will yield free radicals. It is these radicals that will initiate polymerisation of the resin.

Diagrammatic representation of the various types of composite resin

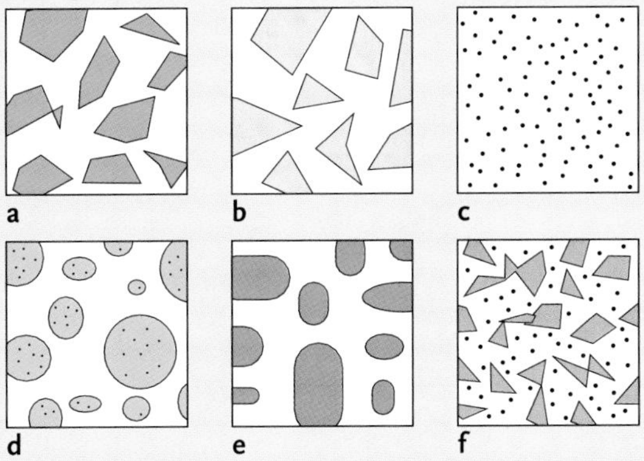

Fig. 9.1 **Diagrammatic representation of the various types of composite resin.** (a) Macrofill. (b) Microfill, splintered prepolymerised particles. (c) Microfill, homogeneous. (d) Microfill, spherical prepolymerised particles. (e) Microfill, agglomerated microfill complexes. (f) Hybrid composite.

Willems classification

Densified composites; midway-filled
Ultrafine midway-filled
Fine midway-filled

Densified composites; compact-filled
Ultrafine compact-filled
Fine compact-filled

Homogeneous microfine composites

Heterogeneous microfine composites
with splintered prepolymerised fillers
with agglomerated prepolymerised fillers
with spherical prepolymerised fillers

Miscellaneous composites
with splintered prepolymerised fillers
with agglomerated prepolymerised fillers
with sintered agglomerates
with spherical prepolymerised fillers

Traditional composites

Fibre-reinforced composites

Fig. 9.2 **Willems classification.** This classification is detailed and complex, but also descriptive.

Other systems

Dual-activated composites have both a light-activated and a chemically activated initiation system and are packaged as two pastes. The light-activation mechanism is used to initiate polymerisation and the chemical-activation is relied upon to continue and complete the setting reaction.

Polymerisation
Composite resins

Summary

Polymerisation
- only 75% of double bonds will be converted, at best, following activation.

Light activation
- between 44% and 75% only. Degree of conversion depends on depth of cure.

Auto-activation
- even conversion throughout restoration to maximum 75%.

260, 261

The free radicals, generated by the initiator system, collide with the carbon–carbon double bonds of the monomer and pair with one of the electrons of the double bond, leaving the other member of the pair free. The monomer molecule itself then becomes a free radical and the process continues. In a chemically activated composite resin, the reaction takes place almost uniformly throughout the bulk of the material. In light-activated systems, the depth to which activation will occur is dependent on a number of factors. It is important to note that much of the resin not activated initially by the light at the time of curing will remain unset.

In both systems, a significant proportion of the methacrylate groups remain unreacted even after some hours. The degree of conversion of double bonds 0.2 mm below the surface of an optimally light-cured composite is between 44% and 75%. Therefore, the quantity of unreacted methacrylate groups is 25–56% and this will be influenced by the concentrations of the different monomers. Greater conversion increases the polymerisation contraction and the only way this can be modified is by increasing the filler loading.

Double bonds remaining at the end of the initial cure decay rapidly over the next 24 hours and become unavailable for future bonding. The half-life of the remaining potentially reactive radicals is only 30–50 hours. This means that most of the chemistry of the setting reaction and the consequent contraction will take place within the first few seconds during light activation and the remainder will be complete within 2 days.

Oxygen inhibition

Polymerisation is retarded in the presence of oxygen, which is taken up by the free radicals. Any resin which comes in contact with air during polymerisation will develop an unpolymerised surface layer as a result of diffusion of atmospheric oxygen into the liquid resin. This 'air-inhibited' layer is thinner (10–20 μm) for the visible light-activated composites than for chemically activated materials.

Unfilled resin-bonding agents

Unfilled resin-bonding agents usually have a chemistry similar to the composite resin produced by that same manufacturer and it is generally recommended that brands should not be interchanged. They have been diluted by additional monomers to provide lower viscosity so that they will more readily wet the surface of acid-etched enamel or glass–ionomer cement, thus improving adhesion. The oxygen-inhibited surface layer is of little significance because the resin will be covered with further increments of composite resin.

Resin fissure sealants

Resin sealants used to fill deep fissures in newly erupted posterior teeth are based on Bis-GMA or urethane dimethacrylate resins. They are available either as one-component, light-activated sealants or in a two-component, chemically activated form; the inorganic filler content will vary from 0 to 40%. Because of the formation of the air-inhibited surface layer, a sufficient thickness of sealant should be applied initially to ensure that, below the surface layer which will be lost, complete polymerisation has taken place in the depths of the fissures.

PROPERTIES

The type of resin matrix, the integrity of the silane coupling of the resin matrix to the inorganic filler, the type and quantity of filler and the filler particle size determine the properties of a composite resin.

Biocompatibility
Response of the pulp

Be aware

Pulp response

Fully polymerised monomers cause no pulp response.

Unpolymerised monomers are a potential hazard.

HEMA is a recognised allergen.

When considering the effect of composite resin on the pulp, it is difficult to differentiate the effect of the components of the composite resin itself, the trauma of cavity preparation, and sequelae such as microleakage at the margin.

Cytotoxicity studies suggest that composite resin which

has been polymerised as far as possible probably causes minimum pulpal irritation. However, incompletely cured resin, because of either the unpolymerised monomers or the surface-active complexes formed between the low-molecular-weight components of the light-activated initiator systems, is a potential hazard. The resin may remain incompletely cured in a restoration if it is placed in large increments or in open dentinal tubules where polymerisation has been inhibited by the presence of air or moisture. HEMA is regarded as an essential component of most of the light-activated composite resins; this is strongly hydrophilic and also strongly allergenic. Even when fully light activated, not all HEMA will be bound, and some will be released with the possibility of an allergic response. It has been shown that HEMA is able to traverse dentine tubules and appear in the pulp tissue and there have been reports of allergic responses.

! Be aware

Microleakage

This is the most significant hazard in restorative dentistry.

Microleakage

Before placement of the restoration, the enamel surrounding the cavity is acid-etched to allow generation of a mechanical bond. Some authorities recommend etching of the dentine as well, to develop a further mechanical bond. There is considerable evidence that acid-etching of dentine, in itself, is not a cause of pulpal inflammation because the acids are buffered by dentine and do not reach the pulp tissue. However, etching the dentine removes the smear layer and opens the tubules, allowing a positive dentinal fluid flow and this leads to an increase in the wetness of the dentine surface. Also, should marginal leakage occur subsequently, the pathway to the pulp will be more open and the pulp will be more susceptible to irritation. Unless the marginal seal of the restoration, particularly on the root surface, can be guaranteed, there is a substantial risk of sensitivity, caries and pulpal irritation resulting from lack of adaptation, microleakage and the ingress of bacteria and their toxins.

It is therefore currently recommended that until reliable techniques and materials are available for resin bonding to dentine, as a general rule:

- dentine should not be etched in vital teeth
- a strong glass–ionomer base should completely cover the dentine of all the cavity walls before acid-etching the enamel margins.

Irritation from activator light

Prolonged exposure of the eye to the 470 nm wavelength visible light has the potential to cause damage to the retina, so a protective shield should be used at all times. The intense visible light generated from some light-activation units has the potential to cause pulpal injury. Temperature rises of 0.5–10°C have been reported through dentine measuring 1–2 mm in thickness; this may lead to pulp damage.

Response of the gingival tissues

Clinical and laboratory evidence shows that tissue cells respond less favourably to composite resin than to glass–ionomer. Incompletely cured resin, particularly in those materials with a low filler content, appears to be a tissue irritant. Also, in the absence of fluoride release, there is no resistance to plaque formation on the surface of a composite resin restoration, so any roughness or porosity will tend to accumulation of plaque.

Water sorption and solubility

Water sorption is higher for microfilled resins (1.5–2.0 mg/cm^2) than for hybrid and macrofilled resins (0.6–1.1 mg/cm^2) because of the larger volume per cent of resin. A limited amount of water sorption may be beneficial to a newly placed composite resin restoration because it will bring about a degree of expansion and help to counteract setting contraction. After completion of the chemistry of the setting reaction, the solubility of the resin is relatively low (0.01–0.06 mg/cm^2).

Variation in the water sorption and solubility of different composite resins is associated with:

- The type and amount of monomers and diluents. Urethane-dimethacrylate-based materials tend to show less sorption and solubility.
- The proportion of filler to resin. The less heavily filled the resin, the greater the proportion of matrix, and therefore the greater the sorption.
- The degree of polymerisation. If the curing time is reduced by 25%, there will be a two-fold increase in sorption and a four-fold to six-fold increase in solubility. Both the long-term durability of the composite and its colour stability will be seriously affected by inadequate polymerisation.

Degradation in the oral environment

In-vivo wear is a complex process and, even in non-load-bearing areas, the surface of a composite resin undergoes degradation in response to chemical, physicochemical and thermal changes. Softening and cracking of the surface enhances the effects of abrasion from load bearing and may result in increased surface porosity. There are a number of factors to be noted, any or all of which may have a bearing on the rate of wear and degradation.

CD 270–274

- Unreacted methacrylate groups degrade more rapidly and may be leached from the resin.
- Hydrolytic degradation of barium or strontium glass fillers may lead to a build-up of pressure at the resin–filler interface, resulting in crack formation.
- Microfilled composites are less susceptible to hydrolytic degradation.

- Water or chemical attack may cause breakdown of the silane coating and failure of the bond between the resin matrix and the filler.
- Rapid thermal changes may also cause breakdown of the silane coating.
- In microfilled composites the bond between the prepolymerised particles and the matrix is a potential site for hydrolytic failure.

Colour stability

In the oral environment composite resin may undergo extensive surface staining, intrinsic colour change or both.

Maximum water sorption will take place in the first 7–10 days after placement, before the completion of the setting chemistry, and strong-staining agents such as tea, coffee or cola drinks may be incorporated into the surface to a depth of 3.0–5.0 μm. In the longer term, surface porosity or roughening of the surface by wear or clinical degradation may lead to the incorporation of stains from drinks and foodstuffs. These problems will be accentuated if there is incomplete curing of the composite resin.

Intrinsic colour change may occur in both chemically activated and light-activated composite resins. Many of the chemically activated materials suffer substantial yellowing within 1–3 years, as a result of oxidation of excess amine from the initiator system, and may require replacement. Visible-light-activated composites lighten in colour and may become more translucent during placement and curing. Further lightening may occur over the next 24–48 hours; this is probably caused by the decomposition of the camphorquinone. In the long term, light-activated composites are relatively colour stable, provided that the resin is adequately cured.

Polymerisation contraction

Composite resins undergo a substantial polymerisation contraction during setting and this may place considerable stress on any union between the restoration and the tooth. Approximate volumetric contraction for the macrofiller-containing materials (hybrid and macrofilled composites) is 1.0–2.5%, and for microfilled composites 2.0–3.5%. For light-activated materials, approximately 60% of the total

contraction takes place within the first minute after photo-initiation; prolonging the activation time from 30 to 60 seconds will increase the total contraction. Because the material closest to the activator light sets first, the contraction will be towards the light, thus tending to pull the resin away from the cavity walls (**Fig. 9.3**).

With chemically activated composites, the contraction develops more slowly and evenly with a tendency to draw towards the centre of the restoration. The result is somewhat less stress at the restoration–tooth interface with a degree of concavity developing on any free surface.

> ### Notes
>
> **Contraction with auto-cure**
> - chemical activation directed towards centre of restoration.
> - occurs slowly and evenly throughout restoration

The polymerisation contraction with either material has a substantial impact on adaptation to dentine, marginal adaptation and marginal seal. In a large cavity, with weakened cusps, there is a potential for cusp deformation leading to post-restoration sensitivity and even fracture at the base of a cusp. Manipulative techniques, such as incremental build-up of light-activated materials in layers of no more than 2.0 mm thickness, can be varied to reduce the clinical effects of this problem. Probably the safest method is the placement of a glass–ionomer base before composite resin build-up. This will reduce the total quantity of composite resin required to restore the cavity and thus reduce the total amount of shrinkage. The lamination technique is discussed in Chapter 8.

> ### Notes
>
> **Contraction with light activation**
> - light activation occurs towards light.
> - 60% occurs within 60 seconds.
> - balance within 2 days.

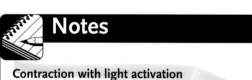

Hybrid or macrofilled composites contract LESS than microfilled.

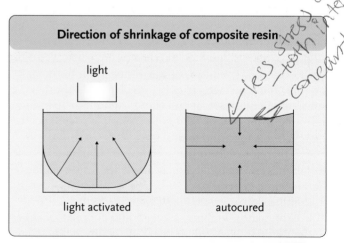

Direction of shrinkage of composite resin

light activated   autocured

less stress at restoration – tooth interface
concavity

Fig. 9.3 Direction of shrinkage of composite resin. A light-activated composite resin shrinks towards the light, putting considerable stress on the weaker bond on the pulpal or axial wall of the cavity. An autocured material tends to shrink towards the centre of the restoration.

Mechanical properties

Hardness

The Knoop hardness number is the usual measure for surface hardness of composite resins. The average over a range of different materials is as follows.

- Hybrid and macrofilled composites – 35–65 kg/mm^2.
- Microfilled composites – 18–30 kg/mm^2.

The surface hardness of a restoration can be increased by 2–4% by additional curing after final completion of occlusal adjustment and finishing procedures.

Wear

Clinical wear of composite resin is a complex phenomenon. In addition to an underlying chemical–hydrolytic degradation of the components of the composite, physical degradation of the surface can be attributed to two other factors.

- Abrasion, associated with indenting and scratching.
- Fatigue, associated with intermittent stresses.

Attempts to correlate clinical wear with specific physical properties have been relatively unsuccessful. Numerous two-body and three-body abrasion tests have been devised to simulate conditions responsible for wear of composite resins in clinical situations, but it has been difficult to predict accurately the wear pattern in the oral environment through the use of these tests.

Regardless of the composite, clinical wear is associated with a roughening of the surface of the restoration, caused partly by scratching of microfilled composites and partly by loss of particles and frictional contact in the case of the macrofilled composites. In load-bearing areas, microcracking may occur on the surface of the restoration and also beneath displaced macrofiller particles. The slightly greater resistance to wear of a heavily filled microfilled composite is consistent with the greater resistance to sliding wear shown by this type of composite.

Wear of enamel opposing a composite in a load-bearing area is related to the type of composite. With coarser filler particles, the scratches will be larger; therefore, the wear on the opposing enamel with be greater. Composites containing quartz fillers cause greater wear of the opposing enamel than those containing barium, strontium or other glass fillers.

Rigidity

The modulus of elasticity indicates the stiffness of a material.

- Microfilled composites – 4–8 GPa.
- Hybrid and macrofilled composites – 8–19 GPa.

The more heavily loaded composites have higher values and about the same stiffness as dentine (18.5 GPa). However, they are substantially less rigid than enamel (82.5 GPa), which is the component of the tooth that they are usually meant to replace.

Fracture toughness

This is a measure of the energy required to propagate a crack within a material; that is, it indicates resistance to crack growth. More heavily loaded composites and those with coarser particles have greater fracture toughness.

- Microfilled composite – 0.7–1.2 MNm$^{-1.5}$.
- Small particle – 0.9–1.3 MNm$^{-1.5}$.
- Larger particle, hybrid and macrofilled – 1.4–2.0 MNm$^{-1.5}$.
- Fibre-reinforced composite – 3.0 MNm$^{-1.5}$.

Fracture toughness tends to reduce over time in the oral environment because of water sorption and degradation.

Creep

Creep measures progressive permanent deformation behaviour under occlusal loading. Microfilled composites exhibit greater creep because they contain a greater proportion of resin matrix than other types. There may also be deformation of any prepolymerised particles (filler blocks). Absorption of water increases creep and decreases creep recovery.

Strength

Measuring the strength characteristics of composite resins, such as ultimate compressive strength and tensile strength, is of uncertain clinical relevance. However, testing the transverse strength, by applying bending forces to a beam of composite, may be useful. Results range from 45 MPa to 125 MPa, with microfilled composites showing the lowest values.

Thermal properties

The thermal coefficient of expansion for composite resins is substantially greater than for the crown of a tooth and can have clinical significance.

- Natural tooth – 11.4×10^{-6}/°C.
- Amalgam – 25×10^{-6}/°C.
- Hybrid and macrofilled composites – $30–40 \times 10^{-6}$/°C.
- Microfilled composites – 60×10^{-6}/°C.

Thermal diffusivity indicates the ability of the material to respond to transient thermal stimuli. Composite resins that contain either glass or ceramic fillers have values similar to dentine despite their relatively high filler contents.

Radiopacity

Radiopaque composite resin restorations enable the clinician to detect secondary (recurrent) caries, particularly at the gingival margins of proximal restorations. Radiopacity of dental materials is measured against aluminium in a standard range of thickness (**Fig. 9.4**).

The radiopacity of composite resins is stable in an aqueous environment and does not decline. Because caries and marginal defects may be detected more reliably with a material of radiopacity similar to that of enamel, the quality of caries diagnosis may be higher for composite resins than for amalgams (**Fig. 9.5**).

Composite resin or tooth	Radiopacity
Occlusin (GC)	5.2
P 50 (3M)	5.0
Ful-Fil (Caulk/Dentsply)	4.8
P 30 (3M)	3.4
Heliomolar Radiopaque (Vivadent)	3.2
Enamel	2.9
Dentine	1.8
Amalgam	21 approx.

Fig. 9.4 The radiopacity of a group of typical composite resins, measured in thickness of aluminium (mm) compared with tooth structure and amalgam. Adapted from Omer *et al.* 1986.

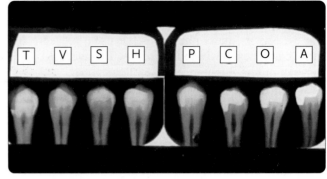

Fig. 9.5 Comparison of radiopacity. T, prepared cavity only; V, Visiomolar (ESPE); S, Sinterfil (Teledyne); H, Heliomolar Radiopaque (Vivadent); P, P 30, (3M Dental); C, Herculite XR (Kerr); O, Occlusin (GC); A, Tytin Amalgam (Kerr).

CLINICAL CONSIDERATIONS

Depth of cure

The only setting reaction which is possible in a light-activated composite resin is that which is initiated by exposure of the resin to light of the required wavelength. There will be no other chemical reaction within the material. By the time of placement, 40–60% of the available resin bonds will have been completed. With most composite resins there will be no more than a 10% improvement from that point and this will occur within the next 2 days.

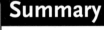
Summary

Light activation
- a maximum of 60% resin bonds will cure immediately on exposure to light.
- a further 10% will cure in the next 2 days.
- remaining resin will not polymerise at all.

Failure to light-activate a composite resin to the full depth of the restoration has important implications for the success and longevity of the restoration. In particular, adhesion to the underlying tooth structure will be at risk if the resin is not fully cured. This applies especially to any margin between dentine and a restoration because, even if the bond to dentine is effective, failure may still occur cohesively within the resin.

A variety of factors influence effective depth of cure:
- Degree of cure decreases with increasing depth.
- Increased time of exposure to the light increases depth of cure. A 40-second cure will penetrate deeper than a 20-second cure.
- The more heavily filled the resin and the larger the particle size the greater depth of cure.
- Microfilled resins will cure to a depth of 2–3 mm, whereas hybrid resins may be cured to a depth of 4–5 mm.
- Lighter shades of material are cured to greater depths.
- Materials that are more translucent are cured to greater depths.
- Light-activator units vary in their light output over time as well as with power fluctuations. The efficiency of each unit should be checked frequently.
- Polymerisation continues at a significant rate for 20 minutes after activation and then more slowly for at least 1 day.
- The tip of the light source should be placed as close as possible to the restoration and should never be more than 4 mm away.
- The depth of cure should be measured from the face of the activator light.
- Curing through tooth structure will reduce the depth of cure to the same extent as curing through a composite resin of similar opacity.

Marginal defects related to occlusal loading

Four types of occlusal margin defects have been identified in relation to composite resin restorations (**Fig. 9.6**):

- Surface fracture of excess composite resin material.
- Crevice formation – ditching, marginal fracture.
- Voids or porosities – incorporation of air between restoration and tooth during placement.
- Wear – progressive exposure of the axially directed cavity wall.

Relatively coarse composites usually exhibit wear at the margins, whereas hybrids tend to chip (crevice formation) as well as wear. Microfilled composites exhibit chipping and surface fracture because of their low fracture toughness, tensile strength and elastic modulus, relatively high polymerisation contraction and thermal coefficient of contraction.

Incremental build-up

Summary

Incremental build-up
- improves depth of cure
- minimises shrinkage
- directs shrinkage towards tooth structure

Polymerisation contraction stresses are responsible for several significant clinical problems. The setting contraction of light-activated composite resin induces stress of approximately 17 MPa at the interface between the restoration and tooth structure, both enamel and dentine. This has the potential to disrupt the mechanical interlock which has been induced by acid-etching and applying a bonding agent (see page 57). However, if the shrinkage can be controlled, subsequent dimensional changes associated with the thermal coefficient of expansion are of little clinical consequence.

A light-activated composite resin cures first at the surface closest to the activating light and shrinks away from other regions. Incremental placement entails placement of the composite in small quantities in selected areas of the cavity and then directing the light-activating unit in such a way that, while curing, the resin will shrink towards the tooth structure rather than away from it. As it is not possible to light-activate excessively any composite resin, it is recommended that the increments be as small as possible and that the light activator be applied from many positions during build-up (**Fig. 9.7**). However, the size and location of the first increment and the direction of the first application of the light are critical to the overall success of the restoration.

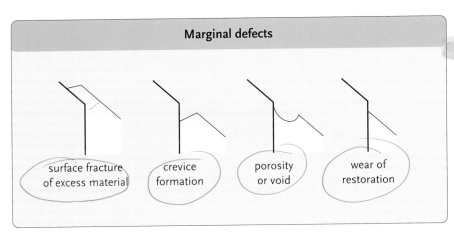

Marginal defects

surface fracture of excess material

crevice formation

porosity or void

wear of restoration

Fig. 9.6 Marginal defects. There are four types of failure which occur at the margin of a composite resin.

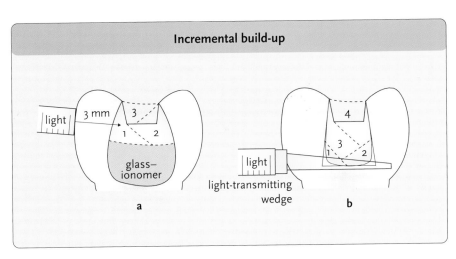

Incremental build-up

light   3 mm   3   1   2

glass–ionomer

light   light-transmitting wedge

4   1   3   2

a   b

Fig. 9.7 Incremental build-up. The lamination technique (**a**) allows for a minimum of composite resin and therefore a reduction in shrinkage problems. (**b**) If the gingival margin is in sound enamel, the entire restoration can be built in composite resin and a light-transmitting wedge will assist in curing the initial gingival increment.

Selection of an activator light

There can be a considerable variation in the efficiency of an activator light and the strength of the light output will decline with time. It is essential for lights to be tested with reasonable frequency and there are meters available for this purpose. Some manufacturers provide a meter built into the machine. A minimum intensity of about 300 mW/cm^2 is necessary to ensure an adequate cure in 40 seconds for the average increment of composite resin. The tip of the light should be at least 10 mm in diameter and must be kept meticulously clean. Note also that there can be a temperature increase of up to 10°C at a depth of 3.2 mm within a 20-second time span during curing and this can be a risk to the pulp. The best defence is a base of glass–ionomer to intercept the temperature rise.

Selection of matrix

To allow optimal light activation of the initial increments of composite resin, it is desirable to use a translucent matrix; there are several types available. Some are precontoured and all can be modified to fit the required circumstances. As the composite resin will not need to be packed into place under pressure it is generally unnecessary to use a matrix retainer such as is usually required for an amalgam. A device such as a 'bitine ring' may offer sufficient support without interfering with placement of the activator light.

Placement of a wedge

If it is necessary to rebuild the contact area when restoring a proximal lesion then it is essential to use a strong wedge to gain separation between the teeth as well as to avoid an overhang. Placement of the wedge during cavity preparation not only protects the gingival tissue and rubber dam, but may also assist by 'stretching' the periodontal ligament and producing a small degree of separation before subsequently placing the matrix.

If both proximal surfaces of the same tooth are to be restored with the one restoration it is logical to build only one side at a time. Place the wedge firmly in one interproximal space and build that surface, then move the wedge to the other interproximal before completing the restoration.

Use of a light-transmitting wedge

There are plastic wedges available with built-in light reflection designed to assist in directing light into the interproximal areas during the initial stages of curing. The amount of light emitted via such wedges is not great and they should not be entirely relied upon for a complete cure. However, it is possible to encourage shrinkage towards the gingival margin to a sufficient degree to justify their use. The alternative lamination technique will eliminate the need because the gingival area will be built in glass–ionomer.

Post-restoration sequelae

Placement of a light-activated composite resin restoration may have several outcomes:

- A tooth that is symptom free.
- A tooth that is sensitive to loading. There may be an intact enamel margin seal but incomplete seal of the dentinal tubules. Movement of dentinal fluid along the tubules (in response to occlusal loading of a weakened tooth) may then stimulate sensory receptors.
- A tooth that is sensitive to thermal and sweet stimuli. There is usually a lack of seal at the enamel or dentinal margins and unsealed dentinal tubules.
- A tooth with fracture of cusps caused by polymerisation contraction in a weakened tooth.

The clinical options to minimise these problems when large composite resin restorations are to be placed include:

- reduction of the total bulk of composite resin by basing the cavity with a substantial quantity of glass–ionomer as a dentine substitute and then replacement of the enamel with careful incremental build-up of composite resin
- restoration using an indirect restoration – a composite resin or ceramic inlay.

RESIN-BONDING AGENTS

It is essential to enhance the adaptation, retention and seal of composite resins to enamel and to dentine (or alternatively to a glass–ionomer base) by the prior application of a resin-bonding agent.

Resin bonding to enamel

Unfilled resin-bonding agents are used to seal the interface between composite resins and acid-etched enamel, thus developing a form of micromechanical retention (Chapter 7, page 57). This union must be resistant to all the stresses associated with curing shrinkage and subsequent function of the restoration. The strength will be dependent upon the strength of the enamel which, optimally, will be well supported by healthy underlying dentine and free of microcracks, which can be generated during cavity preparation. As there is no chemical reaction involved, lack of adaptation, retention or long-term seal may result in microleakage, sensitivity, dental caries and loss of the restoration.

After 15–30 seconds of etching with 37% orthophosphoric acid, the enamel surface will become porous to a depth of 10–20μm and, providing the unfilled resin-bonding agent has a low viscosity, it will penetrate into this surface. The following factors will influence the reliability of the bond.

- Type and concentration of the acid – ideally 37% acid applied for a minimum of 15 seconds.
- Viscosity of the bonding resin – logically a low-viscosity resin will penetrate further than one with a high viscosity.
- Contamination of the enamel after etching – particularly

saliva, although even moisture from exhaled air may reduce the efficiency of the bond.

- Time between resin application and curing – allow a short time (10–15 seconds) for the resin to soak into the enamel.
- Pooling of resin bond at the margins or internal angles represents a weakness in the bond.
- Structure and condition of the enamel at the cavo–surface margin. Microcracks, particularly in unsupported enamel, and already fractured enamel, reduces the efficiency.

Resin bonding to dentine

The goal of a resin–dentine bonding agent is to attach composite resin to healthy dentine and to seal the dentine tubules against the entry of bacteria and their toxins. A successful union will also prevent both inward and outward flow of fluid from either the oral environment or the pulp. It is essential to retain this seal while curing the composite resin restoration because loss of bond will be likely to be associated with post-restoration sensitivity, caries and loss of the restoration.

Until recently, attempts to achieve a reliable seal have been unsuccessful over the long term and there have been wide variations in the results of physical testing *in vitro* and *in vivo*. However, recent improvements in techniques and materials suggest a higher rate of success although the union remains a micromechanical interlock rather than a chemical union, such as that which is available with glass–ionomer. Optimal bonding to dentine requires the removal of all demineralised affected dentine and this is not always desirable. It may mean the removal of dentine that could otherwise be retained, to maintain the integrity of the pulp (Chapter 18). The following principles apply to successful resin–dentine bonding.

- Dentine should be etched to remove smear layer and dentinal tubule plugs using 37% orthophosphoric acid for 15 secs.
- Etching should be sufficient to demineralise the surface layer of both intertubular and intratubular dentine, leaving collagen fibres exposed and available for a mechanical interlock with the resin.
- The surface should be thoroughly washed to remove all remaining etchant.
- The surface should remain wet but not flooded.
- Apply a hydrophilic primer containing acetone, or a similar chemical, to guide and facilitate penetration of the resin adhesive around the exposed collagen fibres.
- Finally, apply the resin adhesive and cure before applying composite resin.

The terms 'conditioning' and 'etching'

It should be noted that the term 'conditioning' has recently been applied rather loosely to the action of 'etching' dentine. The term 'conditioning' was first used in relation to glass–ionomer (Chapter 8, page 80) to differentiate the action of preparing the dentine surface for the ion-exchange adhesion, which is available with that material,

Be aware

'Etching'

used in relation to composite resin

'Conditioning'

used in relation to glass–ionomer

from 'acid etching' the enamel in preparation for a micro-mechanical attachment with resin. It is clear from the above routine that the recommended action for developing union between resin and dentine still requires etching to be successful, so in this text the term 'etching' is retained. There are no untoward implications to be assumed from the use of this definition because it is clear that any low-pH etchant will be effectively buffered before it reaches the pulp tissue and no direct harm is likely to arise.

Components of a resin–dentine bond

Components of a successful resin–dentine bond include:

- Hybrid layer (resin–dentine interdiffusion zone) – a hydrophilic primer and an adhesive bonding agent penetrate approximately $3\mu m$ around and into partly and completely demineralised intertubular dentine on the cavity wall. This layer provides a seal and, perhaps, a little retention for the resin–dentine bond.
- Resin tags – the primer and bonding agent form tags of resin, up to $100\mu m$ long, in the dentinal tubules. Micromechanical bonding on to the partly demineralised walls of the dentinal tubules and the resin tags themselves combine to provide most of the retention achieved by the resin–dentine bond (Chapter 7, page 58).
- Elastic bonding zone – the hybrid layer and the adhesive bonding agent that covers it, provide an 'elastic cavity wall' or 'shock absorber' that assists the bond to resist stresses from polymerisation contraction and functional loading.

Using these materials and techniques it has been shown that bonding to dentine is possible with very high strength *in vitro*. Results *in vivo* also show promise but there are numerous variables in the dentine which also need to be taken into account. Such variables include the distance of the floor of the cavity from the pulp and therefore the relative proportions of intertubular and intratubular dentine (Chapter 7, page 57), as well as the quality and age of the dentine. Also, incremental build-up of the composite resin and the type of resin are important in establishing and maintaining a good bond.

It is apparent that, currently, the most reliable method of uniting dentine and composite resin is through the placement of an intermediate base of high strength glass–ionomer to utilise the ion-exchange adhesion with dentine which is available. The composite resin can then be attached to the glass–ionomer.

POLYACID-MODIFIED COMPOSITE RESINS – 'COMPOMERS'

A new variety of the usual composite resins (comprising resins and inorganic filler particles) is the polyacid-modified composite resin (PAMCR) or 'compomer', which was introduced in the early 1990s. The compomer was introduced as a type of glass–ionomer, with claims that it offered some fluoride release as well as improved physical properties and clinical characteristics However, it has become apparent that, in terms of clinical use and performance, the compomer is best considered as a type of composite resin.

The role of compomers in restorative dentistry remains uncertain and further clinical studies are required to identify specific indications for their use and situations in which they can offer superior performance to composite resins or glass-ionomers of both the traditional or resin-modified types.

Composition and reactions

The compomers presently available contain resins and fillers common to composite resins and glass–ionomers.

The resin component contains functional groups of polycarboxylic acid and methacrylates combined in one molecule. This provides methacrylic groups for cross-linking (as in composite resins) and carboxyl groups to undergo an acid–base reaction in the presence of water and metal ions (as in glass–ionomers).

Fluoride-containing glasses, typical of glass–ionomers, comprise the principal fillers to which may be added glass particles similar to those in composite resins. There may also be other fillers providing additional fluoride release and radiopacity.

The setting reaction in compomers occurs in two stages:

- Stage 1 reaction is typical of light-activated composite resins, forming a resin network enclosing the filler particles. The light-curing mechanism leads to hardening of the material in the cavity.
- Stage 2 reaction occurs slowly after placement in the cavity. Water sorption will occur for up to 2–3 months and, in the presence of carboxyl groups from the polyacid and metal ions from the ionomer glass, there will be a relatively slow ionic acid–base reaction. Hydrogels will form within the resin structure and there will be a slow and low-level release of fluorides.

Adhesion, adaptation and microleakage

Adhesion to tooth structure is micromechanical and requires acid-etching, as for composite resins, and the application of an acetone-containing primer/adhesive. Bond strengths obtained usually approach those achieved by other typical resin bonding systems. Laboratory microleakage studies confirm an adaptation at the cervical margins which is comparable to that of composite resins.

Fluoride release

Although short-term clinical studies have reported no evidence of secondary caries around compomer restorations, independent laboratory studies have generally suggested that fluoride release is limited. Although it is greater than for composite resins, it is significantly lower than for both autocure and resin-modified glass–ionomers. Fluoride release peaks early and then falls rapidly to low levels.

Properties

Findings from clinical studies of longer duration than 3 years are still required. Biocompatibility and fracture toughness of compomers are comparable with those of many composite resins. Their colour matching and optical properties are superior to those of glass–ionomers.

FURTHER READING

Bryant RW. Long-term implications for composite resin restorations. *Ann Roy Aust Coll Dent Surg* 1989; **10**:84–90.

Bryant RW. Direct posterior composite resin restorations. 1. Factors influencing case selection [Review]. *Aust Dent J* 1992; **37**:81–7.

Bryant RW, Hodge K-LV. A clinical evaluation of posterior composite resin restorations. *Aust Dent J* 1994; **39**:77–81

Buonocore M. A simple method of increasing the adhesion of acrylic filling materials to enamel surfaces. *J Dent Res* 1955; **34**:849–53

Craig RG, ed. *Restorative dental materials*. St. Louis: Mosby; 1989.

Fowler CS, Swartz ML, Moore BK. Efficacy testing of visible light curing units. *Oper Dent* 1994; **19**:47–52.

Ironside JG, Makinson OF. Resin restorations; causes of porosities. *Quintessence Int* 1993; **24**:867–73.

Jordan RE. *Esthetic composite bonding: techniques and materials, 2nd ed.* Chicago: Mosby Year Book; 1993.

Lambrechts P, Williams G, Van Herle G, Braem M. Aesthetic limits of light cured composite resins in anterior teeth. *Int Dent J* 1990; **40**:149–58.

Lutz F, Phillips RW. A classification and evaluation of composite resin systems. *J Prosthet Dent* 1983; **50**:480–8.

Martin FE. Composite resin inlays – chairside or laboratory fabrication. *Aust Prosthet J* 1990; **4**(Suppl):13–18.

Mount GJ. Newer restorative materials. *Dent Today* 1989; **5**:1–6; and *Dent Today* 1990; **6**:1–8.

Omer OE, Wilson NH, Watts DC. Radiopacity of posterior composites. *Aust Dent J* 1986; **14**:178–9.

Phillips RW. *Skinner's science of dental materials, 9th ed.* Philadelphia: WB Saunders; 1991 [Chap 12:215–48].

Ruyter IE. Composites – characterization of composite filling materials: reactor response. *Adv Dent Res* 1988; **2**:122–9.

Smith DC, Williams DF. *Biocompatibility of dental materials.* Boca Raton: CRC Press; 1982.

Suzuki S, Leinfelder KF. Wear of enamel cusps opposed by posterior composite resin. *Quintessence Int* 1993; **24**:885–92.

Swartz ML, Phillips RW, Rhodes V. Visible light activated resins – depth of cure. *J Am Dent Assoc* 1983; **106**:634–7

Van Meerbeck B, Peumans M, Verschueren M, *et al*. Clinical status of ten adhesive systems. *J Dent Res* 1995; **73**:1690–702.

Vanherle G, Smith DC. *Posterior composite resin restorative materials.* St Paul, Minnesota: 3M Dental Products; 1985.

Willems G, Lambrechts P, Braem M, Celis JP, Vanherle G. A classification of dental composites according to their morphological and mechanical characteristics. *Dent Mater* 1992; 310–19.

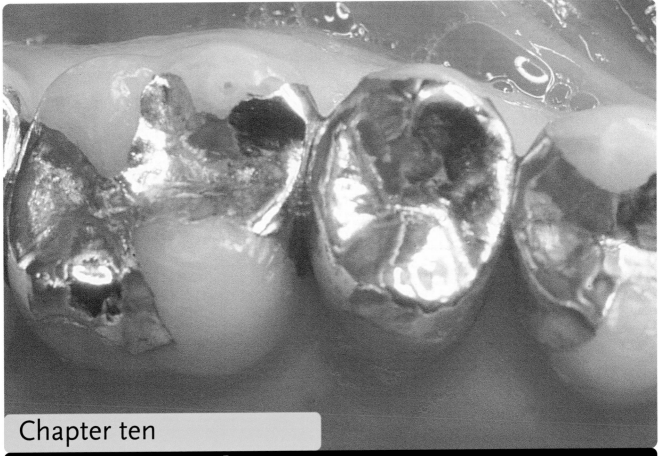

Chapter ten

Dental amalgams

R.W. Bryant

An amalgam is an alloy of one or more metals with mercury.

'Dental amalgam' refers to a particular type of amalgam, which is the most commonly used and one of the oldest dental restorative materials. It is the product of an amalgamation reaction between particles of an alloy, containing varying amounts of silver, copper and tin with mercury.

There is still no adequate, economic alternative for dental amalgam as a restorative material for a moderately sized carious lesion in a high-load-bearing area. The combination of reliable long-term performance in load-bearing situations and small cost per unit is unmatched by any other dental restorative material.

TYPES OF DENTAL AMALGAM ALLOYS

Dental amalgam alloy refers to the combination of metals, such as silver, tin, copper and sometimes zinc, indium, palladium or platinum, as used in dentistry. The particles of the dental amalgam alloy are mixed with mercury to form a dental amalgam. To avoid excessive repetition, the word 'dental' is frequently omitted when reference is made to (dental) amalgam and (dental) amalgam alloy.

Since the 1960s, high-copper amalgams have largely replaced high-silver alloys, which had changed little in composition since the 1890s. Extensive clinical studies have provided information on performance, longevity and reasons for failure; laboratory tests have been developed to obtain a greater understanding of their structure and performance. Amalgams have always been regarded as very tolerant materials which will perform well in the oral cavity in spite of great variations in placement techniques.

However, improvements in methods of prevention and control of caries and consequent modifications to cavity design have resulted in changes in diagnostic concepts, treatment philosophies, restorative techniques and materials. Therefore amalgam is likely to be used less in the future. The potential for allergy to or toxicity from the mercury content has been recognised for many years and intensive investigation and research have been undertaken. Currently, it is apparent that any restriction in the use of amalgam will be related to environmental concerns rather than to the health of individual patients and there appears to be no justification to either cease using it or replace it entirely in the hope of altering a patient's state of health.

A range of amalgam alloys is available commercially and they may be differentiated from each other as follows.

Copper content

Low-copper amalgam alloys have a total copper content of less than 6%. Until the mid-1960s, almost all dental amalgam alloys were of this type.

High-copper amalgam alloys have a total copper content greater than approximately 12% and most modern dental amalgam alloys are in this category. They have superior physical properties and clinical performance, partly because they show low creep and an absence of a tin–mercury (gamma 2, γ_2) reaction phase.

Particle shape and type

There are two particle types depending on method of manufacture (**Figs 10.1** and **10.2**):
1. 'Lathe-cut' refers to the irregularly shaped filings produced by cutting an ingot of alloy on a lathe. Before cutting, the ingot is, by tradition, homogenised to produce an alloy with a single Ag–Sn phase (γ) as well as some regions of Cu_3Sn (ε).
2. 'Spherical' particles are produced by atomising the alloy, whilst still liquid, into a stream of inert gas. They are usually not subjected to a homogenising heat treatment and therefore contain Ag–Sn (β) and Cu_3Sn (ε) dispersed in a Ag–Sn (γ) matrix.

Some alloys contain a blend of lathe-cut particles and spherical particles and, depending on the proportion of each in the mix, the handling properties, particularly 'packability', will be modified.

Zinc content

Alloys containing more than 0.01% zinc are described as 'zinc-containing' and those with less than 0.01% zinc are referred to as 'zinc-free'. Zinc was originally included in the initial melt for an alloy because it acted as an oxide scavenger to produce clean castings of the ingot. Modern techniques of casting into an inert atmosphere have simplified the production of zinc-free alloys. Amalgams that contain zinc appear to exhibit a lower rate of marginal fracture under clinical loading but they tend to exhibit an excessive delayed expansion if contaminated with moisture during placement.

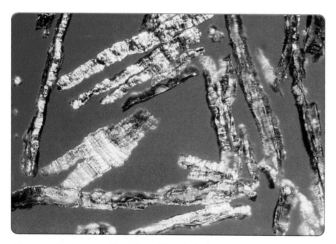

Fig. 10.1 Lathe-cut alloy. The old style lathe-cut particles, which were mixed with a mortar and pestle by hand.

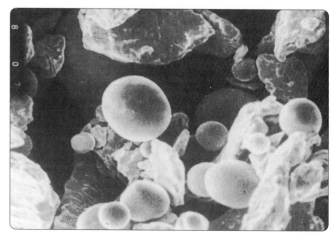

Fig. 10.2 Modern alloy. A modern blend of lathe-cut and spherical particles.

Minor elements

A number of elements, such as indium, palladium and platinum, may be included in the alloy in minor quantities. Although the content of these is usually less than 1%, reference is frequently made to the presence of one of these elements in advertising the alloys.

γ_2 content

Amalgams may be described as γ_2-containing and γ_2-free. Low-copper amalgams contain the Sn–Hg phase, which is called the γ_2 phase to differentiate it from the γ phases of the Ag–Sn and Ag–Hg alloy systems. Several hours after amalgamation, all correctly manipulated high-copper amalgams are γ_2-free.

Packability

'Packability' refers to the resistance offered by the amalgam to the forces of condensation used in placing the amalgam. Amalgams can be described as offering a high or low degree of packability; this will vary according to the size and proportional distribution of lathe-cut or spherical particles. An amalgam containing only spherical particles is relatively 'easy' to pack because it moves readily from under the condenser. Such an amalgam requires the use of a larger packing instrument, but a substantial load is still required to achieve proper adaptation to the cavity and to eliminate as much mercury-rich matrix as possible during the condensation stage.

Classification of alloys and amalgams

Based on the copper content, the shape of the particles and the major elements present in the spherical particles of a blended particle alloy, dental amalgam alloys and their corresponding amalgams can be simply classified into six types.

- Low-copper, lathe-cut (**Fig. 10.3a**)
- Low-copper, spherical
- High-copper, lathe-cut
- High-copper, spherical (**Fig. 10.3b**)
- High-copper blend, Ag–Sn–Cu (**Fig. 10.3c**)
- High-copper blend, Ag–Cu (**Fig. 10.3d**)

The two types of blended particle alloys contain both lathe-cut and spherical particles and the spherical particles which have a high copper content, contain mainly Ag, Sn and Cu, or Ag and Cu.

There has been confusion over the nomenclature given to these different types but the above classification is preferred. The first two have been called 'conventional' or 'silver–tin' and 'high-copper spherical' has been known as 'single-melt high-copper'. Terms such as 'dispersion-modified' and 'Ag–Cu dispersed' have been applied to the last type, and a general label of 'admixed' has been applied to all alloys containing both lathe-cut and spherical particles.

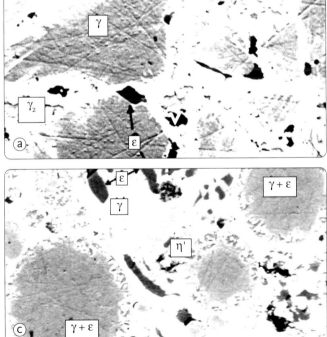

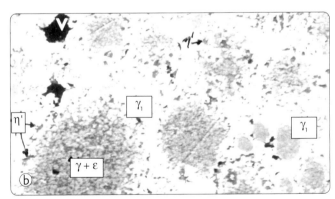

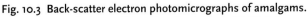

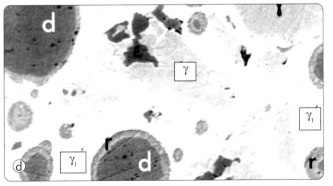

Fig. 10.3 Back-scatter electron photomicrographs of amalgams.
(**a**) Low-copper lathe-cut (New True Dentalloy – SS White)
(**b**) High-copper spherical (Tytin – Kerr) (**c**) High-copper blend, Ag–Sn–Cu (Valiant PhD – Caulk/Dentsply) (**d**) High-copper blend, Ag–Cu (Dispersalloy – Caulk/Dentsply). Bar lines indicate 20 μm. Phases shown are γ, ε, δ, η', γ_1, γ_2, v (void), r (reaction zone, containing γ_1 and η' phases).

AMALGAMATION AND MANIPULATION

Components of the amalgamation reaction
In amalgamation, mercury comes into contact with the surfaces of particles of different types containing different amounts of metals. Approximately 3–5 μm of the surface region of a particle undergoes reaction.

Composition of the alloy
Amalgam alloys differ greatly in their composition, by weight, of metals.
- Low-copper alloys contain approximately 70% Ag, 26% Sn, 3–4% Cu and some minor elements.
- High-copper spherical and high-copper lathe-cut alloys usually contain approximately 41–61% Ag, 28–31% Sn, 12–27% Cu and some minor elements.

Types of particles present
Particles in the alloy may vary according to shape, heat treatment by the manufacturer, size and relative proportions of the different types. These variables will influence the handling, setting rate and properties of the set amalgam.

Initial mercury content
Depending on the shape, size and composition of the alloy particles, the amount of mercury initially required to give a good amalgamation can vary from 40% to 53% by weight. Low-copper microfine lathe-cut particle alloys require a relatively large amount of mercury to be dispensed initially and high-copper spherical alloys require the least. The final mercury content (37–48%) is influenced by the initial mercury content and the clinical technique used when placing the amalgam.

Phases present in unreacted alloy
When mercury reacts with the alloy particles, the metals in the alloy are usually present as phases which approximate stoichiometric composition (**Fig. 10.4**).

Two phases, γ and ε, are present in all unreacted alloys and a third, the dispersant component (d), is only present in the high-copper blend, Ag–Cu type of alloy.

Phases formed by amalgamation
The mercury reacts with the outer 3–5 μm of the surface of the alloy particle and the metals, which are combined together in phases, go into solution in the mercury and then precipitate out in the form of new reaction products. Two of these (γ_1 and η^1) are present in all amalgams and the third product, the γ_2 phase, is only present in low-copper amalgams.

Structure of the set amalgam
Providing the minimal amount of mercury, commensurate with complete amalgamation, is incorporated initially, and then proper condensation techniques are carried out, 35–50% of the final volume of the set amalgam will consist of unreacted portions of alloy particles, held together by the γ_1 phase matrix.

Clinically, amalgams deteriorate with time as a result of corrosion. Corrosion products will be formed within the amalgam as well as on the surface; Sn–Hg phase may be lost from low-copper amalgams. A clinically significant result of corrosion is an increase in the number of voids in the amalgam (**Fig. 10.5**).

Trituration
Trituration of the alloy with the mercury is normally carried out in a mechanical amalgamator. For reasons of variabilty of mix and mercury hygiene, trituration by hand is no longer used. The object is to completely wet the entire surface of the alloy particles with the mercury, to bring about the process known as amalgamation. The efficiency of the machine will be influenced by the speed of the particular unit, the length and type of 'throw' of the capsule in the machine, the presence of a pestle in the capsule and the length of time of mixing.

Fig. 10.4 Composition of the major phases in dental amalgam.

Code	Phase or component	Weight %			
		Ag	Sn	Cu	Hg
γ gamma	Ag$_3$Sn	73.2	26.8		
ε epsilon	Cu$_3$Sn		38.4	61.6	
d dispersant	Ag–Cu eutectic	71.9		28.1	
γ_1 gamma 1	Ag$_2$Hg$_3$ Ag$_{22}$Sn Hg$_{27}$	30.7	1.80		67.5
γ_2 gamma 2	Snx Hgy		82.5		17.5
η^1 eta prime	Cu$_6$Sn$_5$		60.9	39.1	

Amalgamators are made to work at different speeds and the action should be checked periodically. The efficiency can be tested with a trial mix. If, after mixing, the amalgam feels hot or is difficult to remove from the capsule, the mixing time should be reduced. Alternatively, drop the freshly mixed mass on to the bench from a height of approximately 30 cm. If the mix is dry and crumbles, the trituration time should be increased. A well-mixed amalgam should stay together when dropped on the bench but should be a little flattened and retain a wet gloss on the surface. It is unwise to substantially change the trituration time in an attempt to modify working time. Manufacturers control the working time of each alloy and it is preferable to use their recommendation in making a selection.

Summary

Test for correct mix

Over-trituration
- alloy will be hot
- hard to remove from capsule
- shiny wet and soft

Under-trituration
- alloy will be dry
- will crumble if dropped from approximately 30 cm

It is better to slightly over-triturate than to under-triturate an amalgam, since:
- extended trituration may reduce plasticity, shorten working time and increase final contraction

281

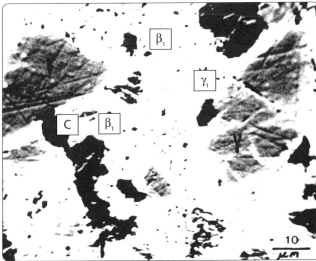

Fig. 10.5 Corroded amalgam. A photomicrograph of a clinically aged amalgam showing evidence of corrosion. C = chloride-containing corrosion product. β_1 = Sn-rich Ag–Hg matrix phase. There is an absence of γ_2 phase, in this low-copper amalgam, which has been replaced by corrosion product.

- reduced trituration may result in incomplete wetting of the surfaces of the alloy particles by the mercury, a weak interface between the matrix (γ_1) and the particles, lower strength, increased porosity, a rougher surface and increased corrosion and loss of surface finish.

Use the lowest possible mercury content, in accordance with the manufacturer's instructions, so that excess mercury does not have to be removed after trituration. However, the dispensing of alloy and mercury and the trituration must ensure that the freshly mixed amalgam has optimal plasticity. Probably no other characteristic has as much influence on the adaptation of amalgam to the cavity wall, optimising the seal and minimising post-restoration sensitivity.

Placement and finishing

Summary

Placement

Place within 3 minutes of beginning mix.

Condense using:
- smooth flat pluggers
- lathe cut – use small pluggers
- blended – use small pluggers
- spherical – use larger pluggers
- use optimal load at all times

After trituration, each capsule of the amalgam should be incrementally placed and condensed into the cavity within 3 minutes. After overbuilding the amalgam beyond the cavity margin, it can then be burnished towards the margins and carved to an approximate occlusal form. At this point the occlusion can be checked and corrected and the amalgam finally burnished again. At a subsequent appointment any necessary final adjustment can be carried out to the occlusal and proximal surfaces. Polishing can be kept to a minimum because developing a mirror finish may bring mercury to the surface. It is sufficient to leave a correctly contoured smooth surface with margins flush with the enamel, an absence of overhangs and a properly shaped contact area.

Purpose of condensation
Condensation refers to the incremental placement of the amalgam into the prepared cavity and compression of each increment into the others to form a continuous homogeneous mass that is well adapted to all margins, walls and line angles. It is best carried out using hand instruments with a smooth flat face which can deliver reasonable force per unit area to the amalgam and compress the layers together. Mechanical condensers are available and reduce the need for application of load. However, they tend to lead to unreliable condensation as well as generation of

heat and mercury vapour, both of which are undesirable. Ultrasonic condensation has also been suggested, but is not recommended because it causes the release of considerable quantities of mercury vapour. The aims of condensation are to:

- adapt amalgam to the margins, walls and line angles of the cavity
- minimise voids and layering between increments within the amalgam
- develop maximum physical properties
- remove excess mercury to leave an optimal alloy: mercury ratio.

Speed of placement

Immediately amalgam is triturated, phase formation commences and the setting reaction is underway. Amalgam must be used in a plastic state, so there should be no delay between trituration and condensation. No amalgam should be placed more than 3 minutes after the start of mixing. Attempting to condense a partly set amalgam into a cavity will result in poor adaptation, reduced marginal seal and a weak restoration.

Moisture contamination

Keep the amalgam completely free from moisture contamination during the entirety of the placement procedures following trituration. The newly mixed alloy must not be touched by bare hands and the cavity must be completely dry and free of gingival seepage or haemorrhage. For preference, work under rubber dam. Inclusion of water during condensation will lead to increase in corrosion and tarnish with a reduction of physical properties. A zinc-containing amalgam will, in addition, develop a delayed expansion.

Placement

Place the amalgam into the cavity in relatively small increments and condense rapidly on to the walls and in to the line angles using a high load of short duration. Pack laterally as well as vertically to ensure complete adaptation, particularly into point angles. Use a smooth-faced condenser of appropriate size.

- Lathe-cut alloy – use small condenser up to one-half cavity width.
- Blended alloy – use small condenser up to one-half cavity width.
- Spherical alloy – use largest condenser to fit the cavity.

Always remove the mercury-rich surface of the last increment before placing a subsequent load and increase the size of the condenser when packing excess beyond the confines of the cavity.

First burnish (precarve burnish)

On completion of condensation carry out a precarve burnish using a large burnisher for 15 seconds. Use light force and move from the centre of the restoration outwards to the margins. This will bring further mercury to the

Notes

Close margins

To close margins and keep them closed:
- first burnish before carving occlusal
- second burnish after completing occlusal carving

surface, which must be removed; it will also improve adaptation to the cavity margins.

Carving

Using remaining enamel as a guide, carve gently from enamel towards the centre. Carving instruments must be of appropriate shape and very sharp so as to create minimum disruption to the amalgam at the margins. Do not carve deep or sharp occlusal anatomy, but take care to maintain marginal ridges and occlusal spillways. Deep, sharply carved patterns on the occlusal surface may look nice, but they act as crack initiators and are undesirable. However, well-defined marginal ridges and lateral spillways will dissipate load from the occlusal table and lead the food bolus away from contact areas.

Always be prepared to adjust the occlusal anatomy of the opposing tooth, including a cusp tip, to avoid developing deep intercuspation between the arches because this may lead to interference during lateral and protrusive excursions and prejudice the longevity of the restoration or the tooth (see Chapter 21, page 243).

Final burnish (postcarve burnish)

Following carving, check the occlusion, particularly in relation to lateral excursions. Now carry out a brief final burnish. Use a large burnisher at a low load and burnish outwards towards the margins to finally adapt the alloy to the marginal enamel on both the occlusal and the proximal surfaces.

Finishing

The restoration should always be finished at a later appointment to allow an opportunity to further adjust occlusal contacts and proximal anatomy and to minimise discrepancies at the tooth–amalgam junction. Do not increase the depth of fissures or increase the angle of the cuspal inclines because this may increase marginal failure over time. The surface does not have to have a high-gloss mirror finish but it should be smooth enough to discourage plaque accumulation. Carry out all polishing procedures under an air–water spray to minimise the generation of heat and the liberation of mercury vapour.

PROPERTIES

Biocompatibility

Be aware

Mercury
Mercury is available in three forms
- elemental mercury (liquid or vapour)
- inorganic compounds
- organic compounds

The only risks from mercury are to the operator, staff and the environment from poor mercury hygiene.

There are no direct risks to the patient

The biocompatibility of amalgam has been the subject of extensive investigation, particularly in relation to the presence of mercury. Available evidence indicates that, for patients, the placement and presence of amalgam restorations does not constitute a health hazard except in the rare case of hypersensitivity. Hazards to dental staff related to dental amalgam are discussed in greater detail in Appendix 1, but it is appropriate at this point to discuss the relevance of amalgam toxicity in the dental practice. There is concern, some of it appropriate, that mercury in dental amalgam may pose threats to the health of patients, to the health of dental care providers and to the environment. From the toxicological viewpoint there are three forms of mercury.
- Elemental mercury (liquid or vapour).
- Inorganic compounds.
- Organic compounds.
It is useful to consider these in turn, since each is very different from the other.

Elemental mercury
Liquid mercury is absorbed relatively poorly across skin or mucosa. Most mercury that is absorbed becomes charged (ionised) before it reaches the blood. Ionised mercury is excreted well through the kidneys and urine. The old practice of 'hand mulling' dental amalgam after mixing, but before insertion into the cavity, resulted in only one documented case of kidney failure – in a long-term dental assistant who demonstrated high renal mercury levels. There is no known risk to patients from liquid mercury. Droplets of mercury that may be swallowed are poorly absorbed; most mercury passes harmlessly in the faeces. A small fraction may be taken up because a surface coat of mercuric chloride will form on the mercury while it is in the stomach, but it is usually readily cleared by the kidneys. Some religious cults swallow large amounts of mercury and collect it from their faeces for re-use without apparent harm.

Mercury vapour
Mercury vapour is less benign because it is rapidly absorbed into the blood via the lungs and remains uncharged, and therefore highly lipid soluble, for several minutes. During this time it can cross the blood–brain barrier where it becomes charged and exits the extra-cellular fluid of the brain and returns into blood much more slowly. This means that mercury levels can accumulate in the brain in those exposed to mercury vapour at high levels for a long time. At high tissue levels, neural enzyme systems become impaired, thus leading to impaired brain function. Low levels may cause restlessness, tremors, or loss of concentration but, at higher levels, insanity and death may occur. The industrial risks of mercury vapour are well studied. There are definite risks to dentists and their staff if poor mercury 'hygiene' is practised in the dental setting and mercury vapour levels are allowed to rise. Appropriate measures for mercury hygiene are described in Appendix 1. The levels of mercury vapour to which dental patients are exposed, even those patients with teeth extensively restored with amalgam, are well below levels known to pose risks to health.

Inorganic compounds of mercury
Dental amalgam contains several different inorganic mercury compounds, but they are of low or very low toxicity and are apparently harmless when swallowed. They are poorly absorbed, do not accumulate in body tissues and are well excreted. In fact some inorganic mercury compounds are used as topical antibacterials, making use of their very low toxicity and poor absorption into the body. Sulphur is used to 'control' spilled liquid mercury because mercuric sulphide forms when the two elements come into contact and this is of no environmental concern.

Organic compounds of mercury
Some organic compounds of mercury are highly toxic at low concentrations but none are known to form in the oral environment through dental amalgam use. There is a valid concern that waste water from dental offices containing organic mercury compounds can add to mercury levels in surrounding water resources such as the sea and rivers. Microorganisms inhabiting sediment on the sea floor can synthesise inorganic compounds such as mercuric chloride, which may then enter small forms of sea life. The food chain may then concentrate the compounds into larger fish, which are subsequently caught and ingested by humans, causing severe illness and death. Although the principal source of mercury in waste water is industries other than dentistry, it is important that the dental profession recognises the risk and behaves responsibly in this regard.

Concerns of patients
Unfortunately some health practitioners may advise their patients that mercury from dental restorations causes a variety of ill-effects or, alternatively, that removal of all amalgam restorations will result in a cure

for serious medical conditions. The US National Institutes of Health in 1991, the Swedish Medical Research Council in 1992, the US Public Health Service in 1993 and the Swedish Board of Health and Welfare in 1994 all found that there was no evidence of ill-health resulting from the use of dental amalgam, with the exception of relatively rare and localised allergic reactions on adjacent mucosa. There is also no evidence of improvement in health following amalgam removal. As is made evident elsewhere in this text, amalgam remains the most satisfactory economic restorative material now available for moderately sized defects in posterior teeth and, at present, there is no satisfactory alternative available for long-term restorations.

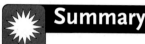

Summary

Corrosion

All amalgams always corrode in one of the following ways:
- tarnishing
- crevice corrosion
- corrosion fatigue
- galvanic corrosion

High-copper types show controlled corrosion

Conventional types corrode more rapidly

Corrosion

Corrosion is defined as the electrochemical destruction of a metal by reaction with its environment. All amalgam restorations undergo at least one of four types of corrosion.

Tarnishing

Surface corrosion causes tarnishing by the oxidation of the Sn–Hg phase in low-copper amalgams or the copper-containing phases in high-copper amalgams, with the formation of a film of oxides, sulphides and hydroxides. Polarisation may also take place with breakdown of the film and formation of a corrosion product followed by pitting and roughening of the surface.

Crevice corrosion

A differential oxygen concentration cell may arise at the margin of a restoration resulting in the surface facing the tooth becoming cathodic in relation to the outer surface of the restoration. Selective attack on phases in the amalgam and the release of tin and copper result in the formation of tin- and copper-containing corrosion products as well as products containing Ca, Cl, Fe, S and Zn. These products will become lodged in the crevice and will seal the interface, producing the so-called self-sealing of the amalgam to tooth.

Corrosion fatigue

This occurs particularly at the margins. Fine branch-like penetrations, having the appearance of fatigue cracks, extend along the grain boundaries of the γ_1 matrix phase in regions subjected to deforming occlusal loads.

Galvanic corrosion

Contact between dissimilar metals or alloys in an electrolyte may lead to galvanic corrosion. Contact between amalgam and cast gold, between amalgam and prosthodontic alloys, and between fresh amalgam and old amalgam may be a cause. It is possible to note, in selected patients, occasional sharp pain or rapid pitting and roughening of amalgam restorations. This is generally self-limiting through the corrosion process; the symptoms will subside over a period of 1 or 2 days.

The γ_2 phase is the phase most susceptible to corrosion in low-copper amalgams. The process extends through the restoration via the γ_2 phase, between grains of γ_1 phase and through voids. In high-copper amalgams the η', d, ε (and possibly the γ_1) phases appear to corrode concurrently. Corrosion is a slower process in high-copper amalgams and extends by way of grain boundaries of the γ_1 phase.

Creep

Creep is progressive permanent deformation under loading. Low-copper amalgams show high creep values of greater than 2.5% and this is associated clinically with greater marginal fracture.

The presence or absence of the γ_2 phase is the principal factor influencing creep. The presence of the γ_2 phase allows the γ_1 phase grains to slide under load, particularly when the γ_1 grains are small. High-copper amalgams, with no γ_2 phase, show less than 0.2% creep after 7 days.

Strength

The importance of the strength of an amalgam in determining clinical success or failure is uncertain, although it has been suggested that the results of particular strength tests may be representative of certain clinical situations. Compressive strength and transverse strength values are shown in **Figure 10.6** for products that are representative of four amalgam types. There appears to be a considerable gain in physical properties over the first 7 days but it must be noted that the clinical results obtained in any given situation will be entirely dependent upon operator variables.

High-copper spherical amalgams have the highest strength of all amalgams at 1 hour after placement and this may be of clinical importance if the restoration is to be subjected to early load. However, they are not fully set at this time and it is unwise to subject a new restoration to undue load or to immediately prepare the restored tooth for a crown. The tensile strength is only about 20–38 MPa after 1 hour, so there is a need for care when checking the occlusion. After 7 days, the strength of high-copper amalgams is substantially greater than that of low-copper amalgams. The transverse strength relates directly to the final mercury content and this may be of clinical importance in large restorations that are to be subjected to heavy occlusal loads.

Rigidity

High-copper amalgams are more rigid than low-copper amalgams, approaching close to the modulus of elasticity of enamel (about 82.5 GPa). This is significant when considering longevity of a restoration and will account, in part, for what appears to be considerably better results being achieved with modern high-copper amalgams.

Fatigue strength

This is the response to repeated loading at relatively low sub-fracture loads for extended periods of time and is related to resistance to creep. Low-copper amalgams with high creep values exhibit slowly developing crack formation because the amalgam bends over an extended period of time before final sudden fracture. In contrast, high-copper amalgams, showing low creep, take extended periods of time before fracturing and, if fracture does occur at all, it is preceded by very little bending.

Thermal properties

Typical values for the linear coefficient of thermal expansion and the thermal diffusivity of amalgam, composite resin, glass–ionomer cement and tooth structure are given in **Figure 8.25** (page 84).

The clinical experience of sharp sensitivity to cold stimuli, particularly during the first 3–5 weeks after placement, is usually associated with incomplete initial adaptation, resulting in a lack of marginal seal of the amalgam. Sealing the dentine tubules by placement of a varnish or resin bond may minimise the sensitivity. Alternatively, placement of a glass–ionomer lining will both seal the tubules and allow fluoride release. Post-insertion tenderness can also be associated with an occlusal interference or prematurity.

Dimensional change

Most amalgams show a small degree of dimensional change on setting but this can be exaggerated if they are not correctly handled during clinical placement. Although most well-manipulated high copper amalgams exhibit a very minor contraction on setting, this is thought to have only minimal clinical significance. Optimal adaptation to the cavity walls and margins is principally associated with ensuring optimal plasticity of the mix, reduced surface roughness of the amalgam and excellent condensation into the cavity.

Zinc-containing amalgams, particularly low-copper amalgams, may exhibit an excessive delayed expansion, commencing after 3–5 days, which may continue for several months, reaching in excess of 400 μm. This appears to be the result of incorporation of water during clinical handling, leading to an electrolytic reaction between the water and zinc and other anodic elements present. Hydrogen gas will be generated within the amalgam, which will then expand and may cause considerable pain and, possibly, even split tooth structure.

Figure 10.7 shows a comparison between several commonly used alloys that have been stored either dry or in water. The clinical implications are even more significant because of the potential for inclusion of water or other oral fluids without the clinician being aware of this. If zinc-containing alloys are being placed, water contamination must be considered as a possible cause of prolonged post-insertion pain.

Amalgam type	Compressive strength in MPa 1 hour	1 week	Transverse strength in MPa 1 week	Modulus of elasticity (GPa)	Static creep (%)
Low-copper lathe cut	155	390	139	41	2.5
High-copper spherical	325	590	148	53	0.1
High-copper blend, Ag–Sn–Cu	190	570	142	56	0.1
High-copper blend, Ag–Cu	190	500	122	52	0.2

Fig. 10.6 Significant physical properties. The physical properties of dental amalgams that are in common use are listed. The clinical significance is uncertain and careful placement is imperative if the figures shown are to be achieved for the oral cavity.

Amalgam	Type	Dry 3 month (μm)	Wet 1 week (μm)	Wet 3 month (μm)	Zinc (%)
Low Cu – lathe cut	N	–13.3	+39.1	+286	0.93
High Cu – spherical	T	–15.2	–9.2	–11.7	0.03
High Cu – blend, Ag–Cu–Sn	V	–9.2	–8.4	-13.3	0.04
High Cu – blend, Ag–Cu–Sn	P	–0.4	+3.0	+5.5	0.18
High Cu – blend, Ag–Cu	D	–12.5	+2.1	+26.6	0.97

N = New True Dentalloy (SSWhite)
T = Tytin (Kerr)
V = Valiant PhD (Caulk/Dentsply)
P = Permite C (SDI)
D = Dispersalloy (J&J)

Fig. 10.7 Effect of water contamination.
This shows the serious side-effects of contamination with water during condensation of an amalgam, particularly if the alloy contains zinc.
Adapted from Nelson and Mahler, 1990.

CLINICAL CONSIDERATIONS

Marginal adaptation and seal
In the first few weeks after placement, amalgam may exhibit a lack of marginal adaptation which, permits microleakage of fluids and microorganisms between the restoration and the cavity wall. This may be associated with marginal deterioration, accumulation of debris, recurrent caries, post-restoration sensitivity or pulpal reactions.

Manipulative techniques influencing adaptation
The following manipulative factors will all have a bearing on the efficiency of the initial marginal seal.
- Over-trituration may result in reduced plasticity and excessive contraction while setting.
- Improved plasticity of the amalgam enhances adaptation.
- Good condensation is essential to adapt the amalgam to the cavity walls.
- Spherical amalgams can be condensed using larger condensers and do not require the same load to achieve optimal physical properties.
- Lathe-cut and blended-particle amalgams require smaller diameter condensers and more care and a heavier load to achieve the optimal degree of adaptation.
- Both precarve and postcarve burnishing of the margins improve adaptation.

Self-sealing
After 48 hours, a well-placed amalgam restoration will begin to exhibit a reduction in leakage that can be attributed to the formation of corrosion products at the amalgam–tooth interface (crevice corrosion), a process which is termed 'self-sealing'. Thereafter, the restoration experiences periods of intermittent microleakage and re-sealing.

Low-copper amalgams seal within 2–3 months, but high-copper amalgams corrode less and therefore take 10–12 months to provide a comparable seal.

Clinical techniques to enhance marginal seal
A number of techniques have been used to minimise or prevent the initial marginal leakage or to seal the dentinal tubules beneath the amalgam. These involve the use of:
- Copal resin varnish. Apply two thin coats of a copal resin varnish to the cavity walls and margins before placing amalgam and it will gradually dissolve, beginning at the cavo-surface, over 2–3 months. As the varnish dissolves out the gap will be filled with corrosion products from the amalgam and dissolution of the varnish will cease.
- The use of chemically activated or light-activated bonding or luting agents, to achieve 'bonded amalgams', may seal the cavity walls against microleakage. They also offer some degree of adhesion of amalgam to dentine and enamel. This is further discussed in the subsequent section on 'Bonded amalgams'.

Notes

Marginal seal
Microleakage is a hazard so marginal seal is important.
- corrosion will seal in 3–12 months
- copal varnish will wash out and allow corrosion
- resin bond will seal long term
- glass–ionomer will seal dentine and release fluoride

- Glass–ionomer linings placed under an amalgam will seal the dentinal tubules and release small quantities of fluoride, but will not affect the enamel margins or enhance the seal at the margin.
- Oxalate solutions, such as potassium oxalate, can be applied to the cavity surface to reduce the permeability of the tubules and possibly seal the dentine. The crystals thus deposited will not wash out but will allow deposition of corrosion products.

'Bonded' amalgams

During the 1990s some clinicians began to routinely bond amalgam restorations to both enamel and dentine. After preparation of the cavity, the enamel and dentine can be etched using a conventional etchant, and a chemically cured resin bonding agent applied to the walls of the cavity. Amalgam is immediately condensed into the cavity before the resin bond has cured with the intention to adapt the resin to the walls and develop a mechanical interlock between the resin and the amalgam.

To date, there is encouraging evidence from laboratory studies suggesting that the system works well, but further clinical studies, extending beyond 2 years, are required to provide convincing evidence.

The advantages claimed for bonded amalgam restorations are as follows.

- Conservation of tooth structure. There is less need to prepare specific retentive elements in the cavity design.
- Retention of complex restorations may be enhanced overall.
- Resistance to cusp fracture appears to be enhanced in laboratory studies. However, clinical evidence is still required to substantiate this concept.
- Elimination of postinsertion sensitivity is claimed by some operators, but controlled prospective studies have not yet supported this claim. Lack of universal acceptance may be because of variations in factors such as plasticity of the amalgam used as well as variations in condensation techniques with different operators.

There are other factors which may be regarded as disadvantages for this technique:

- Clinical difficulty of application of the more viscous bonding agents which are the ones identified in the laboratory as being the most effective.
- Lightly filled resin bonding agents with a high thermal coefficient of expansion tend to pool at the gingival margin resulting in a higher potential for microleakage.
- Excess resin bond and amalgam tend to blend at the margins of the cavity during condensation and make carving difficult.
- Clinical studies do not extend beyond about 3 years so longevity is not established and common modes of failure are not understood.

It is suggested that, until further clinical evidence is available, the technique of amalgam bonding should be used with caution. It may be wise to limit its use to extensive and complex restorations in conjunction with the usual methods of auxiliary retention.

Marginal fracture of amalgam

Marginal fracture has also been referred to as 'marginal breakdown', 'ditching' and 'crevice formation' (**Figs 10.8** and **10.9**). The problem has been widely researched and discussed and several restorations exhibiting different amounts of marginal fracture are shown in **Figures 10.10** and **10.11**. Regardless of the type of amalgam, marginal fracture increases with time. The rate of increase is greater for low-copper amalgams than for high-copper amalgams. Marginal fracture correlates poorly with further caries, unless the crevice exceeds $300\,\mu m$ in width, so care must be exercised in making the decision to replace an amalgam restoration when the margin looks less than ideal. Few amalgams look perfect beyond 3–5 years, but the presence of active caries is the only justification for replacement.

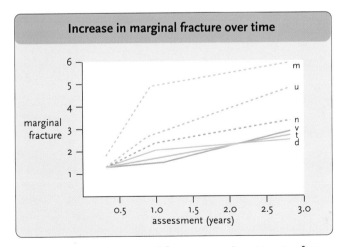

Fig. 10.8 **Increase in marginal fracture over time.** M, microfine low-copper lathe-cut; U, low-copper spherical; N, fine-particle low-copper lathe-cut; V, high-copper blend Ag–Cu–Sn; T, high-copper spherical; D, high-copper blend Ag–Cu.

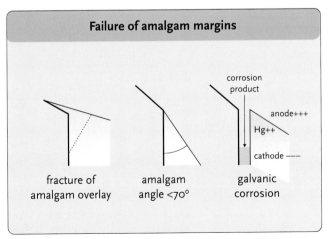

Fig. 10.9 **Failure of amalgam margins.** The main reasons for failure of an amalgam–tooth interface. Usually, corrosion products will seal the interface and recurrent caries is unlikely to arise.

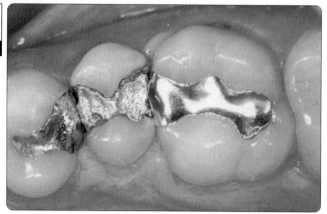

Fig. 10.10 Various margin failure. Three amalgams showing different degrees of marginal failure – reasons unknown.

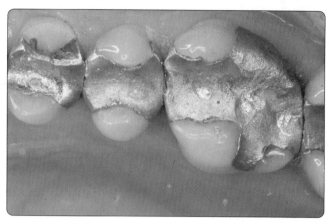

Fig. 10.11 Marginal failure. Three amalgams showing marginal failure believed to be the result of over-polishing. The first bicuspid has lost the buccal cusp.

Clinical techniques to prevent marginal fracture

A number of factors influence the development of marginal fracture. These include the following.

- Excess amalgam, left lying over the occlusal or proximal surface through failure to carve correctly, is subject to fracture and may result in marginal ditching.
- The angle of the cavo–surface margin of an amalgam restoration should be greater than 70° and the cavity should be designed to allow for this.
- On completion of packing, burnish the margins both before and after carving to improve marginal adaptation.
- Where possible, design the cavity to avoid undue stress on the margin of a restoration because amalgam is subject to plastic deformation (creep) and 'corrosion fatigue'.

Bulk fracture of amalgam

Bulk fracture of amalgam restorations is a common cause of replacement during the first 5 years after placement. Although physical strength as well as resistance to corrosion and plastic deformation is of importance, the operator-related factors of cavity preparation (inadequate bulk or thickness of amalgam) and manipulation of the amalgam in the cavity are the major factors which lead to early failure (Chapter 22, page 247). Fractures at the isthmus of Site 2, Size 2, 3 and 4 restorations can generally be attributed to inadequate cavity preparation. High-copper amalgams exhibit less evidence of early bulk fractures than low-copper amalgams.

Lamination of amalgam for deep cavities

A difficult clinical challenge is to restore a proximal box in a posterior tooth which extends beyond the cemento-enamel junction, without incorporating an overhanging margin somewhere in relation to the gingival margin of the cavity. Placement of an adequate matrix is difficult and supporting that matrix sufficiently to withstand proper condensation of amalgam is a further challenge. Attempts

to remove the overhang subsequent to matrix removal are rarely completely successful.

A lamination technique similar to the one proposed for composite resin is an alternative and is discussed in Chapter 8, page 90.

Repair of amalgam restorations

Occasionally there is a need to add fresh amalgam to existing amalgam that has been retained and now forms a portion of the walls of the newly prepared cavity. Alternatively, addition of more amalgam may be required at the initial appointment.

A bond of up to 50% of the unrepaired strength can be obtained when a repair is carried out subsequent to the first appointment. However, additions carried out within the initial appointment can achieve a bond strength of up to 75% of the unrepaired strength. The preparation for the new amalgam should meet all the usual requirements for depth and mechanical retention.

Sometimes it is adequate to simply repair a broken margin rather than replace the entire restoration, keeping in mind that replacing the restoration will almost invariably involve further loss of tooth structure and pulpal irritation. Particularly if the margin is not under direct occlusal load it may be sufficient to open conservatively, to make sure there are no hidden caries, and then seal the margin with a glass–ionomer. Choose the strongest available material and condition the surface with 10% polyacrylic acid for 10 seconds before placement.

Factors contributing to strength of repair

The factors that contribute to the reduction of the strength of the bond between the new and the old amalgam include the presence of porosity and γ_2 phase at the junction, inadequate condensation and, possibly, contamination of the surface of the existing amalgam. This surface should be freshly cut and free of saliva and debris. Use of a mercury-rich mix of the new amalgam does not appreciably improve the strength of the bond and it represents unacceptable mercury hygiene. Where possible use a high-copper spherical amalgam as the repair material.

Galvanic effect

Patients may complain of a metallic taste following placement of an amalgam restoration. This is caused by a rapid, short-lived corrosion that takes place between the new restoration and other older restorations in the vicinity of either amalgam or gold. The galvanic effect is mediated by the saliva and produces an electric current of sufficient intensity to elicit a metallic taste or even pain. Within a few hours, after the formation of a layer of corrosion products, the current is much reduced and the taste is usually no longer of concern. Sealing the new restoration with either a varnish or resin sealant may be indicated to restore patient comfort and confidence. Amalgams of the high-copper blend, Ag–Cu type, have greater initial corrosion than other high-copper amalgams because of the presence of γ_2 phase for up to 1–3 hours.

CLINICAL PERFORMANCE OF AMALGAM RESTORATIONS

A large number of longitudinal clinical studies and cross-sectional surveys have been conducted to examine all aspects of the clinical performance of high-copper and low-copper amalgams.

286–294

Surveys have reported 50% survival times for Site 1 restorations of more than 19 years, for Site 2 restorations of 24 years, and for complex Site 2, Size 3 and 4 restorations, replacing at least one cusp, of 11.5 years. Recent studies of high-copper amalgams report a failure rate after 5 years of only 2–3% and 10-year survival rates of 75–91%. These results must be compared with survival rates of low-copper amalgams of 39–80%.

Early failures of amalgam restorations are largely iatrogenic and can be reduced by more careful attention to cavity preparation and proper manipulation of the amalgam. The replacement of restorations can also be delayed by:

- instituting proper preventive measures – routine fluoride application
- reducing marginal fracture by developing an amalgam margin angle close to 90° in the original cavity design
- careful cavity design to avoid placing occlusal load directly on to restoration margins (Chapter 11)
- using a high-copper amalgam
- careful diagnosis to minimise unnecessary intervention. Particular care should be taken in diagnosing marginal failure because this rarely leads to further caries and replacement of the entire restoration will invariably lead to further loss of tooth structure, weakening of cusps and pulpal irritation.

FURTHER READING

Bonella E, White SM. Fatigue of resin bonded amalgam restorations. *Oper Dent* 1996; **21**:122–6

Eames WB. Mercomania strikes again. *Oper Dent* 1984; **9**:77–8

Eley B. *Dental amalgam; a review of safety* [Occasional paper. November 1993: issue 3]. London: British Dental Association; 1993.

Gjerdet NR, Hegdahl T. Porosity, strength and mercury content of amalgam made by different dentists in their own practice. *Dent Mater* 1985; **1**:150–3.

Greener EH. Amalgam – yesterday, today and tomorrow. *Oper Dent* 1979; **4**:24–35.

Hamilton JC, Moffa JP, Ellison JA, Jenkins WA. Marginal fracture not a predictor of longevity for two dental amalgam alloys: a 10 year study. *J Prosthet Dent* 1983; **50**:200–2.

Hawthorne W, Smales R, Webster D. Long-term survival of restorative materials in private practice [Abstract]. *J Dent Res* 1994; **73**:747.

Mahler DB, Nelson LW. Factors affecting the marginal leakage of amalgam. *J Am Dent Assoc* 1984; **108**:51–4.

Mahler DB, Marantz R. The effect of the operator on the clinical performance of amalgam. *J Am Dent Assoc* 1979; **99**:38–41.

Markley M. Durability of amalgam restorations. *Dent Outlook* 1984; **10**:45–7.

Markley MR. Silver amalgam. *Oper Dent* 1984; **9**:10–25.

Mjor IA, Smith DC. Detailed evaluation of 6 class II amalgam restorations. *Oper Dent* 1985; **10**:17–21.

Mount GJ. The condensation of amalgam by a group of general practitioners. *Aust Dent J* 1972; **3**:222–7.

Nelson LW, Mahler DB. Factors influencing the sealing behaviour of retrograde amalgam fillings. *Oral Surg Oral Med Oral Path* 1990; **69**:356–360.

Phillips RW. *Skinner's science of dental materials, 9th ed.* Philadelphia: WB Saunders; 1991 [Chap 17–18].

Piperno S, Barouch E, Hirsch SM, Kaim JM. Thermal discomfort of teeth related to the presence or absence of cement bases under amalgam restorations. *Oper Dent* 1982; **7**:92–6.

Wing G. The condensation of dental amalgam. *Dent Pract* 1965; **16**:52–9

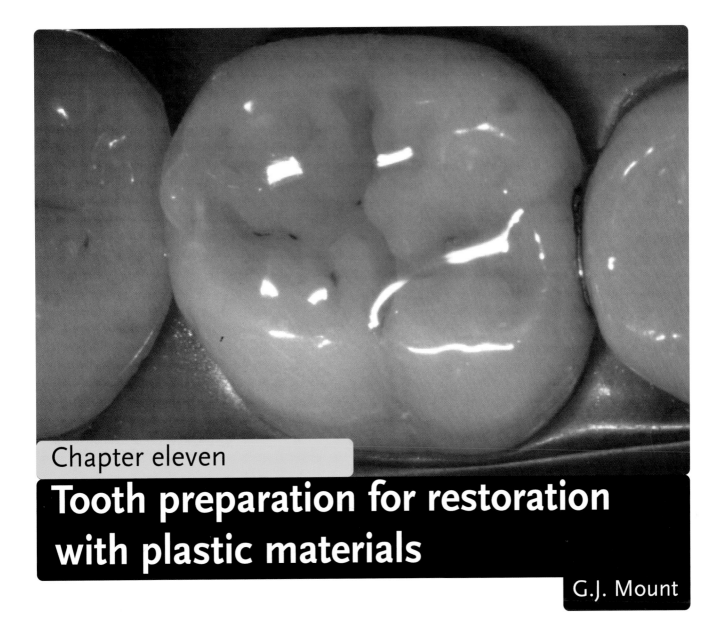

Chapter eleven

Tooth preparation for restoration with plastic materials

G.J. Mount

When preventive measures and remineralisation fail and a carious lesion has progressed into the dentine there is a need to remove the infected dentine, and possibly some of the affected dentine as well, to eliminate cavitation and avoid further accumulation of plaque. In most situations, this will involve removal of a certain amount of enamel to achieve access but it must be noted that both enamel and dentine are capable of being remineralised to some extent and therefore conserved.

The principle of minimal extension is encouraged to allow maximum preservation of natural tooth structure. The proposed cavity classification is designed to make the most of the potential for healing, although it is accepted that a considerable proportion of restorative dentistry is carried out to replace failed restorations. In this case, cavity design is complicated by existing loss of tooth structure.

FISSURE SEAL TREATMENT OF ENAMEL DEFECTS

Fissure sealing or fissure protection is regarded properly as a preventive treatment rather than a restoration but is included for discussion here because it generally utilises normal restorative materials – composite resin or glass–ionomer.

On many occasions, particularly in communities where there is no systemic fluoride available, posterior teeth will erupt showing a pattern of rather deep convoluted fissures on the occlusal surface. The cross-sectional anatomy of these fissures is difficult to predict when viewed from the occlusal but, in many cases, there will be a narrow opening from the occlusal surface that will reduce to a width of less than 200 μm before opening out again just short of the dentino-enamel junction. In a high number of cases, over time, plaque will gather within such a fissure and eventually cause demineralisation of the enamel walls followed by caries in the dentine (**Figs 11.1** and **11.2**). Prevention of caries is the preferred management, so obturation of the fissure shortly after the eruption of the tooth and before demineralisation is desirable so that the tooth structure is sealed and protected.

Indications for placement of a sealant

Obviously, not all fissures need to be sealed. Particularly in fluoridated communities, many teeth will erupt with very shallow fissures and it is highly unlikely that they will ever become carious. It is suggested that there are three 'stages' which should be considered before a decision is taken.

Fissure at risk

In a young patient with newly erupted teeth, the fissures in some of those teeth may appear deep and convoluted. If the community is not fluoridated or the patient is in a high caries risk category, the fissures should be considered at risk and sealed.

Suspect fissure

For the patient in an older age group (15–30 years of age), where the fissures have not previously been sealed, it may be wise to do more than use a sealant alone. By this time there may be considerable demineralisation down the walls of the fissure with the possibility of actual cavitation into dentine. If there is any doubt at all, the fissures should be very conservatively opened, as described on pages 128–129 (Site 1, Size 1 lesion; designated #1.1).

Frank cavitation

The early stages of dentine involvement in a Site 1 lesion are not always easy to detect, but if there is a change of colour or texture in the enamel surrounding a fissure, or some doubt about the X-ray interpretation, then a normal restoration is required. (Site 1, Size 2 lesion; designated #1.2, page 130).

Resin sealants

There have been many methods used to seal fissures and prevent the development of active caries, ranging from silver nitrate to lasers. However, the most popular sealant over many years has been resin in various forms, and now glass–ionomer cement is also proving to be valuable.

Resin, either unfilled or lightly filled, was originally used over 20 years ago, and has a long history of success. It is now available in both a light-cured or an autocured form and many resins are tinted for easier identification. Before placement of resin, the enamel should be etched, both to reduce the surface energy of the enamel and to allow development of the usual micromechanical attachment of the resin. Unfortunately, the enamel on the shoulder at the entry to a fissure is often prismless and irregular and may not accept a good etch pattern, so attachment of the resin may be tenuous. Also, it is not possible to flow the resin into the fissure beyond the point where the fissure is less than 200 μm wide. Failure may occur through partial lifting of the

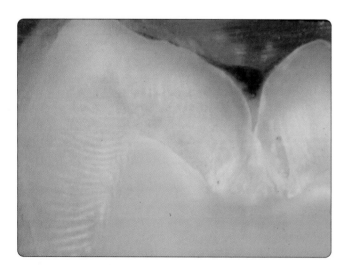

Fig. 11.1 Anatomy of fissures. A simple uncomplicated fissure that does not penetrate the full depth of the enamel.

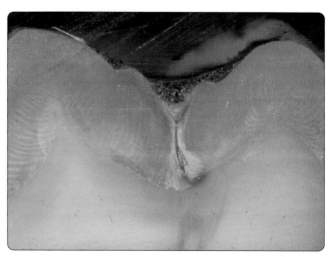

Fig. 11.2 Anatomy of fissures. A more common anatomy where the fissure has demineralised and the dentine is immediately involved.

sealant with exposure of one segment or another of the fissure, allowing the possibility of caries initiation. Despite these possible limitations, the effectiveness of such a preventive measure has been reported to be very high.

Glass–ionomer cement sealants

Glass–ionomer cement is also a very effective sealant for open fissures, although there has not been a great deal of long-term research published. Its value lies in the possibility of developing adhesion to the enamel by an ion-exchange mechanism and, in addition, it has continuing fluoride release. It has the same limitation as resin, inasmuch as it will not flow past the point where the fissure becomes less than $200\,\mu m$ wide (**Figs 11.3–11.6**).

For correct placement, the surface of the tooth should be conditioned with 10% polyacrylic acid for 10 seconds, washed thoroughly and dried lightly. This will remove plaque and pellicle and reduce the surface energy of the enamel to allow the cement to adapt readily and develop good adhesion. A fast-setting Type II restorative cement, autocure or resin-modified, should be mixed with a high powder:liquid ratio, and flowed into the fissure. A lightly lubricated gloved finger can be placed over an autocure cement and finger pressure applied to ensure complete adaptation to the depths of the fissure. Leave the finger in place until the cement has set and then carefully adjust the occlusion, taking care not to dehydrate the cement. A resin-modified cement is a little thinner and will usually flow readily into the fissure, without pressure, in the same manner as a resin seal.

Over time, either the composite resin or the glass–ionomer may wear away as a result of occlusal stress but, with the cement, there will be a fluoride-releasing residue left behind, sealing the fissure for many years. Even if it appears to be lost, resistance to recurrent caries will remain high.

Sealants for the older patient

If a sealant is not placed during the first 2–3 years after eruption, the fissure may be at least partially obturated with an accumulation of pellicle and debris, thus sealing it naturally against further plaque accumulation. However, at a later time the patient may pass through another phase of high caries susceptibility; isolated segments of the fissure may then demineralise and become actively carious. At

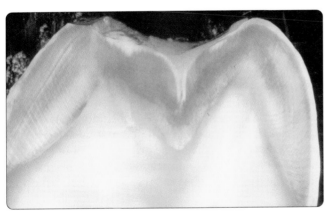

Fig. 11.3 Glass–ionomer seal. A fissure sealed with glass–ionomer. Note that the cement has not penetrated to the full depth.

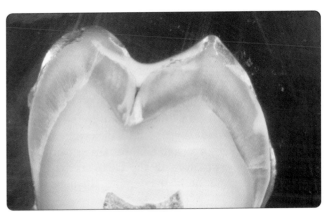

Fig. 11.4 Resin seal. A fissure sealed with resin. Note the seal has not penetrated beyond where the fissure is 200 μm wide.

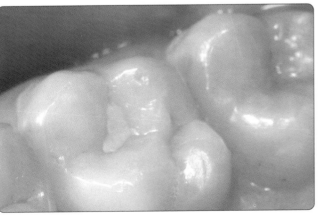

Fig. 11.5 Mature glass–ionomer seal. The seal in the mesial fissure of the upper first molar photographed after 8 years. There was no cavity preparation.

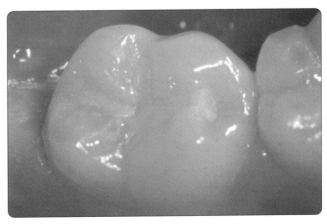

Fig. 11.6 Mature glass–ionomer seal. The seal in a lower molar photographed after 9 years.

this point, once the dentine is involved, a fissure seal alone will probably not be sufficient to protect the tooth and a more traditional restoration may be required, involving removal of carious dentine. Removal of all the remaining fissure system may well not be necessary. The carious area alone may be dealt with in a traditional manner and the remaining fissures sealed as discussed above. The resultant restoration can be regarded as a combination of a fissure seal and a restoration.

PROGRESS OF THE CARIOUS LESION

A carious lesion in enamel will commence as a reasonably broad area of subsurface demineralisation related to an area of plaque accumulation (see Chapter 2, page 14). Progress will be inward towards the dentine, following the orientation of the crystallites, with loss of crystallite surface and central core material, continuing to a considerable depth without loss of overall structure. It is possible for the process of demineralisation to reach the dentine without enamel collapse; that is, without actual cavitation occurring on the external surface of the enamel (**Figs 11.7** and **11.8**). Remineralisation is still possible at this point because of the continuing presence of some crystal structure. However, if cavitation occurs, it will not be possible to prevent plaque accumulation and prevention of further extension of the carious lesion will involve restoration of the surface contour of the enamel.

Once the enamel has been breached, whether cavitated or not, the dentine will be involved in the process of demineralisation in a predictable manner. Caries will progress along the dentinal tubules towards the pulp, with a few 'pioneer' bacteria in the lead, which will initiate the demineralisation. A considerable bacterial invasion will follow causing proteolysis of the collagen matrix and, subsequently, cavitation of the dentine. Remineralisation

is possible early in the development of the lesion but once the matrix has collapsed it will no longer be possible to sustain the replacement of the minerals and cavitation will follow. The breakdown within the dentine can be divided into two identifiable zones.

Infected dentine

The surface layer closest to the oral environment will be heavily infected with a broad mix of bacteria and the collagen matrix will have already collapsed. This is identified as the 'infected' layer and it may be differentiated by an application of basic fuschin dye, which will stain it red. It will be of a relatively soft consistency and can therefore be readily removed with a sharp excavator although its inner limits will often not be clearly defined. Depending on the speed of progress it may be dark brown or black although if it is moving fast it may still be light in colour. It must be noted that, as the lesion penetrates the enamel and involves the dentine, there will be an immediate inflammatory response in the pulp tissue.

Affected dentine

The advancing front of the caries will follow the course of the tubules and the dentine will be demineralised, relatively soft and colourless, but the basic structure of the collagen matrix will still be present and reasonably intact. There will often be a few pioneer bacteria present, but otherwise it will be sterile. This layer is generally regarded as being 'affected' by the carious process and, because the collagen matrix is still present, it may be remineralised to some degree. It is therefore both unwise and unnecessary to remove it entirely, particularly as the pulp immediately subjacent to the approaching caries will be irritated and inflamed by the presence of bacterial toxins and mechanical exposure would almost certainly lead to pulp death. It is better that this layer be regarded as pre-carious and therefore able to be healed.

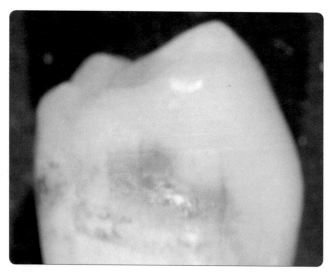

Fig. 11.7 Early carious lesion. The proximal surface of a tooth showing the initial decalcification immediately below the contact area.

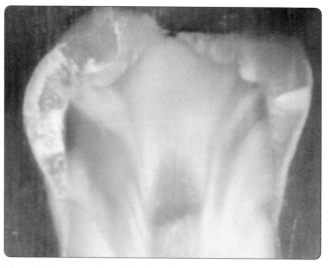

Fig. 11.8 Cross-section of caries. The same lesion cut in cross-section to show the penetration of the demineralisation.

Potential for remineralisation

After the carious lesion has reached the point of frank cavitation, progress will be driven primarily by the bacterial infection. Therefore, if the infected layer is removed and the lesion is completely isolated from the oral environment with an adhesive restoration, which will prevent microleakage, progress may be arrested. Remaining pioneer bacteria left in the affected dentine will become dormant and pulpal irritation will cease. The deep affected layer that had been demineralised will be subject to remineralisation because the collagen matrix will still be relatively intact. In the past, a zinc oxide and eugenol paste was used as the sealant because of its antibacterial properties, but now glass–ionomer is preferred because it completely seals the cavity and releases fluoride, calcium and phosphate ions thus encouraging further remineralisation and healing of the dentine.

Spread of coronal caries

On the occlusal surface, entry will normally be through a fissure and, once the dentine is reached, the lesion will progress down the tubules towards the pulp with a limited amount of lateral spread. Essentially, the depth of penetration will be approximately twice the width of the lesion. Eventually, if the lesion is allowed to continue, the enamel roof will break down and progress will become random (**Fig. 11.9**).

A lesion on the proximal surface will begin as an elliptical area of demineralisation immediately below the contact area between teeth and will spread on a broad front from the surface, narrowing down as it approaches the dentine. Once the dentine is involved, progress will be downwards and inwards along the path of the dentinal tubules in an 's' curve towards the pulp. As the lesion progresses, there will be a degree of lateral spread facially and lingually as well as occlusally that, in time, will undermine the marginal ridge and lead to collapse of the occlusal enamel. Again, penetration will be approximately twice as deep as it is wide until the lesion is quite advanced, at which point progress will become random.

Spread of root surface caries

The progress of caries on the exposed root surface will be different inasmuch as there is no enamel present to confine and direct the initial lesion. Cementum and dentine are mineralised to approximately the same extent. This means they will demineralise at approximately the same rate, and plaque accumulation on the root surface is likely to spread over a relatively large area. The subsequent lesion is usually hard to detect initially; the speed of progress may be rather rapid and the outline of the area may be poorly defined. Demineralisation will follow the dentinal tubules in a similar pattern to that described above and, certainly initially, the collagen matrix will still be present and available for remineralisation (**Figs 11.10** and **11.11**).

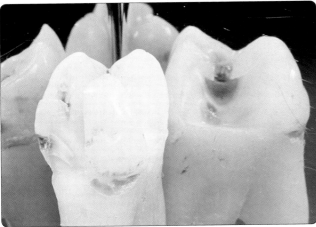

Fig. 11.9 **Progress in dentine.** Note progress of the proximal lesion on the left-hand side as the caries moves down the dentinal tubules towards the pulp. The occlusal lesion also follows the dentinal tubules and is generally twice as deep as it is wide. The enamel lesion is quite narrow until it loses dentine support.

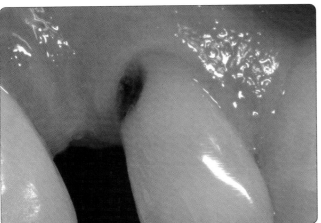

Fig. 11.10 **Root surface caries.** A mature lesion that has been present so long that it has become dark and leathery.

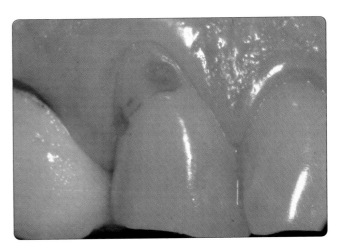

Fig. 11.11 **Root surface caries.** Two lesions on the root of a lateral incisor that are progressing faster than the lesion discussed in figure 11.10 and therefore are not so dark. The full extent of the lesion may be difficult to define.

GENERAL PRINCIPLES OF CAVITY DESIGN

Until recent times, cavities were designed along surgical lines, without an understanding of the action of the fluoride ion and for placement of restorative materials that were difficult to handle, were subject to microleakage and were often not aesthetic. Also, in the absence of adhesive restorative materials, it was regarded as essential to remove all unsupported enamel regardless of its location. More importantly, it was often necessary to remove additional sound tooth structure just to make room for the restorative material, thus defeating one of the prime purposes of restoration; that is, the preservation of remaining tooth structure.

It is very difficult indeed to reproduce the anatomy and appearance of the original tooth with any of the plastic restorative materials. However, now that it is possible to develop long-term adhesion to both enamel and dentine in the oral environment, the way is open for a complete reassessment of cavity design. Although the materials currently available are still not perfect, they are adequate for the restoration of the smaller initial lesions and, in combination, can be used to restore cavities of moderate size.

When placing plastic restorative materials, reproduction of the original anatomy of the tooth is entirely dependent upon the skill of the operator and this will have a considerable bearing on the longevity of the restoration. It is accepted that longevity of conventional plastic restorative materials placed in a traditionally designed cavity is not great: 10–15 years on average. However, in the presence of a better understanding of the caries process and improved knowledge of the function of fluoride, it is now possible to limit the size of a cavity by retaining at least some of the demineralised enamel and dentine and allowing it to heal through remineralisation. Thus, it is possible to retain more natural tooth structure with the expectation of greater longevity and therefore the potential for longer periods between replacements. This leads to the new classification of cavity designs presented below.

A NEW CAVITY CLASSIFICATION

Many of the above comments on the progress of the carious lesion are not new and, in fact, have been known and understood for many years. What has changed is the understanding of the effect of fluoride on the demineralisation–remineralisation cycle as well as the advent of true long-term adhesion with restorative materials. These two factors make it possible to reconsider the classification of carious lesions and cavity designs first rationalised by G.V. Black over 100 years ago. Although his concepts are not entirely outdated, there is certainly a need to reconsider the design of cavities with the prime object of retaining natural tooth structure. The statement opposite is included in recognition of Black's contribution to restorative dentistry and in justification of this proposal for a new classification (**Fig. 11.12**).

The three sites of carious lesions

Carious lesions occur in three sites on the crown or root of a tooth; that is, in those areas subject to the accumulation of plaque (**Fig. 11.13**).
- Site 1 – pits, fissures and enamel defects on occlusal surfaces of posterior teeth or other smooth surfaces.
- Site 2 – approximal enamel immediately below areas in contact with adjacent teeth.
- Site 3 – the cervical one-third of the crown or, following gingival recession, the exposed root.

It is regarded as logical to classify lesions by these sites and then to grade them by size according to the extent of progress. The classification applies equally to both anterior and posterior teeth.

The four sizes of carious lesions

Taking into account the progress of the carious lesion, described above, it is possible to consider restoration in four sizes, regardless of the site of origin of the lesion.

SIZE / SITE	Minimal 1	Moderate 2	Enlarged 3	Extensive 4
Pit/fissure 1	1.1	1.2	1.3	1.4
Contact area 2	2.1	2.2	2.3	2.4
Cervical 3	3.1	3.2	3.3	3.4

Fig. 11.12 Cavity classification. A proposed classification for cavity designs that allows the introduction of smaller, more conservative cavities than are possible with the G.V. Black classification while allowing for the more extensive cavities that are the inevitable end-result of continuing replacement restorative dentistry.

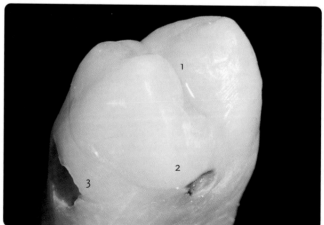

Fig. 11.13 Three sites for caries: 1 Pits and fissures on otherwise smooth surfaces; 2 contact areas on the proximal surfaces of all teeth; 3 cervical margins on the crown or exposed root surface of any tooth.

The G. V. Black concept

When Black defined the parameters for his classification, the cavity designs were controlled by a number of factors, many of which no longer apply. Caries was rampant and the significance of fluoride was not understood. There were limitations in the available instruments for cavity preparation as well as in the selection of restorative materials. The five categories of carious lesion were related to the site of the lesion and to the nature of the intended restoration, but they did not take into account the increasing dimensions of a cavity nor the complexity of the method of restoration. Black suggested that it was necessary:

- to remove tooth structure to gain access and visibility
- to remove all trace of affected dentine from the floor of the cavity
- to make room for the insertion of the restorative material itself
- to provide mechanical interlocking retentive designs
- to extend the cavity to self-cleansing areas to avoid recurrent caries.

The result was that, by today's standards, all such restorations were large. In his designs, Black showed commendable respect for remaining tooth structure as well as occlusal and proximal anatomy but it was necessary to sacrifice relatively extensive areas of enamel to achieve his goals. Other far more effective methods of dealing with a carious lesion are now available. With modern understanding of adhesion and remineralisation it is no longer necessary to remove all unsupported demineralised enamel around the cavity margin, the concept of self-cleansing areas has been discarded and removal of all affected dentine from the axial wall of the cavity is strictly contra-indicated because of the potential for remineralisation and healing.

Many of the old limitations no longer apply and it is now appropriate to think again about the problems presented by a carious lesion. Without in any way denigrating the achievements of Black's concepts and work, fresh thoughts are offered and a new approach to the definition of cavity design is outlined in this text. The proposed classification is designed to simplify the identification of lesions and to define their complexity and is expected to provide benefits for the profession and patients.

- Size 1 – minimal involvement of dentine just beyond treatment by remineralisation alone.
- Size 2 – moderate involvement of dentine. Following cavity preparation, remaining enamel is sound, well supported by dentine and not likely to fail under normal occlusal load. The tooth is sufficiently strong to support the restoration.
- Size 3 – the cavity is enlarged beyond moderate involvement. Remaining tooth structure is weakened to the extent that cusps or incisal edges are split, or are likely to fail if left exposed to occlusal load. The cavity needs to be further enlarged so that the restoration can be designed to provide support to the remaining tooth structure.

- Size 4 – extensive caries and bulk loss of tooth structure has already occurred.

The Size 1 cavity will necessarily be a new lesion and adhesive restorative materials are ideal for restoration under these circumstances. A cavity of Size 2, 3 or 4 may be a new lesion that has progressed to a considerable extent without the patient presenting for treatment or it may be a breakdown of an old restoration that requires replacement. The same basic principles for developing a cavity design will apply in both cases and, for obvious reasons, the larger the cavity the greater the problems in restoration and the shorter the probable longevity of the plastic restorative materials. The selection of the most suitable material for the larger restorations will be dictated by such properties as resistance to fracture and flexure as well as abrasion resistance.

- The use of composite resin will be limited by its shrinkage on setting, whether autocured or light-activated, as well as by the presence or absence of well-supported enamel strong enough to provide adhesion through acid-etching around the entire margin.
- The main limitation for amalgam is its poor aesthetic appeal, although its physical properties are generally adequate for all circumstances.
- Glass–ionomer develops excellent adhesion to both enamel and dentine and has satisfactory aesthetic appeal, but lacks the strength required for restoration of incisal edges and marginal ridges.

To assist in communication, the relationship between Black's classification and the modern site and size concept is shown below.

Site 1, Sizes 1, 2, 3 and 4 – pit and fissure caries

- Cavity located on the occlusal surface of a posterior tooth or any simple enamel defect on an otherwise smooth surface of any tooth.
- Black class I – the smaller Size 1 could not be carried out previously because suitable restorative materials were not available, so the Black classification begins with Site 1, Size 2 (#1.2).

Site 2, Sizes 1, 2, 3 and 4 – approximal lesion commencing in relation to contact areas

- Cavity located on the approximal surface of any tooth (anterior or posterior) initiated immediately below the contact area.
- Black class II – lesions occurring between posterior teeth only. Because of materials limitations there was no equivalent of Size 1, so the Black classification begins with Site 2, Size 2 (#2.2).
- Black class III – cavity located between anterior teeth only. Because of materials limitations there was no equivalent to Size 1, so the Black classification begins with Site 2, Size 2 (#2.2).
- Black class IV – an extension of a class III lesion involving the incisal corner or incisal edge of an anterior tooth. An alternative cause would be traumatic fracture of the incisal corner. Now classified Site 2, Size 4 (#2.4).

Site 3, Sizes 1, 2, 3 and 4 – gingival one-third of the clinical crown or exposed root surface following recession

- Cavity located in the gingival one-third of the crown or exposed root.
- Black class V – this classification does not differentiate lesions on the gingival one-third of the approximal surface (particularly root surface caries) from class II lesions. An erosion/abrasion lesion or a small carious cavity would be a Site 3, Size 1 (#3.1) or Site 3, Size 2 (#3.2) and interproximal lesions would usually be Site 3, Size 3 (#3.3) or Site 3, Size 4 (#3.4).

Cavity design and preparation

It will be noted from the above that the Black's classification did not allow for the Size 1 lesion in either Site 1 or Site 2 because of the absence of adhesive restorative materials. Also, it must be recognised that there is a clear division between restoring a new lesion and replacing a failed restoration. When dealing with new active caries the cavity design should be very conservative, because it is possible to remineralise both enamel and dentine that is only demineralised and not cavitated. Margins need be extended only to smooth surfaces that are capable of remineralisation and the concept of 'extension for prevention' no longer applies. It is often possible to maintain tooth-to-tooth contact interproximally and cavity outline form should be dictated by cavitation only.

On the other hand, in replacement of a failed restoration, the cavity outline is already defined and will often be more extensive than ideal. For these replacement restorations, most of the principles laid down by Black will still apply, if for no other reason than tooth structure cannot be replaced. In fact, for both Size 3 and Size 4 lesions, very little has changed

Whether the problem presenting is a new lesion or replacement of a failed restoration, the limitations of the physical properties of both the remaining tooth structure and the restorative material must be taken into consideration. A small restoration can be reliably supported by remaining tooth structure, particularly in the presence of adhesive restorative materials. In fact, it is claimed that a tooth crown can be restored to full physical strength in the presence of adhesion. However, as the cavity enlarges, the tooth becomes weaker until it reaches a point where the restoration must be placed in such a way that the restorative material itself will support remaining tooth structure. This requires modification to cavity designs and some consideration as to which material to utilise. These factors are taken into account.

SITE 1 LESIONS

Lesions identified under this classification usually commence in fissures on the occlusal surface of a posterior tooth that has not previously been sealed. Pits on the lingual of upper anterior teeth are not uncommon and may also occur on the buccal surface of lower molars and the lingual extension of the distal occlusal groove of upper molars. Erosion and attrition lesions on the occlusal surfaces of posteriors and the incisal edges of anteriors are also included.

Site 1, Size 1 (#1.1)

Small defect in one section of a pit or fissure; it is often combined with placement of a fissure seal on the remainder of the fissure system.

Site 1, Size 2 (#1.2)

Moderate size lesion with most fissures involved or replacement of an existing Black class I restoration.

Site 1, Size 3 (#1.3)

A larger lesion requiring incorporation of protection for one or more cusps in the design.

Site 1, Size 4 (#1.4)

Extensive lesion with one or more cusps already missing.

SITE 1, SIZE 1; designated #1.1

There is no equivalent in the G. V. Black classification.

Preparation

The lesion occurs either on the occlusal surface of a posterior tooth or in relation to a pit on an otherwise smooth surface. It is identified clinically or radiographically or by transillumination as dentine involvement below the enamel in a particular section of the pit or fissure system. Usually, the extent is limited and most of the fissure system is free from caries. Other sections of the fissures may be deep and convoluted and subject to later attack; they require protection through sealing at this time.

Using the very finest tapered diamond point (#200) (**Fig. 11.14**) at intermediate high speed under air–water spray, enter the fissure in the region of the carious attack and open the enamel far enough to determine the full extent of the lesion (**Figs 11.15** and **11.16**). Develop only sufficient access to clean the cavity walls of all of the infected layer of dentine. It is unnecessary to remove the affected, demineralised dentine on the floor of the cavity, but it is essential that the walls are completely clean and free of caries. The enamel margins should be sound and free of microcracks and loose enamel rods.

Having determined the extent of the problem, open and explore the remaining fissure system, as necessary, using the very fine tapered diamond point to ensure there are no further pockets of active caries. Use small round burs (#008 or #012) to clean the walls of infected enamel.

Generally there is no need to penetrate the full depth of the enamel, and retention of some enamel at the base of the fissure will assist in maintaining the strength and structural integrity of the crown of the tooth.

Restoration

Glass–ionomer is the material of choice because of the adhesion and fluoride release available. Use the strongest cement available, either an autocure or a resin-modified cement so long as it is radiopaque and is mixed at a high powder : liquid ratio to ensure optimal physical properties. Condition the cavity with 10% polyacrylic acid to ensure optimal adhesion. Placement of the cement with a syringe is desirable to ensure positive adaptation into the depths of the cavity (**Fig. 11.17**).

- When using an autocure cement it is desirable to apply positive pressure using a lightly lubricated gloved finger-tip as the matrix. Immediately the cement is set, seal the cement with the required resin sealant to maintain the water balance. Trim the occlusion with a round steel bur (#012) at low speed with no air–water spray and seal again to ensure there is no water contamination.
- When using a resin-modified glass–ionomer cement, no matrix is required and there is no need to seal it against water uptake so long as it has been light activated for a minimum of 40 seconds. The restoration can be contoured and polished immediately after light activation at intermediate high speed under air–water spray.

It should be noted that erosion/abrasion lesions on the occlusal surfaces of posteriors and the incisal edges of anteriors should also be recorded in this category (**Fig. 11.18**). As the cavity surface is free of caries and perfectly smooth it should not be instrumented at all and a lamination technique is the preferred restoration. Following conditioning, place a strong glass–ionomer and, if the occlusal load is heavy, laminate with a composite resin (**Figs 11.19** and **11.20**).

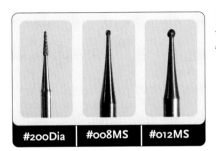

Fig. 11.14 Burs used in the preparation of a #1.1 lesion.

#200Dia | #008MS | #012MS

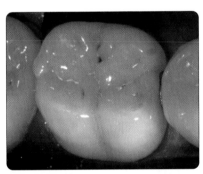

Fig. 11.15 Lesion in the occlusal fissure. Note the small #1.1 lesion in the lingual groove of the lower molar. Dentine involvement was suspected.

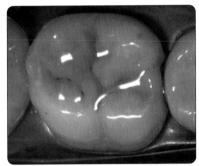

Fig. 11.16 Prepared cavity. The fissure has been explored and caries removed. The conditioning liquid is present to enhance the photograph.

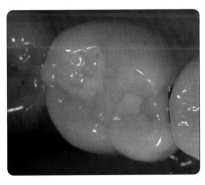

Fig. 11.17 Restored #1.1 lesion. The same restoration recorded 5 years after placement. Note the limited wear over time.

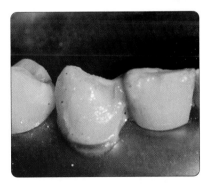

Fig. 11.18 Incisal abrasion/erosion. The mesial incisal corner of the canine shows an abrasion/erosion #1.1 lesion. It requires restoration to protect the tooth and improve lateral excursion.

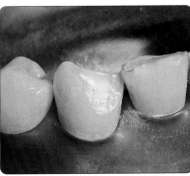

Fig. 11.19 Glass–ionomer cement base for composite resin. Before build-up with composite resin an autocure glass–ionomer base is placed on the dentine. The enamel and cement are then both etched to provide union between both materials.

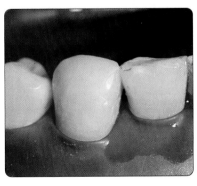

Fig. 11.20 Composite resin build-up. The completed restoration with composite resin adhering to enamel and glass–ionomer cement.

SITE 1, SIZE 2; designated #1.2

G.V. Black classification – Class I.

Preparation

This may be a new cavity but it will often arise through the need to replace an existing restoration, such as an old amalgam 'prophylactic odontotomy', where all of the fissure system has already been involved. A tungsten carbide bur (#140TC) (**Fig. 11.21**) should be used at ultra-high speed to remove old restorations, taking care not to extend the cavity any further than necessary. A tapered or parallel-sided diamond cylinder (#168Dia or #156Dia) at intermediate high speed under air–water spray is then preferred to explore the extent of the problem. Small round burs (#012MS or #016) can be used to remove remaining caries from the walls, but removal of all affected dentine from the floor is not required. Occlusal enamel should be retained, even though it is unsupported, so long as the margins are sound and there are no microcracks. Remaining fissures can be explored with the fine tapered diamond (#200Dia) (**Fig. 11.22–24**).

Restoration

Glass–ionomer cement is the best material for the initial restoration because it can reinforce undermined enamel and it can be laminated as required with composite resin if the occlusal load is excessive (**Figs 11.25–11.27**).

- Use the strongest glass–ionomer available, either a resin-modified or an autocure cement so long as it is radiopaque and mixed at a high powder : liquid ratio to allow for the development of optimal physical properties. A sublining of calcium hydroxide is not required. Condition the cavity and place the cement with a syringe starting at the floor of the cavity.
- Composite resin should not be used alone because of its shrinkage on curing with the consequent risk of microleakage. Lamination over glass–ionomer cement provides a combination of the two materials sufficient to

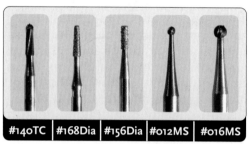

| #140TC | #168Dia | #156Dia | #012MS | #016MS |

Fig. 11.21 Burs used in the preparation of a #1.2 lesion.

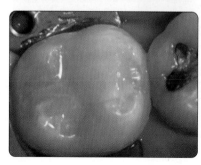

Fig. 11.22 Radiograph of a #1.2 lesion. A bite-wing radiograph of an extensive #1.2 lesion arising from an occlusal fissure on the second molar.

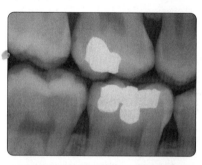

Fig. 11.24 Prepared cavity. The completed cavity. Note the remaining fissures have been carefully explored but not opened as for a traditional design. The cavity conditioner is in place to enhance the photograph.

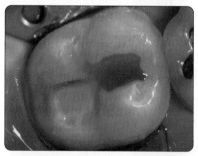

Fig. 11.26 Lamination. The cement has been laminated with composite resin for occlusal support.

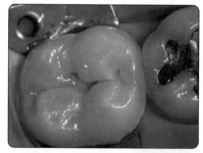

Fig. 11.23 Carious fissure. Note the limited size of the external involvement of the fissure. In the presence of fluoridation the extent of the lesion is often concealed.

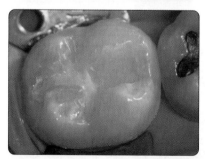

Fig. 11.25 Restoration. The entire cavity has been restored with a glass–ionomer with no sublining required. Because of the extent of the occlusal involvement, the cement has been cut back to allow room for lamination.

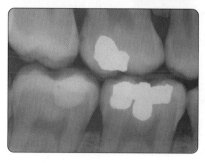

Fig. 11.27 Final radiograph. A final radiograph shows the extent of the restoration. Note the presence of demineralised affected dentine, which is expected to remineralise.

restore the physical properties of the tooth very close to the original conditions.

- If a resin-modified glass–ionomer is to be laminated, it can be cut back immediately and the enamel margins cleaned ready for etching. With an autocure cement, allow time for it to completely set before cutting it back (by approximately 2 mm) to allow room for the composite resin. Render the enamel margins free of

cement and bevel if necessary. Etch the enamel for 15 seconds and, if an autocure cement has been placed, etch the cement at the same time. Wash thoroughly and dry but do not dehydrate. Apply an appropriate unfilled resin enamel bonding agent followed by incremental build-up of the composite resin. After light-curing, adjust the occlusion and polish as required.

SITE 1, SIZE 3; designated #1.3

G.V. Black classification – Class I.

When the cavity reaches this size there will be extensive undermining or breakdown of at least one cusp with the possibility of a split developing at the base. It may be a new lesion involving almost the entire dentine of the crown or it may be an old restoration that has become recurrent.

Preparation

Tungsten carbide burs (#140) (**Fig. 11.28**) should be used at ultra-high speed to remove any remaining old restorative material and the use of a small diamond cylinder (#156) is the best option to open the enamel to determine the extent of the problem. Round burs (#012 or 016) can then be used to remove infected dentine from the walls. Be careful not to remove all affected dentine on the floor of the cavity, to avoid the problems arising from pulp exposure (**Figs 11.29** and **11.30**).

If it is a new cavity resulting from active caries, it may be desirable to carry out an indirect pulp capping as described in Chapter 18, page 213. Open the cavity with a small diamond cylinder (#156), only as far as required, to gain access to the infected dentine then clean the walls only, using a round bur of appropriate size (#012, #016). Seal the cavity with glass–ionomer for a minimum of 12 weeks and then reassess the cavity design when preparing the final restoration. At that stage carefully check all remaining

cusps to determine the need to protect them from occlusal load. If a cusp has a column of sound dentine providing adequate support for the enamel and there is more than one-half of the medially facing cuspal incline still present, it can remain standing without protection.

If a cusp is undermined and the medial incline is subject to occlusal load, it requires protection otherwise it will develop a split at the base. It may be necessary to include retentive elements in the cavity design, such as grooves and ditches placed in remaining sound dentine, using a #168MS to ensure that the restoration is soundly locked in. These two aspects of cavity design are discussed in detail in Chapter 7, page 59.

Restoration

Of the plastic materials, amalgam is the material of choice for such an extensive restoration. Using it, it is easier to build and to carve the occlusal anatomy to the extent required and the wear factor is similar to that of natural tooth structure. Also, amalgam has a superior resistance to flexure and therefore is better able to provide positive protection to the weakened tooth structure. Eventually, it will make a more satisfactory base for the crown which, under these circumstances, will probably be required at a later stage (**Figs 11.31** and **11.32**).

- When using amalgam as the restorative material, a lining of glass–ionomer (≤ 0.5 mm thick) should be placed over the floor of the cavity to minimise thermal exchange. Any greater thickness of lining will reduce the bulk of the restorative material and tend to reduce its physical properties. It may also be desirable to place a resin or glass–ionomer amalgam bond to provide a degree of adhesion between the amalgam and remaining tooth structure (see Chapter 10, page 117).
- The remaining enamel is generally too weak to

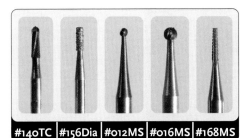

Fig. 11.28 Burs used in the preparation of a #1.3 lesion.

#140TC | #156Dia | #012MS | #016MS | #168MS

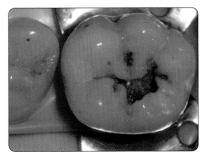

Fig. 11.29 Size 3 cavities: #1.3 lesion. An extensive #1.3 lesion on the occlusal of a lower molar. It is likely that the lingual cusps will need protection.

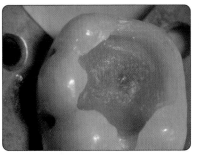

Fig. 11.30 Completed cavity. The cavity is complete; the entire distolingual cusp required a protective design.

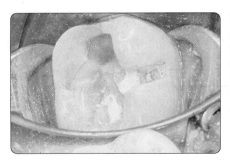

Fig. 11.31 Split cusp. On opening the #1.3 cavity, a split at the base of the mesiolingual cusp became apparent.

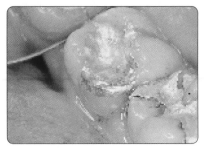

Fig. 11.32 Completed restoration. Because of the extent of the cavity, amalgam was chosen as the restorative material. Note that the mesiolingual cusp has been protected by the restoration.

withstand the stress of the setting contraction of composite resin even when the restoration is built incrementally. It may be possible to use a lamination technique over glass–ionomer, as described in Chapter 8, so long as the occlusal load is not excessive.

- Observe carefully the anatomy of the opposing tooth and be prepared to modify the length of an opposing working cusp to minimise the depth of the inter-cuspation between the two teeth. This will reduce the splitting stress on the heavily restored tooth and help to eliminate undesirable contacts during lateral excursions (see Chapter 21, page 242).

SITE 1, SIZE 4; designated #1.4

G.V. Black classification – Class II.

Preparation

This is an extensive cavity, most likely located in a molar tooth. At this size there will have been a further break-down with complete loss of one or more cusps and full restoration with a plastic restorative material will be complex. Amalgam could be utilised for a reasonably satisfactory restoration, but usually an indirect extracoronal restoration such as a full or three-quarter crown will be required subsequently to restore completely the coronal anatomy and occlusion.

Cavity preparation should be carried out as described above for a #1.3 cavity, using a diamond cylinder (#156) (**Fig. 11.33**) at intermediate high speed to enter the cavity and round burs (#012 or 016) to remove the infected dentine. Old restorative material is best removed using tungsten carbide burs (#140TC) at ultra-high speed.

In those cases where caries is highly active, it may be desirable to carry out the indirect pulp cap technique as described in Chapter 18, page 213.

A protective design for unsupported cusps can be developed using the #168Dia bur as described in Chapter 7, page 59, and retentive elements will be incorporated using #168MS burs.

Restoration

If amalgam is to be used as the restorative material, mechanical interlocks with the remaining tooth structure are essential, using ditches and grooves strategically placed in the gingival area. Generally one or more of the remaining cusps will need protection as described earlier. As there will have been considerable loss of dentine it will be necessary to lay down a lining of glass–ionomer cement about 0.5 mm thick to act as a thermal barrier. It will also be necessary to place a matrix to compensate for the missing enamel wall. Build the amalgam incrementally and condense well. Over-build the occlusal contour and be prepared to adjust an opposing working cusp to minimise the degree of intercuspation and free the occlusion in lateral excursions (**Figs 11.34 and 11.35**).

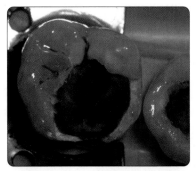

Fig. 11.34 #1.4 lesion. An extensive lesion in a lower second molar. It is apparent the buccal cusp is very weak.

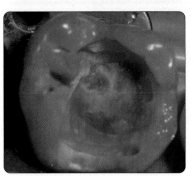

Fig. 11.35 Completed cavity. Retentive grooves have been placed in the floor of the cavity to retain the amalgam.

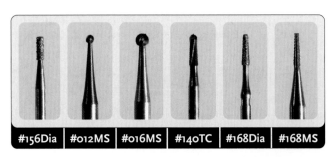

| #156Dia | #012MS | #016MS | #140TC | #168Dia | #168MS |

Fig. 11.33 Burs used in the preparation of a #1.4 lesion.

SITE 2 LESIONS

These are lesions which arise on the proximal surface of either an anterior or a posterior tooth beginning immediately below the contact area.

Site 2, Size 1 (#2.1)
Minimal dentine involvement which has reached a point beyond stabilising or healing through remineralisation. It may be identified by radiography or transillumination.

Site 2, Size 2 (#2.2)
More extensive involvement of the dentine with the marginal ridge weakened or broken down but still sufficient tooth structure remaining to support the restoration. It may be a replacement for a small Black Class II restoration.

Site 2, Size 3 (#2.3)
On a posterior tooth there will be considerable involvement of the dentine with a split at the base of a cusp – or at least the potential for a split – with the need to protect one or more cuspal inclines from occlusal load. On an anterior tooth there will be extensive proximal caries with loss of support for the incisal corner which will be deeply undermined.

Site 2, Size 4 (#2.4)
There will be complete loss of at least one cusp from a posterior tooth or loss of part of the incisal edge of an anterior tooth as a result of either caries or trauma.

SITE 2, SIZE 1; designated #2.1

There is no equivalent in the G.V. Black classification.

The initial lesion commences in the enamel immediately below the contact area and extends facially and lingually in an elliptical shape controlled by the extent of the contact area. It will generally not involve the contact area nor undermine the marginal ridge or incisal corner to any extent until it has progressed to Size 2. It is often possible, therefore, to maintain the entire proximal surface of enamel. Early demineralisation can penetrate the full depth of the enamel but, providing the prism structure does not collapse, the enamel can be remineralised sufficiently to regain its original physical strength. It may be stained and disfigured but, following removal of the infected dentine within and sealing with a fluoride-releasing glass–ionomer, the proximal wall may remineralise and remain intact.

If enamel caries has progressed to the extent that there is actual cavitation of the enamel, there may be a need to tunnel to the exterior, to a limited extent, through the enamel cavity so that the cavitation can be obturated; this will eliminate further plaque retention, but the remainder of the proximal wall can remain intact. In the presence of fluoride released from the cement, as well as external topical application of fluoride, remineralisation will support and reinforce the enamel and prevent further breakdown.

All of these considerations apply to both anterior and posterior teeth; three different approaches can be considered for these lesions depending upon their position in relation to the marginal ridge or the presence of a lesion in the adjacent tooth.

Internal occlusal fossa ('tunnel')
When the enamel lesion is at least 2.5 mm apical to the crest of the marginal ridge, the simplest and most conservative approach is through the occlusal fossa just medial to the marginal ridge using the 'internal occlusal fossa' or 'tunnel' approach. The initial access for this lesion should be as small as possible through the occlusal fossa to preserve natural tooth structure. Maintenance of the original proximal contour, with a normal contact area, is desirable so removal of enamel should be minimal. The entry should begin just medial to the marginal ridge with careful preservation of remaining enamel.

'Slot cavity'
If the lesion is close to the marginal ridge, and a 'tunnel' approach is likely to leave the ridge too weak to be maintained, access can be gained through the marginal ridge itself. This design has been called a 'slot cavity' and is probably more commonly used in anterior teeth.

Proximal
Finally, if the adjacent tooth already has a Site 2, Size 3 or Size 4 lesion prepared in it with the entire proximal surface missing there may be direct access to the Size 1 lesion through a proximal approach. The occlusal surface can remain intact and a very conservative cavity can be designed to remove the caries only. In view of the normal direction of progress of the dentinal caries, the marginal ridge will generally not be involved or weakened at all.

SITE 2, SIZE 1; internal occlusal fossa ('tunnel') #2.1

Preparation

In posterior teeth, use a small tapered cylinder diamond bur (#168) (**Fig. 11.36**) under air–water spray at intermediate high speed. Begin in the occlusal fossa just medial to the marginal ridge. Enter the enamel aiming towards the expected carious lesion. Usually, the tactile sense available at this speed will allow the operator to feel when the lesion is entered. Approach carefully, observing progress under magnification and good illumination until the defect is identified. Now turn the same bur into a more upright position, encroaching into the marginal ridge area to a minimum extent, to enlarge the cavity and improve visibility. Lean the bur facially and lingually to create a funnel-shaped access cavity to the lesion. The entry will now be approximately triangular in outline with the apex towards the central occlusal fossa and the base along the medial aspects of the marginal ridge. The carious dentine will now be directly visible and can be removed with small round burs (#008 or 012). It may be necessary to use a bur with a long shank to ensure that the walls and the gingival floor are in sound dentine so that a good seal can be developed around the entire circumference. Note that the removal of all affected dentine on the axial wall is unnecessary, particularly if there is a risk if exposing the pulp. Glass–ionomer will seal and isolate the area, after which the dentine will remineralise (**Figs 11.37–40**).

The extent of the proximal enamel defect will become clear at this point and a decision can be made on the presence or absence of enamel cavitation. If the enamel is only demineralised and not cavitated it should be left alone to be supported and remineralised through the cement. If the enamel is already cavitated, or needs to be broken through, a short length of standard metal matrix should be placed interproximally and wedged into place to protect the adjacent tooth. Small round burs (#008) and small fine hand instruments can be used to complete the cavity design. It is usually possible, with magnification, to see the gingival enamel margin, but access to the occlusal margin is more difficult. However, it is only necessary to remove the seriously cavitated enamel because remaining demineralised enamel around the cavity margin will remineralise (**Figs 11.41–44**).

No specific retention design is required because an adhesive restorative material will be used for restoration.

If, at this point, it appears the marginal ridge is cracked or severely compromised, a decision may have to be made to remove the marginal ridge; that is, the cavity may have to now be classified as a Site 2, Size 2 lesion (#2.2) and modified accordingly.

In anterior teeth, access to the lesion is similar to that described for a posterior tooth and can be gained through either the labial or lingual enamel. However, because no restorative material can be regarded as completely permanent, it is much better to approach from the lingual side, thus preserving the labial enamel and minimising aesthetic problems in the future. An approach from the labial side will occasionally be necessary because of crowding of the teeth with consequent overlapping and difficulty of gaining both access and visibility, particularly when the lesion is in a lower anterior tooth.

Enter the lesion with a tapered diamond cylinder (#168) at intermediate high speed under air–water spray just medial to the marginal ridge. Extend very conservatively, both incisally and gingivally, to disclose the extent of the problem while maintaining the proximal enamel. Remove caries with small round burs only (#008). There is no need to develop specific retentive elements because normally, simply cleaning the cavity will produce some degree of undercutting. If the proximal enamel is not cavitated in the area of the initial lesion, leave it intact so that it can remineralise. In the presence of cavitation, clean the defect with care while protecting the adjacent tooth with a short length of metal matrix strip as described above. Do not extend any further than is essential to eliminate plaque retention because the remaining enamel will remineralise. The presence of undermined enamel is of no consequence because it will be supported by adhesion to the restorative cement (**Figs 11.45, 46**).

Restoration

Glass–ionomer is the material of choice for the restoration of both anterior and posterior teeth, with the option of lamination with composite resin if the load-bearing area of the restoration involves the occlusal support against the opposing tooth. Condition the cavity as usual. Wash and dry it but do not dehydrate the tooth.

If using a Type II.1 resin-modified glass–ionomer cement, ensure it is radiopaque and mixed at a high powder :liquid ratio, preferably capsulated for automated mixing. Use a short length of mylar strip as a matrix and wedge it lightly into place to ensure good proximal contour. Place the cement in two increments using a syringe. Tamp the first increment into the depths of the cavity using a small dry plastic sponge. If the enamel is cavitated, watch to ensure that some excess cement is extruded through between the matrix and the tooth. Add the second increment and tamp again to ensure firm adaptation to the entire cavity wall. Light-activate the cement from

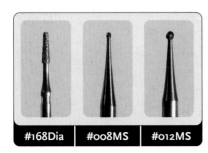

Fig. 11.36 Burs used in the preparation of a #2.1 lesion using the internal occlusal fossa approach.

#168Dia | #008MS | #012MS

several directions for a minimum of 60 seconds. As soon as the cement is set, remove the matrix and trim the restoration to a satisfactory occlusion. Apply a surface glaze to seal the cement as discussed on page 77.

If an autocure cement is to be placed, use the strongest available. If aesthetic results are important, a Type II.1 cement can be used, but it will need to be sealed to maintain the water balance as soon as the matrix is removed because these cements remain susceptible to water loss and water uptake for several hours after placement. The restoration must be covered immediately after removal of the matrix, with a very low viscosity, single-component, light-activated resin bond. Trim any excess cement with a sharp blade and adjust the occlusion if necessary with a round bur (#016) at slow speed with no air–water spray. Add further resin bond to ensure adequate isolation of the cement from the oral environment; finally, light-activate the resin.

Whichever cement is used, if the occlusal involvement of the cement is thought to be too great or there is labial exposure of the glass–ionomer and the aesthetic results are less than ideal, the cement should now be cut back, using a small diamond cylinder (#156) under air–water spray, sufficient to allow room for lamination with composite resin. Regard the cement as a dentine substitute and remove it to a depth of approximately 2 mm only, sufficient to expose the entire enamel wall. Bevel the enamel as required and acid etch it for 15 seconds only. When using an autocure cement, the cement should also be etched for the same timespan. Wash well and apply an enamel-bonding resin. Build the composite resin incrementally to full contour and, after polymerising fully, trim and polish as required.

Because it will take up to a week for a glass–ionomer cement to mature and achieve its final colour and translucency, it is desirable to delay a decision to use lamination to improve aesthetics for that length of time.

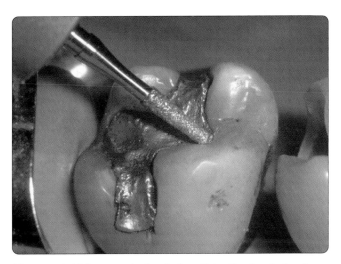

Fig. 11.37 Initial approach, #2.1 lesion. Enter the #2.1 lesion from the occlusal fossa aiming towards the lesion. Watch carefully until the lesion is identified.

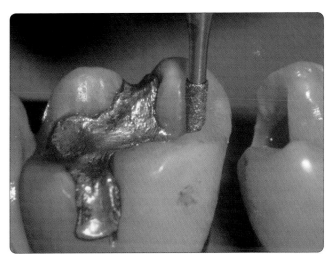

Fig. 11.38 Gain access. Turn the bur vertical and lean it buccally and lingually to 'funnel' the cavity for visibility.

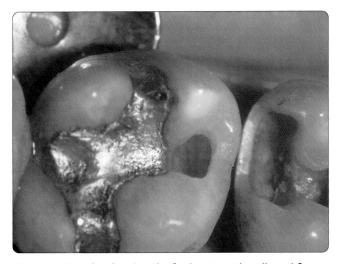

Fig. 11.39 Completed cavity. The final cavity with walls and floor cleaned but axial wall left untouched.

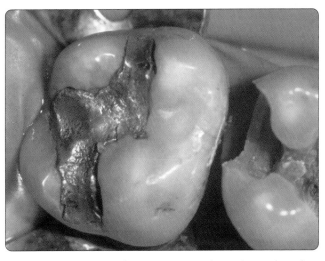

Fig. 11.40 Restoration. Place a matrix, condition the cavity and syringe the glass–ionomer into place.

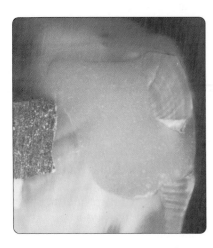

Fig. 11.41 Sectioned tooth. The same tooth as in figure 11.40, sectioned mesiodistally, to show restoration in place. Note demineralised enamel around the glass–ionomer cement which will remineralise.

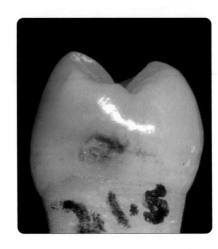

Fig. 11.42 Proximal lesion. A proximal lesion on an extracted tooth to be prepared as if *in vivo*.

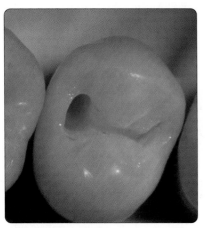

Fig. 11.43 Prepared cavity. The cavity completed. Note 'funnelled' entry and minor occlusal fissure extension which is optional.

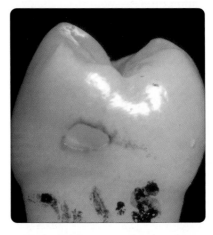

Fig. 11.44 Completed proximal. The proximal lesion following preparation. Note the remaining demineralised enamel around the cavity.

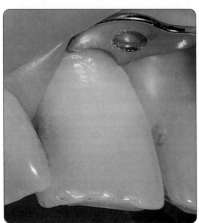

Fig. 11.45 Anterior 'tunnel'. There is a small #2.1 lesion below the contact at the distal of the upper central incisor.

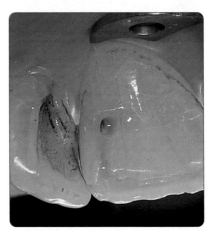

Fig. 11.46 Completed 'tunnel'. The cavity is complete. Note that the proximal enamel remains intact except for a small break just below the contact area similar to a posterior 'tunnel'.

SITE 2, SIZE 1; slot cavity #2.1

There will be occasions when the carious lesion commences high on the proximal surface of a posterior tooth leaving less than 2.5 mm of the marginal ridge occluso-gingivally, or it may be cracked or otherwise very weak. Under these circumstances, it may be wise to approach the lesion through the marginal ridge and produce a small box-form cavity sufficient to eliminate the lesion but not extended beyond the demineralised enamel. It is often possible to maintain a contact with the adjacent tooth on the facial margin, lingual margin or both, thus facilitating the maintenance of a relatively normal contact area between the two teeth.

Preparation
Open into the lesion using a fine tapered diamond bur (#168) (**Fig. 11.47**) at intermediate high speed under air–water spray to maintain a good tactile sense. Extend carefully until the extent of the carious lesion is clearly visible. Gentle use of a gingival margin trimmer will allow careful extension without damage to the adjacent tooth. Remove caries with small round burs (#008 and 012) and make clean margins around the entire circumference. If possible, maintain a contact with the adjacent tooth (**Figs 11.48–51**). Do not extend medially more than halfway through the marginal ridge or the cavity design may have to be modified further (see Site 2, Size 2 – #2.2, below).

Restoration
In the absence of heavy occlusal load, a resin-modified or Type II.2 glass–ionomer alone is generally sufficient. Use a short length of mylar strip as a matrix wedged firmly into place between the teeth. Condition the cavity as usual and syringe the cement to place using a fine tip on the syringe or capsule. Light-activate adequately, contour, polish and glaze. If the occlusal load is heavy, it may be wise to cut the cement back about 2 mm and laminate it with composite resin.

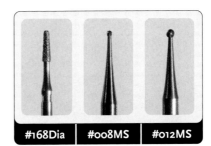

Fig. 11.47 Burs used in the preparation of a #2.1 lesion using the slot cavity technique.

#168Dia | #oo8MS | #o12MS

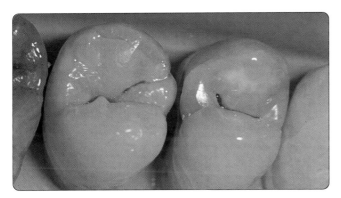

Fig. 11.48 'Slot cavity' #2.1. There is a small #2.1 lesion high on the proximal surface of the first bicuspid. The preferred approach is via the marginal ridge.

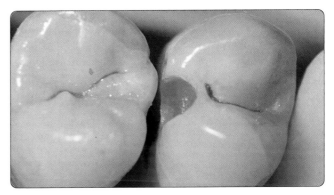

Fig. 11.49 Finished cavity. The completed slot cavity from the occlusal view.

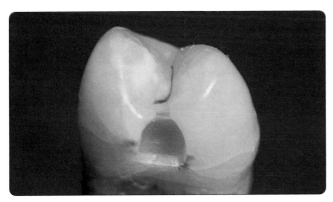

Fig. 11.50 Proximal aspect. The same cavity after removing the tooth from the model viewed from an occlusal angle.

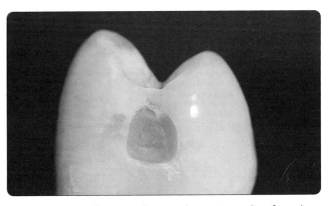

Fig. 11.51 Proximal aspect. The complete cavity outline from the proximal. Note there is still some demineralised enamel beyond the margin which will remain.

SITE 2, SIZE 1; proximal approach #2.1

Occasionally, the preparation of a larger Site 2, Size 3 or Size 4 cavity will allow good access and visibility to the proximal surface of an adjacent tooth with a Site 2, Size 1 lesion. Restoration of this cavity is relatively straightforward without the need to involve the marginal ridge or approach through the occlusal fossa.

Preparation

Use a small tapered diamond cylinder bur (#168) (Fig. 11.52) at intermediate high speed under air–water spray. Access to the lesion and the entry angle will be dictated and controlled to some degree by the cavity in the adjacent tooth but, as the caries is progressing into the

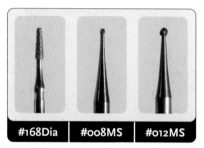

| #168Dia | #oo8MS | #o12MS |

Fig. 11.52 Burs used in the preparation of a #2.1 lesion using the proximal approach.

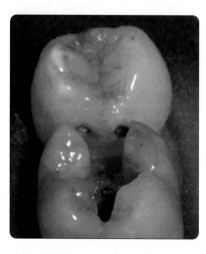

Fig. 11.53 Proximal approach #2.1. A small #2.1 proximal lesion becomes accessible through a traditional cavity prepared in the adjacent tooth.

dentine in an apical direction and normally does not undermine the marginal ridge at this size, there is no problem removing all the infected layer without involving the marginal ridge. Remove the enamel as far as is necessary to achieve access to the caries. Use a small round bur (#008 or 012) with a long shank to clean the cavity, particularly around the full circumference of the walls. A retentive design is not required, although the walls will generally be slightly undercut (Fig. 11.53).

Restoration

It is essential that the restorative material be radiopaque to avoid subsequent radiographic confusion as to whether a lesion is restored or not. A resin-modified glass–ionomer can be used, but there may be problems with access for the activating light. As the restoration is not under load and aesthetics is not usually a problem, a Type II.2 autocure cement is the material of choice. Condition the cavity as usual and place a small piece of matrix strip interproximally, lightly supported with a wedge. Syringe the cement into place and apply the matrix firmly over the cement to ensure positive adaptation. As soon as the cement is set, the matrix can be removed and the cement contoured and polished before proceeding with the adjacent restoration (Fig. 11.54).

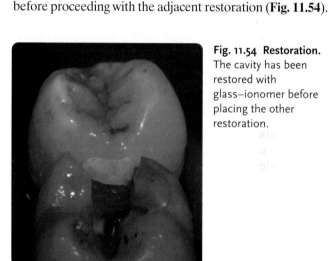

Fig. 11.54 Restoration. The cavity has been restored with glass–ionomer before placing the other restoration.

SITE 2, SIZE 2; designated #2.2

G.V. Black classification – Class II (posterior), Class III (anterior).

A new proximal lesion may be more extensive than a minimal lesion before it is identified with the marginal ridge and proximal surface broken down or so weakened that the previous cavity design is no longer valid. The extent of the cavitation of the proximal enamel will dictate the classification and, ultimately, the outline form of the cavity. There is no need to remove sound enamel, particularly from the gingival floor, just because it is undermined following

removal of caries. The enamel at the gingival is not under occlusal load and can be retained, thus keeping the restoration margin out of the gingival crevice. Also, there is no need to develop dovetail retentive elements on the occlusal of a posterior tooth or the lingual of an anterior tooth, because an adhesive restorative material is to be placed that does not require mechanical interlocks. The final proximal outline form will often be curved rather than dovetailed, and the generation of sharp point and line angles is strictly contraindicated because the angles complicate the placement of the restorative material and may lead to stress concentration, resulting in further failure of tooth or restoration.

For a replacement restoration following breakdown of a previous restoration, or the elimination of amalgam in favour of a more aesthetic material, the same basic rules will apply, but the cavity will generally be somewhat larger and already extended further than necessary for a modern Site 2, Size 2 cavity (#2.2). It may be verging on a Site 2, Size 3 (#2..3) cavity and a decision will be required on the final design and classification once the cavity is nearing completion.

The decision as to which plastic restorative material to use in a given situation is discussed in Chapter 16 and the final cavity design will depend on the selection. If amalgam is the material of choice for restoration of a posterior tooth, inclusion of the occlusal fissures is usually required because it is difficult to complete an amalgam restoration part-way along a fissure. The preparation of an occlusal extension is not relevant to retention of the restoration as a whole inasmuch as each section of an amalgam restoration must be individually self-retentive rather than rely on any one section to retain another. In fact, if a proximal lesion can be restored without involving the occlusal fissures at all, then a small proximal box alone may be adequate.

If restoring with amalgam, the main retentive form in the proximal box should be placed within the dentine at the gingival floor as well as in the facial and lingual walls as discussed in Chapter 7, page 59. If the separate sections of the restoration are individually self-retentive, there will not be failure at the narrow isthmus that joins the occlusal extension to the proximal box.

On the other hand, if composite resin, glass–ionomer or both are to be used for the restoration there will generally be no need to open the occlusal fissures any further than recommended for a fissure seal or a #1.1 restoration and there will be no need for a retentive design to be included in the proximal box. Removal of the caries and extension of the cavity outline to include all the cavitated enamel will be sufficient. Weakened enamel around the proximal box, particularly along the gingival floor, can be supported and reinforced with glass–ionomer, but facial and lingual enamel must be soundly based on dentine if it is to be a significant factor in retention and prevention of micro-leakage when placing a composite resin restoration.

In anterior teeth there is no fissure involved, so a slot-preparation is all that is required. Remove the demineralised enamel and infected dentine only and, if possible, avoid removing the entire contact area. Unsupported enamel will be maintained through adhesion with the restoration.

Preparation

For the new lesion, access should be gained with a small diamond cylinder (#156) (**Fig. 11.55**) under air–water spray at ultra-high speed beginning just medially to the margin-al ridge and aiming towards the carious lesion. Extend facially, lingually and medially with the same bur only as far as is necessary to expose the extent of the caries. If restoring with amalgam, extend the preparation along the full extent of the occlusal fissure system with the same diamond cylinder, thus producing an extension approximately 1 mm wide, to the full depth of the enamel and just into the dentine, with parallel walls to allow adequate condensation of the amalgam. When restoring with composite resin, the fissure system may be opened with a very fine diamond point (#200) sufficient only to ensure there is no further carious lesion. There is no need to remove enamel just to make room for more composite resin.

Remove the caries with small round burs (#008 to 012) at a low speed. Clean the facial and lingual walls and the gingival floor, but leave affected dentine on the axial wall to be remineralised. Cavity outline can now be completed, often with hand instruments such as gingival margin trimmers, removing cavitated enamel only. Further extension to the facial or lingual is unnecessary and the walls need not be free from contact with the adjacent tooth. Retain as much gingival enamel as possible to keep the gingival margin of the restoration out of the gingival crevice, even if the enamel is undermined and weakened following removal of the caries. Because this enamel is not subjected to occlusal load, it can be supported and reinforced through adhesion with glass–ionomer. Weakened and unsupported enamel should not be involved in adhesion using composite resin with the etching technique because it is likely to fail under the setting contraction of the resin.

If the cavity is being modified for replacement of a failed restoration the outline form will already be dictated by the previous cavity design. Remove old metal restorations at ultra-high speed with a tungsten carbide bur (#140) taking care not to enlarge the cavity. Ditch the metal and break it out in pieces. Refine the cavity using a diamond cylinder (#156) at intermediate high speed for improved tactile sense. Remove caries and old lining material at low speed (#012). If amalgam is to be placed again, mechanical retention must be provided in the gingival one-third of the crown, using a tapered fissure #168 mild steel bur.

If composite resin is to be placed, mechanical retention is not required because adhesion will be obtained with the enamel through acid-etching. If there are minor under-cuts already present following removal of caries, these should be restored with glass–ionomer rather than by removal of further tooth structure (**Figs 11.56–11.58**).

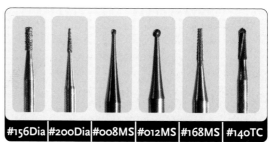

Fig. 11.55 Burs used in the preparation of a #2.2 lesion.

#156Dia #200Dia #008MS #012MS #168MS #140TC

Restoration

If amalgam is the material of choice for restoration and the caries has progressed to a point further than half way to the pulp chamber, a lining or a base should be placed on the axial wall to act as a thermal barrier. A layer of glass–ionomer, hand mixed or capsulated at a 1.5 : 1.0 powder: liquid ratio, should be flowed over the surface, in a layer no greater than 0.5 mm thick, as thermal insulation.

The cavity and the lining should be covered by a single application of copal varnish or a resin or glass–ionomer amalgam bonding agent. Copal varnish is expected to wash out over a short period of time and this will allow the deposition of corrosion products to seal the interface. The amalgam bonding agents are expected to provide some degree of adhesion between the amalgam and the tooth structure but the strength will be limited to the tensile strength of the resin or cement. A matrix can now be placed, wedged sufficiently firmly to develop a degree of separation between adjacent teeth, and the amalgam condensed to place. An alloy containing a high percentage of copper with spherical particles is easier to condense and shows moderately superior physical properties (see Chapter 10, page 115) (**Fig. 11.59**).

If the final restoration is to be composite resin it should always be placed using a lamination technique over a glass–ionomer base (see discussion on lamination in Chapter 8). Note that a sublining of calcium hydroxide is unnecessary because the glass–ionomer will provide a seal that is proof against microleakage and it is sufficiently biocompatible to cause no lasting pulpal response.

For those same reasons, the choice for final restoration may be glass–ionomer alone without lamination. In fact, the only reason for covering with composite resin would be in situations where the occlusal load is expected to be too great for the glass–ionomer to remain without support. This may be the case when restoring a posterior tooth, but will be rare in an anterior tooth (**Figs 11.60, 11.61**) and many deciduous teeth can be safely restored with glass–ionomer alone.

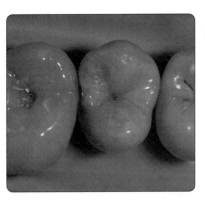

Fig. 11.56 Moderate #2.2 lesion. A #2.2 lesion, distal of second bicuspid, to be prepared for adhesive restoration.

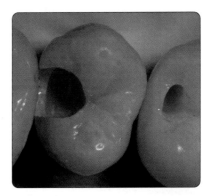

Fig. 11.57 Finished cavity. Note minimal involvement of occlusal fissure.

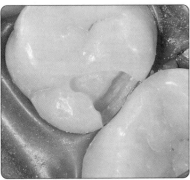

Fig. 11.58 Conventional #2.2 cavity. A conventional amalgam cavity. Note the mechanical interlock at the gingival.

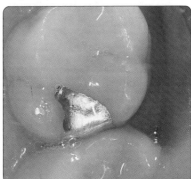

Fig. 11.59 Completed restoration. The completed amalgam restoration. The tooth structure gives full support to the amalgam.

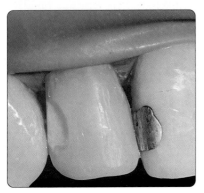

Fig. 11.60 Anterior #2.2 lesion. Old resin #2.2 restorations being replaced from the labial.

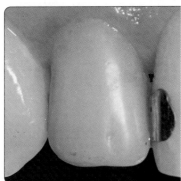

Fig. 11.61 Completed restorations. Completed glass–ionomer restorations.

SITE 2, SIZE 3; designated #2.3

G.V. Black classification – class III (anterior), class II (posterior)

Site 2, Size 1 and Size 2 lesions (#2.1 and #2.2) in both anterior and posterior teeth have been described together, because all principles and procedures are the same for both situations. However, when discussing larger Site 2 lesions (#2.3 and #2.4) in posterior teeth, which have a potential for split cusps or total loss of cusps, the preparation and restoration phases will be described separately, principally because anterior teeth do not have cusps with their associated potential for fracture.

#2.3 lesions in anterior teeth

This lesion represents an extension of the Site 2, Size 2 (#2.2) lesion in an anterior tooth which has weakened the incisal corner. The lesion may be relatively minor with adequate healthy enamel around all the margins onto which to develop mechanical adhesion with composite resin through acid etching of the enamel. However, with extensive caries or replacement of old approximal restorations, the enamel at the gingival margin may be weak and friable and not able to be relied upon for retention of the restoration. Under these circumstances, it will be desirable to use a glass–ionomer as the dentine substitute and laminate over that with composite resin because the cement does not have sufficient fracture toughness to support the incisal corner on its own. Depending upon the degree of tooth loss, this restoration may be followed at a later date by full crown preparation and under those circumstances it is desirable to have sound adhesion to remaining tooth structure for the original restoration so that it will remain in place during further preparation.

Preparation

Gain access very conservatively, using a #168Dia (**Fig. 11.62**) retaining all possible enamel even though unsupported by dentine. Remove all remaining unsatisfactory old restorative material using a #140TC and remove caries from the walls with small round burs (#012, 008). There is no need to remove all affected dentine from the axial wall. Retention through mechanical interlocks, such as dovetail extensions in the lingual enamel, is both undesirable and unnecessary because adhesive restorative materials will be placed and all possible natural tooth structure should be retained. Smooth all enamel margins and remove friable enamel rods using a fine sintered diamond (#223). Bevel as required to enhance retention with the composite resin. Undermined enamel should be supported with glass–ionomer and it will then provide a degree of retention to composite resin. If composite resin alone is to be used the enamel must be well supported with sound dentine around the full circumference.

Pins are contraindicated because they are very difficult to disguise completely within the restorative material and may result in an unsightly shadow being cast through the restoration. They are also likely to lead to microleakage in the future. There will be occasional exceptions to this where there is extensive tooth loss but under those circumstances an extracoronal restoration is probably indicated (**Figs 11.63** and **11.64**).

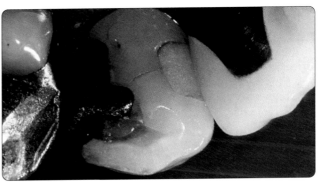

Fig. 11.63 Anterior #2.3 lesion. Old amalgam restoration, distal of canine, to be replaced.

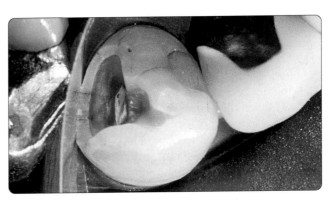

Fig. 11.64 Cavity design. Completed cavity. Note retention of labial enamel to be supported by adhesive restoration.

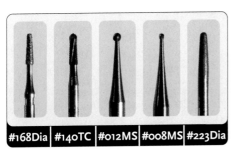

Fig. 11.62 Burs used in the preparation of a #2.3 lesion in anterior teeth.

| #168Dia | #140TC | #012MS | #008MS | #223Dia |

Restoration

If there is a satisfactory enamel margin around the full circumference of the cavity, it will be sufficient to cover and protect the exposed dentine with a glass–ionomer as a dentine substitute. The micromechanical attachment of the composite resin to enamel through acid etching will then retain the restoration. Etch the enamel only, apply a thin layer of a low-viscosity enamel resin bond, blow off the excess with dry air and light activate.

If the cavity is extensive and the gingival enamel is either insufficient or too weak to sustain adequate adhesion the restoration should begin with a glass–ionomer as a dentine substitute. The cement should be the strongest possible with a high powder:liquid ratio, preferably capsulated, to ensure optimal physical properties. As soon as the cement is set it can be cut back to expose the enamel margins and make room for the composite resin. Rebuild the contact area in composite resin but leave the gingival extension of the proximal box in glass–ionomer. Etch the enamel and apply a thin film of a low-viscosity enamel–resin bond. It is desirable, in extensive cavities, to develop enamel bonding on both the labial and the lingual to enhance the overall strength of retention of the restoration.

Build the composite resin incrementally, beginning with the lingual surface, and use a hybrid composite resin for optimum strength (**Figs 11.65** and **11.66**).

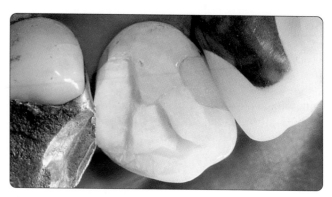

Fig. 11.65 Glass–ionomer cement base. Restoration with glass–ionomer cement, cut back to allow space for composite resin, etched for adhesion.

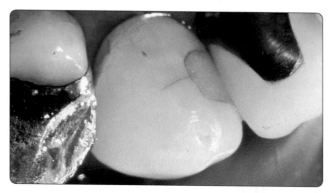

Fig. 11.66 Completed restoration. Composite resin laminate over glass–ionomer cement adhering also to enamel.

#2.3 lesions in posterior teeth

In a posterior tooth, as the carious lesion becomes more extensive, the remaining tooth structure becomes progressively weaker until the point is reached where the restoration must be relied upon to provide some support to the tooth rather than the reverse. Initial opening of an occlusal fissure into dentine will double the length of the cusps and development of a proximal box will tend to double the length again. Occlusal load on the cuspal inclines produces flexure in the cusps which, on many occasions, later lead to symptoms of pain on pressure because of the development of a split at the base of the cusp. Ultimately, there is likely to be total failure, with loss of tooth structure in bulk (note discussion on protective cavity designs in Chapter 7, page 62).

Preparation

The steps for preparation of a protective restoration are as follows. Open the cavity conservatively using a small diamond cylinder bur (#156) (**Fig. 11.67**) at ultra-high speed under air–water spray. To remove an old restoration use a tungsten carbide bur (#140), also at ultra-high speed. Remove all remaining caries around the walls (#012, 016), but be conservative with affected dentine on the axial wall. At this point, determine the extent of the problem and decide if remaining tooth structure requires protection.

Identify a split at the base of a cusp if it is present.

For a cusp that is split or at risk, modify the cavity outline by leaning the facial or lingual wall outwards in a straight line from the gingival floor to just beyond the cusp tip using a #168Dia bur at intermediate high speed, as described in Chapter 7, page 64. Note that this technique can be used to provide protection for any weakened or undermined tooth structure. Support for one-half of a cusp or a single cusp is relatively straightforward, but all four cusps on a molar can be protected at once if necessary. However, maintenance of full height on at least one cusp gives an indication of the original occlusal height

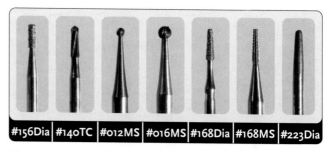

#156Dia | #140TC | #012MS | #016MS | #168Dia | #168MS | #223Dia

Fig. 11.67 Burs used in the preparation of a #2.3 lesion in posterior teeth.

and simplifies replacement of the remainder to normal occlusal anatomy.

Retention can now be achieved using the principles as laid down in Chapter 7. The #168MS is preferred for the preparation of all retentive elements and the #223 fine sintered diamond is useful to refine enamel margins (**Figs 11.68–11.73**).

Restoration

Cavities in this category are usually large, and placement of a lining or a base as a barrier and for thermal protection is desirable.

Because of the large size of the cavity, amalgam is generally the material of choice. Line the cavity with a thin layer of glass–ionomer with a low powder content. Condense the amalgam carefully and overfill the cavity by 1–2 mm above each cusp. Allow it to set briefly before beginning to carve back. Release the amalgam from the matrix band first with a fine probe until the enamel can be seen below the amalgam overbuild. Shape the buccal and lingual contour before attempting to carve the occlusal surface. The original cusp height can be used as a guide for nonworking cusps, but care must be taken to maintain the height of the working cusps while developing the occlusal anatomy. When adjusting the occlusion with the opposing tooth, be prepared to adjust the opponent as well as the new restoration to avoid deep intercuspation. This is the correct time to relieve lateral stresses on the cusps as well as eliminate interference in lateral excursions while maintaining a correct centric occlusion relationship between the arches.

If composite resin is preferred for the restoration, glass–ionomer should be placed as a base or dentine substitute with the resin laminated over to replace the enamel. The details of the lamination technique are discussed in full in Chapter 8, page 88, and success will depend on careful application. Clearly, by the time a tooth is in this condition, an extracoronal restoration would have been advisable but there may be many reasons for avoiding or delaying this move (**Figs 11.74, 11.75**).

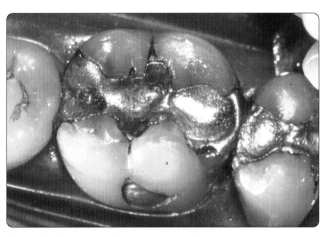

Fig. 11.68 #2.3 lesion. The tooth is sensitive to pressure suggesting that there is a split under some of the cusps.

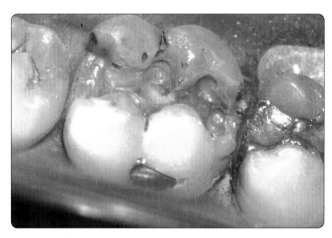

Fig. 11.69 Weakened cusps. The amalgam has been removed revealing a split beneath the lingual cusps.

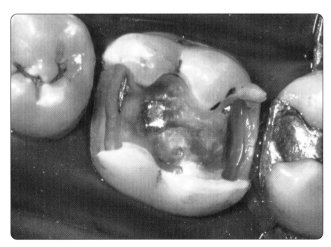

Fig. 11.70 Split revealed. Following modification of the cavity design the split can be clearly sighted. The cusps require support from the restoration.

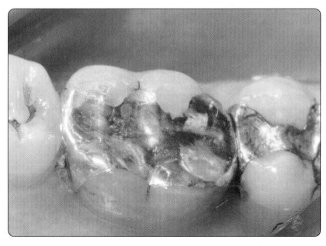

Fig. 11.71 Protective restoration. A view from the lingual showing the extent of the cusp protection.

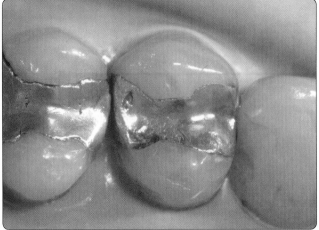

Fig. 11.72 #2.3 lesion to be restored with resin. An amalgam restoration requires replacement and the lingual cusp is rather weak.

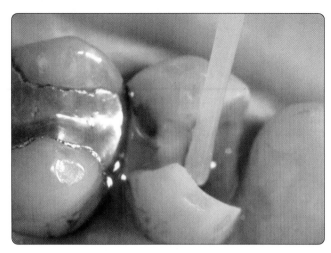

Fig. 11.73 Cavity design. The final cavity design showing some protection for the lingual cusp.

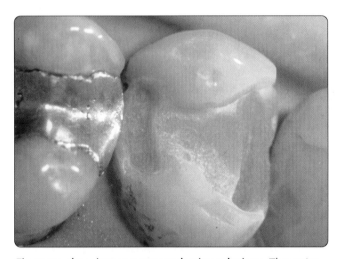

Fig. 11.74 glass–ionomer cement dentine substitute. The cavity was restored with glass–ionomer cement, then cut back to make room for lamination with composite resin.

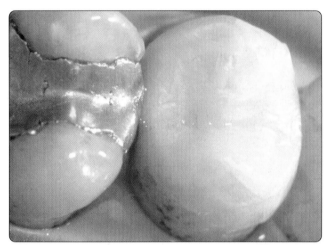

Fig. 11.75 Final restoration. The final restoration with composite resin lamination to protect the glass–ionomer cement and reinforce the remaining cusps.

SITE 2, SIZE 4; designated #2.4

G.V. Black classification – class IV (anterior), class II (posterior).

2.4 lesions in anterior teeth

These lesions are often caused by trauma, with loss of a major section of the incisal half of the crown. They can also follow extensive caries or breakdown and extension of a #2.3 restoration. In most cases, the occlusal load will not be heavy and the problems of restoration mainly revolve around restoring aesthetic appeal.

Preparation

After traumatic fracture, there will be very little preparation required. Exposed dentine should be protected as soon as possible with a strong glass–ionomer, which can subsequently remain as a base at the time of restoration. The enamel margins should be bevelled (#223) (**Fig. 11.76**) to ensure optimum adhesion with composite resin as well as to blend the union to tooth structure to ensure acceptable aesthetic appeal.

For an extensive carious lesion or replacement of an old restoration, care must be taken to preserve as much of the original enamel as possible. Correct access can be achieved using a #168 or #156. Unsupported enamel can be supported to some degree with glass–ionomer, so trim the margins to a smooth finish. Remove caries (#012) from around the walls only and leave affected dentine on the axial wall for remineralisation. Avoid the use of pins for retention because of likely future problems such as micro-cracks in dentine and a shadow cast by the pin (**Figs 11.77** and **11.78**).

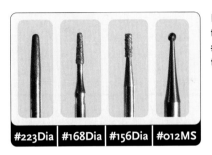

Fig. 11.76 Burs used in the preparation of a #2.4 lesion in anterior teeth.

#223Dia #168Dia #156Dia #012MS

Restoration

Composite resin is the only material that can be used successfully under these circumstances, but a base of glass–ionomer is desirable to act as a dentine substitute and provide reliable adhesion. Restore the entire cavity with a high-powder-content reinforced or resin-modified glass–ionomer and fully light activate as required from all directions. Cut the cement back to expose all the enamel margins, except possibly the gingival margin if there is no enamel left or it is too weak to allow retention with the composite resin. Bevel the enamel to develop optimum adhesion with the resin and to smooth over the aesthetic transition of enamel to composite resin. Build the composite resin incrementally, following the lamination technique described in Chapter 8, page 88. Begin with a hybrid resin on the lingual for optimum strength and laminate with a microfil resin on the labial to enhance the aesthetics. Colour matching with these restorations is a challenge, but modern packaging of the materials allows for artistic mixing and blending of various shades and types of composite resin (**Figs 11.79–11.82**).

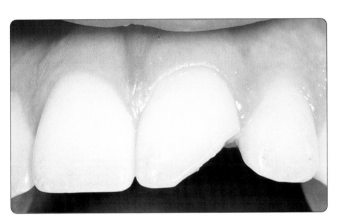

Fig. 11.77 Traumatic fracture: #2.4 lesion. The upper right central incisor was fractured by trauma. Dentine is exposed but not the pulp.

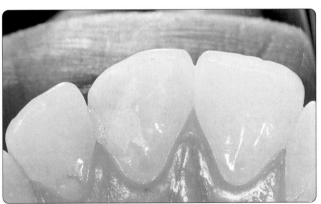

Fig. 11.78 Glass–ionomer cement base. A glass–ionomer cement base was applied as an emergency procedure and left in place for 1 week until both the tooth and the patient were stable.

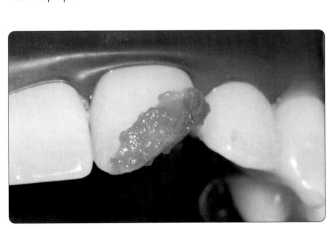

Fig. 11.79 Lamination with resin. After 1 week, the surface was freshened and the enamel lightly bevelled. Both were etched to allow development of adhesion to the enamel and the glass–ionomer cement.

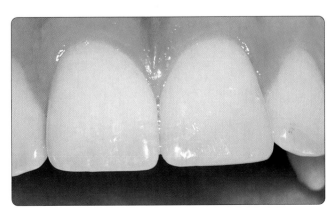

Fig. 11.80 Completed restoration. The incisal corner was built up with composite resin.

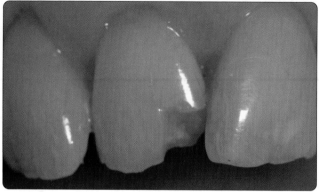

Fig. 11.81 Failure of weakened incisal corner, #2.4 lesion. The incisal corner of the upper right central incisor was undermined by an old #2.2 resin restoration. This was removed and replaced with glass–ionomer cement first.

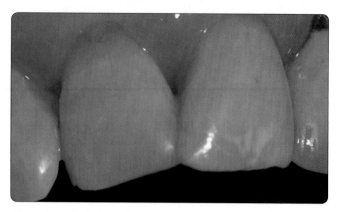

Fig. 11.82 Rebuilt incisal corner. Subsequently the incisal corner was laminated with composite resin.

#2.4 lesions in posterior teeth

Restoration of a #2.4 cavity in a posterior tooth poses further problems when an entire cusp has failed, either from extensive carious attack or as the result of a split, and it generally leaves at least one margin close to the epithelial attachment. Cavity design is then very similar to that described above for the #2.3 cavity except that rebuilding to the correct occlusal height is complicated by the lack of guidance from the missing cusp.

Preparation

Open the cavity and remove all traces of the old restoration using a small diamond cylinder (#156) (**Fig. 11.83**), or tungsten carbide bur (#140) as indicated, at ultra-high speed under an air–water spray. Remove all caries around the walls to determine the extent of the problem (#012, 016). Remain conservative, and retain affected dentine on the axial wall and pulpal floor. Retain any cusp that is based on sound dentine and treat as described for a #2.2 cavity design. Cusps that are undermined or split should be protected as suggested in the design for a #2.3 cavity. Retention must be developed in the gingival floor wherever possible, using ditches and grooves cut with a small tapered fissure bur (#168) as described in Chapter 7, page59

(**Fig. 11.84**). Refine and polish the margins using a fine sintered diamond #223.

Restoration

In these extensive cavities, amalgam is the material of choice because of its superior strength and lack of flexibility. Placement of a matrix may be complex, and adequate condensation will be time consuming. Overbuild in the first place and carve back to the correct anatomy. Carve the facial and lingual aspects in relation to protected or restored cusps first. Pay particular attention to the interproximal contour because it is very easy to develop overcontours in such extensive restorations and at the same time difficult to develop the correct anatomy in contact areas.

There are limitations to the use of composite resin, particularly for restoration of molars, for a number of reasons. There will be minimal sound enamel available for the development of acid-etch adhesion, particularly at the gingival margin, so problems of microleakage may be difficult to overcome. Glass–ionomer can be utilised as a dentine substitute as described in the lamination technique in Chapter 8, page 88, but it also requires support from remaining tooth structure (**Figs 11.85–11.89**). The setting shrinkage of a light-activated composite resin can be compensated for, to some degree, by incremental build-up but, in an extensive restoration, this becomes more and more difficult and time consuming and the total shrinkage may be too great. Also, fatigue under cyclic loading as well as long-term water uptake of the present generations of bis-GMA resins is such that the breakdown under occlusal load may be greater than can be tolerated and may limit longevity of the restoration.

However, the demand for an aesthetically acceptable restoration means that the lamination technique will be the method of choice, particularly for bicuspids, providing the occlusal load is not excessive.

| #156Dia | #140TC | #012MS | #016MS | #168MS | #223Dia |

Fig. 11.83 Burs used in the preparation of a #2.4 lesion in posterior teeth.

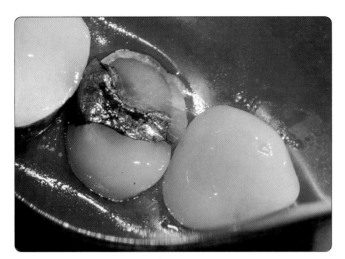

Fig. 11.84 Lost buccal cusp, #2.4 lesion. The buccal cusp of the upper first bicuspid failed in the presence of a relatively small #2.2 amalgam.

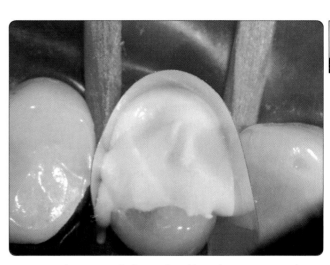

Fig. 11.85 Placement of a base. The old amalgam was entirely removed and the cavity restored almost completely with glass–ionomer cement.

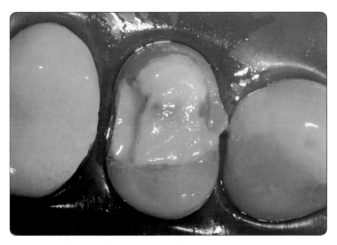

Fig. 11.86 Shaping the base. The glass–ionomer cement was cut back sufficiently to make room for lamination with composite resin. Remaining enamel was lightly bevelled where possible.

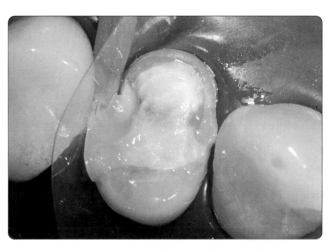

Fig. 11.87 Begin composite rebuild. A small length of mylar strip was placed and wedged on the distal only and the resin carefully built incrementally.

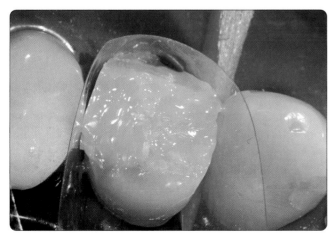

Fig. 11.88 Incremental build-up. The mesial was wedged and built after completion of the distal.

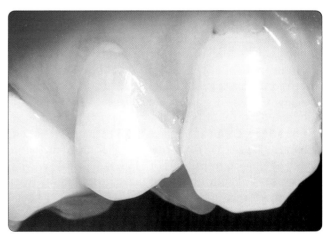

Fig. 11.89 Completed restoration. A buccal view of the completed build-up.

SITE 3 LESIONS

Site 3 lesions occur in the gingival one-third of the crown or on the exposed root surface of any tooth. Lesions can occur on the open surfaces (facial or lingual) in relation to the contours of the gingival tissue or interproximally, well below (and not related to) the contact area following gingival recession.

Caries can occur anywhere around the full circumference of a tooth as a result of lack of hygiene and plaque accumulation. The carious lesion may have an enamel margin around the full circumference but the usual cavity in this area has an occlusal (incisal) margin in enamel and a gingival margin in dentine.

Root surface caries also occur anywhere on the root surface following gingival recession. If it occurs interproximally, this lesion will be well below, and unrelated to, the contact area. It will also be classified as a Site 3 lesion and restoration will generally be undertaken, depending on access and convenience, from the facial or lingual rather than from the occlusal aspect.

Abrasion/erosion lesions should also be included in this category. There are three possible causes as discussed in Chapter 4 and it is desirable to determine the cause and eliminate it at the time of treatment otherwise the erosion may continue around the restoration.

SITE 3, SIZE 1; designated #3.1

G.V. Black classification – class V.

Preparation

A carious lesion is usually found at the gingival margin associated with a high caries rate and poor oral hygiene routines. A decision will need to be made as to whether remineralisation and improved hygiene will be sufficient to stabilise the situation or whether a restoration should be placed. If a restoration is required, it is sufficient to remove the carious dentine only, using small round burs (#008 or #012) (**Fig 11.90**). Occasionally, if the enamel is very friable, it may be necessary to extend the cavity out into the enamel, but there will be no need to remove all the white lesion representing demineralised enamel. Use a small diamond cylinder (#156) at intermediate high speed under air–water spray for limited extension. With placement of glass–ionomer, the state of the enamel is not important because the continuing fluoride release will encourage remineralisation. If the cavity is to be restored with composite resin, the outline will need to be extended to reach sound, fully mineralised enamel, which can be safely etched to provide micromechanical attachment. Because an adhesive material will be used for restoration it is unnecessary to develop a retentive design.

No instrumentation is required for the restoration of an erosion lesion (**Fig 11.91**). Take care to avoid damage to the gingival tissue because haemorrhage will interfere with adhesion. Control of gingival seepage and haemorrhage can be achieved with an application of trichloroacetic acid (Chapter 14, page 177). Alternatively, placement of a short length of gingival retraction cord into the gingival crevice may assist by slightly displacing the soft tissue away from the cavity.

Restoration

The material of choice is a Type II.1 restorative aesthetic glass–ionomer, either autocure or resin-modified, because the aesthetic result is very similar to that which can be achieved with composite resin and the adhesion and fluoride release are superior. An autocure cement can be used, and in many cases the aesthetic result will be adequate. Alternatively, if the colour and translucency is not entirely satisfactory, the cement can be laminated later with composite resin.

An erosion/abrasion lesion should be cleaned with a brief scrub of pumice and water on a small rubber cup to remove the pellicle. Do not use proprietary prophylactic pastes, whether they contain fluoride or not, because they tend to leave a smear layer that will interfere with the adhesion and the ion exchange. Either an erosion lesion or a carious cavity should then be conditioned with 10% polyacrylic acid for 10 seconds, washed thoroughly and dried lightly.

A resin-modified cement can then be placed, contoured and adapted with a translucent matrix, light-activated for 20 seconds, and the matrix removed. Light-activate for at least a further 20 seconds to ensure complete activation. Contour and polish immediately with very fine diamonds under an air–water spray. Finally, apply a thin coat of the appropriate glaze to seal any remaining surface porosities and scratches.

When using an autocure glass–ionomer, prepare the cavity as above. Use a cement with a high powder:liquid ratio, preferably capsulated, and place it with a syringe. Apply a soft tin matrix to adapt the cement well to the surface of the tooth and leave it to set for approximately 4 minutes. As soon as it is set, remove any excess cement from around the matrix, lift off the matrix and immediately

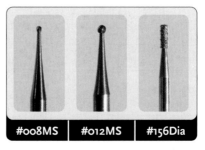

Fig. 11.90 Burs used in the preparation of a #3.1 lesion.

| #008MS | #012MS | #156Dia |

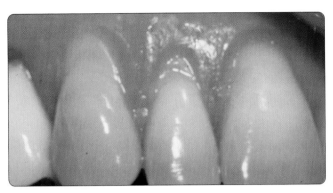

Fig. 11.91 Erosion lesions, #3.1. Erosion lesions at the gingival of the central, lateral and canine were restored with glass–ionomer.

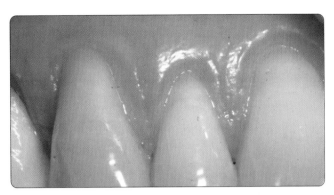

Fig. 11.92 Restorations after 8 years. The same restorations as shown in Figure 11.91, 8 years after placement.

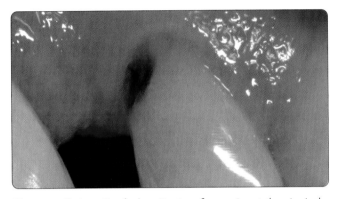

Fig. 11.93 Carious #3.1 lesion. Root surface caries at the gingival of the lateral incisor requires repair.

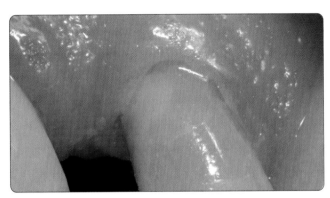

Fig. 11.94 Restoration after 5 years. The same restoration as shown in Figure 11.93, 5 years after placement.

cover the cement with a generous layer of a single-component, very low viscosity resin–enamel bond to stabilise the cement and avoid water uptake or water loss. If required, trim the cement further using a sharp blade only, but do not contaminate with water. Develop a reasonable contour and cover with additional resin bond to complete the seal. Light-activate the bond and trim the gingival margin if there is an excess of sealant remaining. Complete the contour and polish after a minimum of 1 week later. Seal again with a low-viscosity resin to cover porosities and scratches (**Figs 11.92–11.94**).

If, after a few days, the aesthetics of the glass–ionomer is unsatisfactory, it can be trimmed back with a fine diamond bur (#223) under air–water spray to allow for lamination with composite resin. Clean all the enamel at the occlusal margin and bevel it lightly so as to develop optimum micromechanical union. Etch the enamel and the cement for 15 seconds, wash thoroughly and dry lightly. Apply a thin layer of an enamel–resin bonding agent, blow off the excess and light-activate. Build the composite resin incrementally beginning at the gingival margin.

SITE 3, SIZE 2; designated #3.2

G.V. Black classification – class V.

The #3.2 lesion is similar to the #3.1 except that it is somewhat more extensive and possibly more complex to restore. It will normally be a large carious lesion on the facial or lingual surface of a tooth, arising from poor oral hygiene technique in the presence of rampant caries. It will be seen occasionally in patients with xerostomia.

Preparation

Follow the routine as described above, taking care to retain as much natural tooth structure as possible. Note the potential for remineralisation of both enamel and dentine.

Use round burs (#012, #016) (**Fig. 11.95**) at a low speed to remove infected dentine from the walls and leave

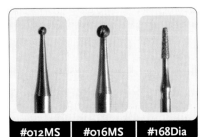

Fig. 11.95 Burs used in the preparation of a #3.2 lesion.

| #012MS | #016MS | #168Dia |

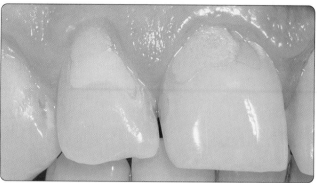

Fig. 11.96 Replacement of resins. Old #3.2 composite resins on labial of the central and lateral need replacement.

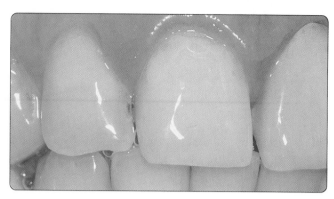

Fig. 11.97 Restoration. The two lesions shown in figure 11.96 were restored with glass–ionomer cement. The lateral was subsequently laminated with composite resin.

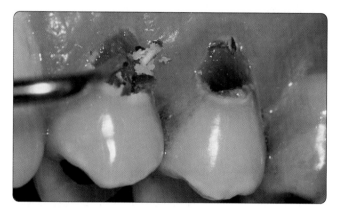

Fig. 11.98 Rampant caries, #3.2 lesion. Rampant caries present on both bicuspids.

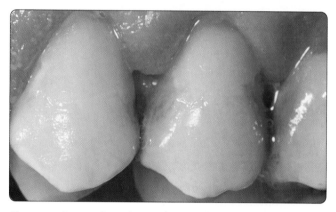

Fig. 11.99 Restoration. The two lesions shown in figure 11.98 restored with glass–ionomer only.

affected dentine on the axial wall. Use small diamonds (#168) at intermediate high speed to define the enamel outline but remain very conservative with demineralised enamel.

Restoration
Glass–ionomer is the material of choice and it can be either resin-modified or autocured depending on the ability to gain full access for light activation. Always condition the cavity with 10% polyacrylic acid for 10 seconds before placement. Use the cement at a high powder:liquid ratio for optimal physical properties, place carefully and always use a matrix to apply pressure for complete adaptation (**Figs 11.96– 11.99**).

SITE 3, SIZE 3; designated #3.3

G.V. Black classification – class V.

This category represents approximal lesions that have developed either as primary root surface caries after gingival recession or recurrent caries at the gingival margin of an existing restoration that is satisfactory in all other respects. Replacement of the entire original restoration may not be necessary; a conservative approach for the maintenance of the maximum amount of remaining tooth structure might be made from the facial or lingual side depending upon the position of the carious lesion. Aesthetic appeal will seldom be a problem, but access may be limited. Placement of rubber dam will be of assistance and a minor gingivectomy by electrosurgery or laser treatment may be justified.

Preparation
If there is a risk to the root surface of the adjacent tooth, place a short length of metal matrix band and wedge it lightly into place before beginning cavity preparation.

Use a small tapered diamond cylinder (#168) (**Fig. 11.100**)at intermediate high speed under air–water spray and approach the lesion from the most occlusal portion of the caries aiming gingivally towards the most gingival extent of the cavity. Open conservatively, sufficient to

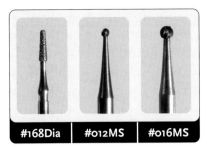

Fig. 11.100 Burs used in the preparation of a #3.3 lesion.

#168Dia   #012MS   #016MS

459–466

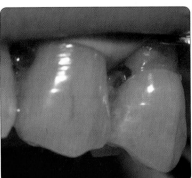

Fig. 11.101 Root surface caries, #3.3 lesion. There is a #3.3 lesion on the root surface at the mesial of the first bicuspid.

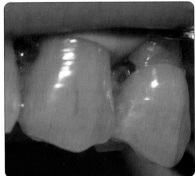

Fig. 11.102 Initial approach. Entry is gained from the occlusal margin aiming upwards and inwards towards the lesion.

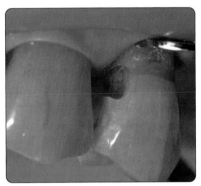

Fig. 11.103 Final cavity design. Refine the cavity with small round burs, cleaning the margins only and leaving the axial wall alone.

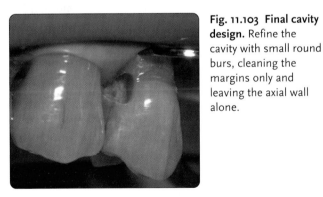

Fig. 11.105 Place the restoration. A resin-modified glass–ionomer was placed and light-activated from both labial and lingual.

achieve reasonable visibility. Carry out a gingivectomy if required and control haemorrhage with trichloroacetic acid. Remove caries around the walls and gingival floor with small round burs (#012, #016), with long shanks if required, and define the cavity outline. Proceed with caution on the axial wall because demineralised-affected dentine can be remineralised and can therefore remain covering the pulp so long as the margins are sealed. It is often difficult to identify a pulp exposure in such a cavity and care should be taken to avoid one. Whenever possible, retain a wall of tooth structure on the side opposite the access cavity because this will facilitate construction of a matrix and the ultimate placement of the restoration (**Figs 11.101–103**).

Restoration

A radiopaque autocure glass–ionomer is the material of choice because of its adhesion and fluoride release. The fast-setting Type II.2 cements are useful under these circumstances but, because they tend to lack translucency, aesthetic appeal may be a problem. A resin-modified cement can be placed where activator light access is not a problem. Condition the cavity with 10% polyacrylic acid and place a matrix and wedge it. If using a metal matrix, apply a light coat of a separator such as an unfilled resin. Syringe the cement into place in two increments. Tamp each into place with a small plastic sponge. Wrap the matrix around the tooth and allow the cement to set. Trim carefully to ensure there is no overhang or overcontour (**Figs 11.104–11.106**).

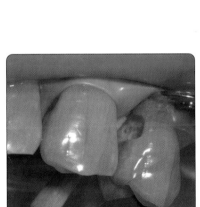

Fig. 11.104 Matrix. Use a short length of mylar strip as a matrix, supported lightly with a wedge. Condition the cavity with 10% polyacrylic acid for 10 seconds.

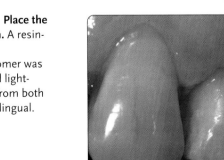

Fig. 11.106 Completed restoration. The completed restoration immediately after removing the rubber dam.

SITE 3, SIZE 4; DESIGNATED #3.4

G.V. Black classification – class V.

This category represents a combination of two or more cavities around the cervical margin of any tooth. The typical situation is likely to appear around a lone-standing lower canine where a labial #3.2 lesion is joined by another #3.3 lesion on the distal side and possibly even another #3.2 on the lingual side. Treatment remains similar to that for an individual lesion but is more complex to carry out.

Preparation

Retain as much natural tooth structure as possible, paying particular attention to the axial wall of the cavity. The demineralised affected dentine can often be remineralised and, if possible, should not be removed. Follow the recommendations under the 'atraumatic restorative treatment' technique (Chapter 18, page 213) where indicated.

Clean the walls only, using the small tapered diamond #168 (**Fig. 11.107**), and maintain as much enamel as possible. Remove infected dentine from the walls using small round burs (#012 or #016) taking care to maintain the axial wall. Condition the cavity as usual before placement of the cement (**Fig. 11.108–11.111**).

Restoration

Glass–ionomer is the material of choice because of adhesion properties and fluoride release. The greatest problem will be to construct a suitable matrix to facilitate placement of the cement. One technique is to cut a soft tin matrix to shape and then cut a small hole in an appropriate position, through which it is possible to syringe the cement. The matrix can then be placed and held with green-stick compound or a similar substance and left in place until the cement is set.

An alternative technique is to use a resin-modified cement and build the restoration incrementally with careful light-curing at each stage (**Figs 11.112** and **11.113**).

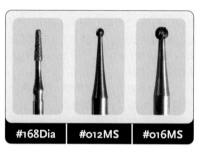
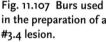

| #168Dia | #012MS | #016MS |

Fig. 11.107 **Burs used in the preparation of a #3.4 lesion.**

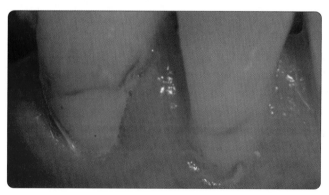

Fig. 11.108 **Complex cervical restoration, #3.4 lesion.** An old composite resin restoration is failing and requires replacement.

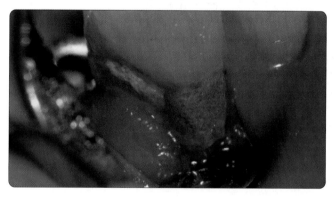

Fig. 11.109 **Lingual view.** A lingual view of the same tooth shown in Figure 11.108 showing general failure around to the lingual.

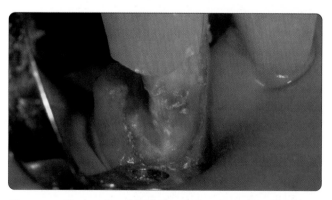

Fig. 11.110 **Final cavity – labial.** The final cavity outline from the labial.

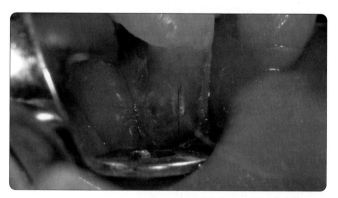

Fig. 11.111 **Final cavity – lingual.** The lingual view of the cavity. The axial wall consists of affected dentine that will later remineralise and that will therefore not be removed.

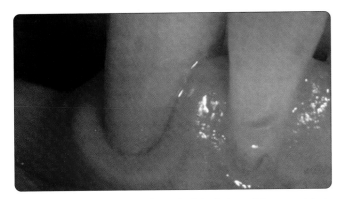

Fig. 11.112 Finished restoration. The labial view of the completed resin-modified glass–ionomer restoration 2 years after placement.

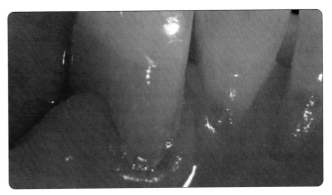

Fig. 11.113 Lingual view. A lingual view of the completed restoration 2 years after placement.

FURTHER READING

Black GV. *A work on operative dentistry; the technical procedures in filling teeth.* Chicago: Medico-Dental Publishing Company; 1917:5.

Cavel WT, Kelsey WP, Blankenau RJ. An in-vivo study of cuspal fracture. *J Prosthet Dent* 1985; **53**:38–42.

Doukoudakis S, Doukoudakis A. Amalgam onlay restoration. *J Prosthet Dent* 1991; **66**:493–7.

Evans JR, Wetz JH. The pinned amalgam restoration. Part 1 [Review]. *J Prosthet Dent* 1977; **37**:37–41.

Hasselrot L. Tunnel restorations: a three-and-a-half-year follow-up study of class I and II tunnel restorations in permanent and primary teeth. *Swed Dent J* 1993; **17**:173–82.

Hunt PR. A modified class II cavity preparation for glass–ionomer restorative materials. *Quintessence Int* 1984; **15**:1011–18.

Hunt PR. Micro conservative restorations for approximal carious lesions. *J Am Dent Assoc* 1990; **120**:37–40

Khera SC, Chan KC, Rittman BRJ. Dentinal crazing and interpin distance. *J Prosthet Dent* 1978; **40**:538–43

Knight GM. The use of adhesive materials in the conservative restoration of selected posterior teeth. *Aust Dent J* 1984; **29**:324–31

McCullock AJ, Smith BGN. In-vitro studies of cuspal movement produced by adhesive restorative materials. *Br Dent J* 1986; **161**:405–9.

Morand J-M, Jonas P. Resin-modified glass–ionomer cement restoration of posterior teeth with proximal carious lesions. *Quintessence Int* 1995; **26**:389–94.

Mount GJ. The use of amalgam to protect remaining tooth structure. *N Z Dent J* 1977; **73**:15–20.

Mount GJ. The three stages of the amalgam cavity. *Aust Dent J* 1978; **23**:75–80.

Mount GJ. Minimal treatment of the carious lesion. *Int Dent J* 1991; **41**:55–9.

Outhaite WC, Garman TA, Pashley DH. Pin *versus* slot retention in extensive amalgam restorations. *J Prosthet Dent* 1979; **41**:369–400.

Papa J, Wilson PR, Tyas MJ. Tunnel restorations [Review]. *J Esthet Dent* 1992; **4**(Suppl.):4–9

Plasmans PJJM, Willi PR, Vrijhoef MMA. The tensile resistance of extensive amalgam restorations with auxilliary retention. *Quintessence Int* 1986; **17**:411–4.

Plasmans PJJM, Kustors ST, De Jonge BA *et al.* In-vitro resistance of extensive amalgam restorations using various retention methods. *J Prosthet Dent* 1987; **57**:16–20.

Roydhouse RH, Richardson AS. The current clinical status of fissure sealants. *J Canad Dent Assoc* 1972; **38**:219–20.

Santos AC, Meiers JC. Fracture resistance of premolars with MOD amalgam restorations lined with amalgambond. *Oper Dent* 1994; **19**:2–6.

Shillingburg HT, Jacobi R, Brackett SE. Preparation modifications for damaged vital posterior teeth. *Dent Clin North Am* 1985; **29**:305–26.

Simonsen RJ. Cost effectivness of pit and fissure sealant at 10 years. *Quintessence Int* 1989; **20**:75–84.

Starr CB. Amalgam crown restorations for posterior pulpless teeth. *J Prosthet Dent* 1990; **63**:614–9.

Zenker JEA, Baratieri I, Monteiro S, Andrada MAC, Vieira LCC. Clinical and radiographic evaluation of cermet tunnel restorations on primary molars. *Quintessence Int* 1993; 24:783–91.

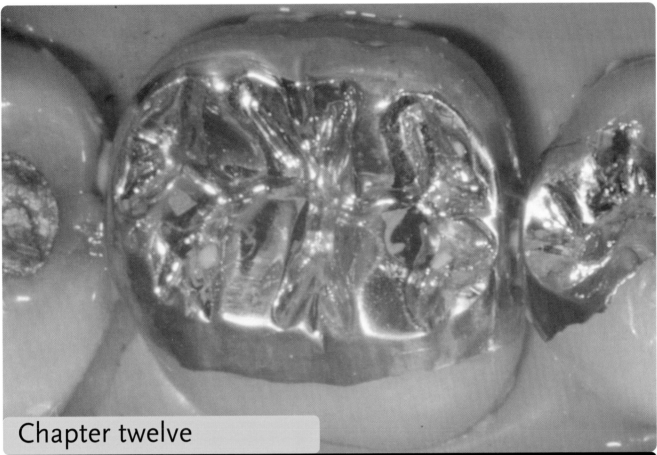

Chapter twelve

Rigid materials used in tooth restoration

D. Southan

This chapter deals with the rigid materials that can be used in the restoration of teeth following caries or fracture.

Because the materials are themselves as rigid and inflexible as the tooth, the techniques used for the construction of the restoration are almost invariably indirect, meaning that a model replica of the tooth or teeth must be constructed first and the restoration then constructed from the model, on the laboratory bench. Although this is a time-consuming procedure and requires a number of steps, each of which is subject to human error, the end result, when properly carried out, is the closest possible reproduction of original correct dental anatomy that can be achieved.

Structures can be described as rigid or flexible. A rigid material has a high modulus of elasticity and can resist high stress without permanent deformation. Rigid substances are almost perfectly elastic and many behave in a brittle fashion at room temperature.

The rigidity of any structure is controlled by the inherent elastic modulus of the material, the thickness of the structure and its shape. Otherwise, rigid materials can be made flexible when the relative dimensions of the body are changed. A long, thin glass rod can be flexible, whereas a thick slab of the same material behaves in a rigid fashion. Ductility is the antithesis to rigidity. Ductile substances can be permanently deformed easily at room temperature. Ceramic materials are rigid – pure gold is ductile.

FACTORS TO CONSIDER IN THE SELECTION OF RIGID MATERIALS

The physical properties of a tooth are the result of its complex composite structure and the manner in which it is supported within the bone by the periodontal ligament. The enamel–dentine complex displays a brilliant marriage of hard tissues with differing rigidity. Enamel, the harder mantle, with a modulus of elasticity approaching 100 GPa, is supported by a base of dentine, with a modulus of elasticity of 14–28 GPa. The Vickers pyramid hardness number for enamel is about 300, whereas that of dentine is only about 60. When teeth are vital and sound they are rigid and their composite structure endows them with a high resistance to fracture and, in function, teeth do not deform permanently.

Intact, a tooth is ideally suited for physiological function; this involves dynamic change in its form and, with normal function, the dentition wears without loss of vertical dimension, strength or efficiency.

Physical factors

However, teeth are prone to some structural loss caused by attrition and erosion. If hard dental tissue is lost from disease or trauma, this delicate balance may be severely upset. When a tooth loses both its enamel and its dentine foundation from caries, its physical integrity as well as its biological integrity is compromised. The major requirement when replacing lost tooth structure is to replace form and function in the most satisfactory manner. As discussed previously, the plastic restorative materials are satisfactory in small lesions but, as the problem of restoration of form and function becomes more extensive, the need to employ rigid materials increases in an attempt to reinstate the original anatomy and function of the tooth.

Biological factors

Another important factor in selecting a restorative material is the biocompatibility of the material. This embraces the surface chemistry, texture and toxicity as well as the physical and optical properties.

In the past, pure gold foil was used with a high degree of success to restore proximal and facial cavities in teeth. This is a ductile material which can be cold-welded at room temperature, so it can be condensed into well-defined undercut areas in dentine and worked over bevelled enamel cavo–surface margins. A successful restoration is held in compression by the stressed dentine and its surface is work-hardened during the burnishing process. However, there is a risk in attempting to retain such a ductile material in stressed dentine. Initial adaptation to bevelled margins may be achieved, but the seal may be lost through permanent deformation of the restoration under load.

Therefore, rigid materials should be employed where function without permanent deformation is required. On the other hand, when using relatively fragile aesthetic restorative materials such as a porcelain veneer or metal–ceramic complexes, a rigid foundation is essential.

The following are the materials most commonly used for the construction of rigid restorations.

NOBLE METAL ALLOYS

There are a number of sound reasons for the selection of noble metals and their alloys for the restoration of teeth. Principally, they resist oxidation and are not attacked by acids. Seven metals meet this definition: gold, platinum, palladium, rubidium, ruthenium, osmium and iridium; however, only the first three of these are used in dentistry, and their inert properties are of great value in the hostile environment of the mouth.

Pure metals are generally very soft and can be easily shaped and worked. Gold, platinum, silver, aluminium, copper and tin have been used in dentistry because they can be permanently bent or shaped. However, this ductility is not acceptable in load-bearing restorations and, to remedy this, metals are combined with one another to produce alloys with more acceptable properties for the task in hand. In 1907, Taggert patented a dental casting process using a lost-wax technique. The development of gold alloys suitable for dentistry followed around 1917–20, but standards and specifications were not established by the American Dental Association until the mid-1930s.

Selection of alloys for crowns and bridges should be based on a rational appraisal of the properties relevant to the intended use of the alloy, which are:
- physical and chemical properties
- biocompatibility
- ease of handling
- compatibility with ceramics.

Dental gold alloys

There are essentially four types of gold alloy that have been developed for dental use with diverse properties designed for particular tasks.

Type I (A or soft)

These alloys contain up to 10% silver and 5% copper, and should only be employed in low-stress situations, such as proximal and facial cavities, under no occlusal load. They are relatively soft and easily burnished, and cannot be heat treated. They melt at 900–1000°C and are cast in a gypsum-bonded investment mould that has been heated to 700°C. Their essential properties are:
- proportional limit – 85 MPa
- elongation to failure – 25%
- maximum hardness – 75 BHN (Brinell Hardness Number).

Type II (B or medium)

These alloys contain up to 15% silver, 10% copper, 1% platinum, 4% palladium and 1% zinc, but never less than 78% noble metals. They are readily burnished and can be employed for most types of inlays. They melt at 920–980°C

and are cast in a gypsum-bonded investment mould that has been heated to 700°C. Their essential properties are:
- proportional limit – 160 MPa
- elongation to failure – 24%
- maximum hardness – 100 BHN.

Type III (C or hard)
These alloys contain up to 26% silver, 11% copper, 3% platinum, 4% palladium and 1% zinc, but never less than 78% noble metals. Quenching after casting will soften the metal to allow for burnishing; heat treatment will reharden the casting. They are ideal for crowns and bridges or when a thin section of metal is required for protection of underlying tooth structure. They melt at 900–1000°C and are cast in a gypsum-bonded investment mould that has been heated to 700°C. Their essential properties are:
- proportional limit – 195 MPa (as cast); 290 MPa (heat treated)
- elongation to failure – 20% (as cast); 10% (heat treated)
- maximum hardness – 140 BHN (as cast); 179 BHN (heat treated).

Type IV (D or extra hard)
These alloys contain up to 20% silver, 16% copper, 4% platinum, 5% palladium and 2% zinc, but never less than 75% noble metals. They are used principally in partial denture construction. They melt at 850–950°C and are cast in a gypsum-bonded investment mould that has been heated to 700°C. They are subject to heat treatment and their essential properties are:
- proportional limit –360 MPa (as cast); 585 MPa (heat treated)
- elongation to failure – 15% (as cast); 10% (heat treated)
- maximum hardness – 150 BHN (as cast); 230 BHN (heat treated).

High gold content alloys for metal–ceramic techniques
The standard gold-containing alloy for metal–ceramic restorations contains about 85% gold with approximately 6% platinum and 5% palladium. The metals are carefully proportioned to control thermal expansion and contraction and contain additives of up to 1% silver and traces of indium, iron and tin to promote hardness, proper oxide formation and controlled grain growth. The coefficient of thermal expansion needs to be compatible with the porcelain, and they require a yield strength and Brinell hardness in the range of Type IV casting gold. The melting point should be 1200–1250°C. A phosphate-bonded investment is used and the casting should be cooled slowly for maximum hardness and strength. Their essential properties are:
- proportional limit – 265 MPa
- elongation to failure – 3%
- maximum hardness – 150 BHN.

Heat treatment of alloys
As noted above, not all alloys are subject to modification of properties through heat treatment but, under certain conditions, this can be a valuable asset. For example, when using a type III alloy for a gold inlay, it may be sufficiently soft after casting to allow a degree of burnishing along the margins, on the model or in the mouth, to correct minor deficiencies. Then, after polishing, it can be heat treated and hardened just before cementation. The following are the standard procedures required for successful heat treatment of alloys.

Softening
Heat to red heat (700°C) to produce a disordered solid solution and immediately quench in water. Because the solid solution remains disordered, dislocations in the lattice can move and the alloy can be shaped by mechanical deformation.

Hardening
Heat to red heat (700°C) and then allow temperature to fall and hold at about 420°C for 10 minutes before bench-cooling. This allows an ordered solid solution to form a super-lattice, which interferes with dislocations. Hardness and proportional limit are raised and elongation and ductility are reduced.

Fracture process in gold alloys
Gold alloys can be tough. This is the property that allows such alloys to absorb the energy of fine cracks – that threaten constantly to spread and lead to complete rupture – generated by the stresses and strains imposed upon them. The classic means of controlling crack propagation in metals is to relieve the concentration of stress by glissile dislocations. The property of toughness endows gold alloys with a clinical dynamism so that, in thin section, they resist high occlusal loading without catastrophic fracture. Such a property is not available in ceramics.

Gold alloys may therefore be employed in high-stress situations where aesthetic considerations are minor and relatively thin sections in the restoration are necessary or desirable. The alloy selected for a given situation must be rigid enough to resist permanent deformation. In the presence of deformation there could be marginal leakage that would be difficult to detect until the tooth had sustained gross damage. For restorations under heavy stress, use an alloy with a high modulus of elasticity and include some form of buttressing to increase the thickness in selected sections of the cavity design.

Balancing ductility against rigidity
The ability to be able to vary the balance between the properties of ductility and rigidity in gold restorations is very valuable. Accessible margins can be burnished onto a cavo-surface bevel with ductile alloys but not when using rigid alloys. However, a balance can be achieved by softening the alloy and burnishing the margin and then heat treating it to strengthen and harden it again before cementation.

PORCELAIN

Porcelain is used for the construction of aesthetic restorations such as jacket crowns, inlays and laminated veneers; it can be used alone or in conjunction with metal alloys, which can be incorporated as a foundation or reinforcement. It is the most biologically and aesthetically acceptable material available to dentistry. It is basically a pigmented glass crystal composite. Most modern dental porcelains consist of homogenised, fritted powders with short, low-temperature sintering cycles; that is, they are 'low fusing'.

Vitreous matrix

The vitreous matrix of dental porcelain is a silicate glass, which can be regarded as an inorganic product of fusion that has cooled to a rigid state without crystallising. Silica (SiO_2) is the prototype of the glass-forming oxides; the constituent Si^{4+} ion is small, highly charged and just fills the space between four oxygen atoms. If the chemical composition of the melt does not provide sufficient oxygen ions to permit the formation of independent SiO_4 groups, the tetrahedra must share oxygen ions; it is this sharing of oxygens that is the main reason why silicate melts polymerise. On cooling, the polymerisation increases the viscosity of the melt very rapidly and finally leads to a rigid three-dimensional network. Because of the high charge of the silicon ion, SiO_2 produces open structures. Glass is not a chemical compound in the ordinary sense of the word, inasmuch as its unit cell is infinitely large, and consequently there is no restriction with regard to relative numbers of chemically different atoms, providing always that the valences are balanced.

Aluminosilicate glass

In moderate amounts, Al^{3+} can replace Si^{4+} in vitreous structures, so the matrices in dental porcelains are aluminosilicate glasses. They contain a major percentage of silica, and are characterised by their high softening temperatures. Al^{3+} ions form AlO_4 tetrahedra with similar dimensions to SiO_4 tetrahedra, and these groups are the characteristic structural elements in aluminosilicate glasses $[Al^{3+}(O^{2-}/_2)_4]$. The AlO_4 tetrahedra have negative charges, which neutralise the charges of univalent cations that are accommodated in the interstices between tetrahedra in a continuous network. In a sodium aluminosilicate glass, the binding force between an Na^+ ion and the surrounding network is weak. It is represented by the whole tetrahedron.

$$Na^+[Al^{3+}(O^{2-}/_2)_4]^-$$

Therefore, the matrices of dental porcelains can be regarded as three-dimensional random networks of SiO_4 and AlO_4 tetrahedra with alkaline earth ions acting as modifiers of the network (**Fig. 12.1**).

Most of these are highly vitreous because of the presence of aluminosilicate glass particles with variable compositions. The cations included in the particles can be K^+, Na^+ and Ca^{2+}.

($K_2O.Al_2O_3.6SiO_2, Na_2O.Al_2O_3.6SiO_2, CaO.Al_2O_3.2SiO_2$) Dispersion strengthening with alumina improves their physical properties; the thermal expansion of some porcelains has been increased by raising the potassium content such that leucite ($K_2O.Al_2O_3.4SiO_2$) is precipitated in the glassy matrix. This will raise the thermal expansion to match that of a metal alloy, which can be placed underneath as a supporting framework. However, it also opacifies and weakens the porcelains.

Optical properties and aesthetics

Dental porcelain can be highly translucent and this makes it very valuable and versatile as a dental restorative material. It consists of crystals of alumina, quartz, or both, suspended in a vitreous matrix containing pigment and pores. The matrix in metal–ceramics supports leucite crystals ($K_2O.Al_2O_3.4SiO_2$), pigment, opacifiers and minor gaseous inclusions; it is the reflection and refraction of light at the interfaces between phases that scatters the light. The degree of scattering is a function of the relative refractive indices of the different phases, their particle sizes, shapes and volume concentrations. Porosity and the presence of pigment and crystalline inclusions have a marked opacifying effect.

The fracture process in dental porcelain

Dental porcelains are brittle materials, but this is not necessarily synonymous with weakness. Because of the strength of the silicon–oxygen bond and the absence of grain boundaries, the vitreous matrices of dental porcelains have a high intrinsic tensile strength. The approximate elastic moduli of the various types of porcelain is listed below.

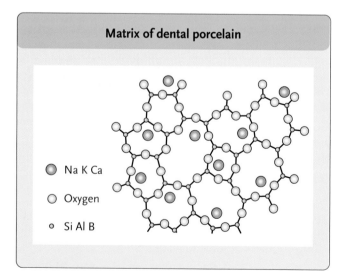

Matrix of dental porcelain

- ⬤ Na K Ca
- ◯ Oxygen
- ∘ Si Al B

Fig. 12.1 Matrix of dental porcelain. A two-dimensional model of a three-dimensional random network of SiO_4 and AlO_4 tetrahedra. B^{3+} ions may also be involved and, sometimes, Ca^{2+}, Na^+ and K^+ will be present to modify the network.

Elastic modulus (E)
- Quartz-bearing dental porcelains – 57 GPa
- Aluminous body materials – 63 GPa
- Aluminous core materials – 99 GPa

Roughly, a strain of 0.1–0.2 is required before a plane of atoms is completely removed from the attractive force of its neighbours. Rupture, then, would be expected at a maximum stress of 0.1–0.2 E. The theoretical strength would be about 5.7–11.4 GPa for a porcelain with an elastic modulus of 57 GPa. However, the measured strength of various dental porcelains ranges from about 50 MPa to 100 MPa. This discrepancy arises because dental porcelain is almost perfectly elastic; hence its measured strength is strongly dependent upon the presence or absence of surface defects and flaws.

Fracture propagation

Fracture occurs in tension and is caused by stress concentration at the tip of a surface flaw. Classic stress release at the crack tip in metals takes place by glissile dislocations. This is not possible in a vitreous material where fracture occurs when the applied stress produces a stress at the flaw tip equal to the intrinsic strength of its matrix. This would occur at the most severe flaw present in the stressed region, one that could magnify the macroscopic stress by two orders of magnitude. Once initiated, the extension of the crack is ensured by the applied stress and the increasing stress–concentration factor of the growing crack (**Fig. 12.2**). The presence of flaws in dental porcelain is by far the most important factor in determining its practical strength. Other factors, such as varied chemical composition of the matrix and the presence of internal voids, may have a direct influence on measured strength, but these are of minor interest.

Static fatigue

Exposure to water reduces the strength of dental porcelain, causing delayed failure. This phenomenon, called 'static fatigue', is a property of glasses generally and is similar to stress corrosion cracking in metals. However, fatigue of glass differs appreciably from fatigue of metals. No structural change can occur in glass before failure and glass does not fatigue under cyclic loading any faster than it does under a static load.

Delayed failure in glasses has been attributed to a stress-enhanced chemical reaction between the glass and water; this is likely to occur primarily at the tips of surface cracks where stresses are high. Water reacts with glass, destroying the Si–O network, and hydroxyl ions attack the siloxane bonds of the network structure.

$$OH^- + R\text{–}Si\text{–}O\text{–}Si\text{–}R \Rightarrow R\text{–}SiOH + R\text{–}SiO^-$$

The silanolate groups formed by this reaction are strongly basic and can be hydrolysed by water to form silanol groups and hydroxyl ions.

$$R\text{–}SiO^- + H_2O \Rightarrow R\text{–}SiOH + OH^-$$

Crack propagation is believed to be influenced markedly by the crack tip hydroxyl ion concentration. Catastrophic failure occurs when the crack length becomes critical; that is, when it is able to magnify the macroscopic stress to a stress equivalent to the theoretical strength of the vitreous matrix at the crack tip. Also, in the presence of water, the amount of energy required to rupture the silicon–oxygen bond between two silica tetrahedra is diminished by a factor of about 20. Atomic studies of fracture suggest the possibility for controlling the strength of brittle materials by designing surface coatings to block the opening of the crack and restrict the passage of small molecules, such as water.

The concept of an endurance limit, or a load that a specimen will withstand indefinitely, is important. There is an intermediate stress at which the tendencies to sharpen the crack by 'stress corrosion' and to blunt it by ageing are just balanced; this may account for the existence of an endurance limit in dental porcelain.

Clinical implications

The relatively thin sections of porcelain in a dental crown are supported mostly on a base of dentine (E = 14–18 GPa) and the intervening cement film (E = 9.1 GPa). However, dentine has only a limited ability to support a restorative material because of its relatively low elastic modulus (**Fig. 12.3**); a strain of only 8–10 μm/cm in dental porcelain is required before it fractures.

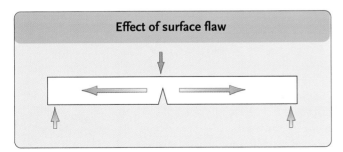

Fig. 12.2 Effect of surface flaw. Diagram shows how a surface flaw in a brittle material magnifies an observed macroscopic stress into a high microscopic stress.

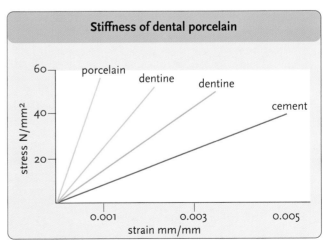

Fig. 12.3 Stiffness of dental porcelain. A graph showing the relative stiffness of dental porcelain compared with dentine and an average type of dental luting cement.

The endurance limit of porcelain may be low enough to be below the functional loading experienced by a crown; thus, when dental porcelain is subjected to loads that are, initially, sub-destructive but above its endurance limit, its behaviour will be unpredictable. Any loading above this limit could be harmful and it should be noted that intermittent overloading may lead to a reduction in the endurance limit.

It seems that bending stresses are of major importance in ceramic restorations and, in order to increase their reliability in service, they need to be either well supported or stiffened.

Methods of manufacture of porcelain restorations

There are two important techniques for the manufacture of dental restorations in porcelain alone. The first involves swaging a platinum matrix on to a model of the tooth and then building the porcelain on the matrix. The crown and the matrix can then be removed from the model for placement in the furnace. The second method requires the construction of a model in a refractory plaster, onto which the porcelain can be built directly; being of a suitable refractory material, the model itself can be placed in the furnace. A third method of supporting porcelain on a metal foundation will be discussed on page 163.

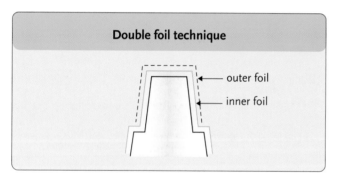

Double foil technique

outer foil
inner foil

Fig. 12.4 Double foil technique. The inner foil is laid down in the traditional style with an apron around the cervical shoulder. The outer foil is then laid over that and cut short by approximately 0.5 mm from the shoulder. The outer foil remains in place permanently attached to the porcelain.

Fabricated on single platinum foil matrix

This technique requires the construction of a pure platinum foil matrix directly on to a model of the prepared tooth. The model must be very strong because the action of swaging the platinum is relatively vigorous to ensure proper adaptation. A strong model is generally produced by copper plating the impression before pouring a model in a resin or hard stone. The platinum is then swaged on to the copper model and a porcelain slurry can be built up on the matrix.

The original technique was to swage a single layer of platinum on to the dye and use a tinner's joint on the lingual to produce a relatively accurate representation of the tooth preparation. After completion of the firing cycles the platinum was peeled out from the inside of the crown. Generally, the fit of the crown on the tooth was still sufficiently accurate, leaving space for a thin, even layer of cement to lute the crown to place.

Fabrication on double platinum foil matrix

A modification to the above procedure is to swage a second layer of platinum foil over the first and cut it back to clear at least 0.5 mm from the gingival shoulder. The second bonnet can be plated with tin and will thus become firmly attached to the porcelain, so that the second layer of platinum is retained within the finished crown (**Fig. 12.4**).

One of the greatest weaknesses in porcelain crowns is the potential for the inclusion of porosities, which will lead to crack propagation (**Fig. 12.5**). Using the platinum foil techniques for construction the porosities occur as sub-surface polymorphic pore strata at the internal surfaces. They communicate with the surface through relatively small openings and may be largely responsible for high cement retention. The concentration of the defects is unpredictable, but there is a predilection for surface porosities near the gingival shoulder (**Fig. 12.6**), and empty spherical bubbles within glass may cause a stress concentration of about 2.

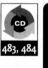

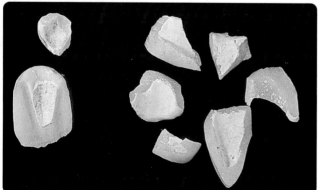

Fig. 12.5 Fractured crowns. Cement clings to sections of fractured porcelain crowns held there by mechanical interlock with the minor porosities in the surface.

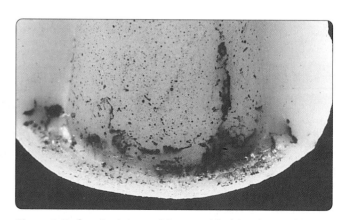

Fig. 12.6 Defects in the porcelain. Lampblack has been rubbed into porosities and defects on the inner surface of a porcelain crown. Note the concentration at the gingival.

Probable fracture process

In the fracture process it is probable that most cracks start from the inner surfaces, especially at or near the gingival margins. In the vicinity of the cervical shoulder, flaws tend to become flattened and polymorphous and these have stress concentrating powers greater than spheres, and are, therefore, up to twice as dangerous as flaws elsewhere of the same shape and size. After condensation, there must be intimate contact between the glass and the foil to achieve optimal adaptation or bonding after sintering. Poor adaptation of aluminous core porcelain to the platinum matrix is a major problem because the aluminous particles are unreactive, even at the core firing temperatures, and are unlikely to bond to the platinum foil, whether it is tin coated or plain.

Fabricated on a pervious refractory matrix

The use of a pervious refractory die for producing porcelain crowns will limit the occurrence of internal faults and will still consistently produce crowns that are precisely adapted to the prepared tooth.

Following the preparation of a master die of the crown preparation, it is coated with a predetermined and accurate layer of 'relief' to allow room for the luting cement, and an impression is taken in vinyl polysiloxane. A duplicate die is then made in a phosphate-type investment that contains no carbon. Appropriate thermal expansion is achieved by mixing 3.5 ml of distilled water with 25 g of investment powder. The die must be pervious to allow for condensation of core porcelain slurry down onto its surface by absorption of the suspension medium through its body. It must also have a thermal expansion that is similar to that of alumina.

The next step is to construct a high-fusing ceramic core or framework, upon which further applications of more translucent, lower fusing porcelain can be made. The core must be dimensionally stable at moderate firing temperatures and, at the same time, it must provide an optically acceptable background for the crown. Aluminous porcelain is satisfactory when it is filled with enough chemically bound, appropriately sized alumina crystals, providing it is fired properly.

Function of core build-up

The function of the core material is not to impart additional strength to the crown, but to provide a stable framework for subsequent applications of more translucent, lower-fusing, aluminous porcelain.

When the full-thickness core build-up is fired for the first time large cracks must appear in it if the internal surface of the core is to be free of defects. The cracks are then filled with a thin, high-fusing core slurry, right down to the porous die, by absorbing the suspension medium through the die. No extra thickness should be added to the framework at this stage and the cracks ought to be healed completely at the second firing. Hold the core at a high temperature (1150°C) and at atmospheric pressure (without vacuum) for

10–15 minutes to allow optimal condensation of the glassy matrix to occur around the impediment provided by the skeletal, refractory alumina grains.

Strengthening processes available for dental porcelain

All successful methods of strengthening glass without significantly interfering with its translucency have required the introduction of a compressive stress at the surface to offset the tensile stress developed under a load or impact. With these techniques the intrinsic strength of glass is employed indirectly, because a high compressive stress at the surface can only be sustained by a comparable internal tensile stress (**Fig. 12.7**). The following two methods can be employed to strengthen dental porcelain.

Dispersion strengthening

As noted above, toughness in metals is achieved by controlling crack propagation because the concentration of stress at the tip of a crack is relieved by glissile dislocations. However, there are other heterogeneous biological materials that are tough and nonductile, such as wood, bone and teeth, which do not relieve stress through glissile dislocation. What appears to be common to these composite substances is that they contain large numbers of interfaces, or planes of potential cleavage, that provide numerous weak interfaces across the path of a tensile crack, and prevents it from propagating by a simple process of increasing stress concentration. Glass–alumina composite systems function in this way. However, opacity is a feature of all heterogeneous systems and presents a severe practical limitation to the use of this method in the dental field.

In aluminous porcelains, the alumina-reinforcing phase is prefritted with the glassy phase to improve the bond with the glassy matrix and these glass–crystal composites behave as constant strain systems with rupture strength dependent on their elastic moduli. Core materials with 45–50% alumina have an elastic modulus of around 99 GPa.

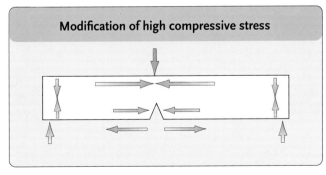

Fig. 12.7 Modification of high compressive stress. Diagram showing how a high compressive stress at the tip of a surface crack can modify the effect that a low tensile stress at the surface has in this region.

Chemical strengthening

Although flaws throughout the body of a crown are capable of initiating fracture, it is those at the surface that have the greatest effect. The magnitude of the tensile stress at the tip of a surface crack determines whether or not fracture will occur. It follows that prevention of fracture under a particular load requires the production of a definite compressive stress at the tip of the crack (**Fig. 12.7**). The strength of aluminous dental porcelain can be trebled by chemical treatment and the endurance limit can be increased by at least the same factor.

Chemical strengthening can be carried out by replacing cations in the surface layers of the vitreous matrix with larger ions while the matrix remains below its transformation region and is, therefore, capable of supporting the compressive stress developed. This is called low-temperature ionic crowding. Sodium ions in the matrix can be replaced by larger potassium ions by immersing the porcelain crown in a bath of molten potassium nitrate (**Fig. 12.8**) The technique is as follows.

- Characterise the finished crown and adjust the occlusion. Glaze it to the stage at which it is ready to be cemented.
- Place the crown onto a mound of analytically pure crystalline potassium nitrate powder held in either a small porcelain crucible or a stainless steel container. The internal parts of the crown should be packed with the powder to ensure that it sinks into the melting salt and does not float on the surface.
- Place the container into a cool furnace and raise the temperature slowly to 500°C. Aluminous porcelain should never be heated quickly since cracking can occur because of the different coefficients of thermal expansion of the core, dentine and enamel porcelains. The crown must remain completely submerged.

- Hold the temperature at 500°C for 6 hours.
- Remove the crown from the solution and allow it to drain in the furnace.
- Remove the crown from the furnace and cool to room temperature, then wash in warm water.
- The crown is ready for cementation. A limited amount of occlusal adjustment can still be done without significant detriment to its strength.

Under no circumstance should a chemically strengthened crown be fired again because there will be deeper migration of ions from the crowded ionic surface layer, creating tensile stresses at the surface.

Effect of strengthening processes on translucency

Translucency is the ratio of the intensity of the transmitted light to that of the incident light. Opacity is the reciprocal of the translucency and optical density is the common logarithm of the opacity. The translucency of a body is defined as the fraction of incident visible light from a specified source that is transmitted through or from that body. Generally, all processes designed to strengthen porcelain tend to increase opacity. The original intensity of the incident light is reduced in several ways between incidence and final emergence. Some reflections occur at the entry face, although a portion of the light may be absorbed within the body by the glass or by other components. Scattering of light within the body diminishes the intensity of the emerging beam because some of the light is reflected in a backward direction.

Reflection and refraction of light at the interfaces between phases scatter the light so the degree of scattering is a function of the relative refractive indices of the different phases, particle size and shape and volume concentrations. Both porosity and dispersion strengthening will increase opacity but chemical strengthening has little effect.

Effect of surface abrasion on strength

Chemically strengthened dental porcelain has a low optical density–strength coefficient and this is highly desirable for an aesthetic restoration. Cutting a scratch in the tensile surface of porcelain weakens it considerably, particularly for untreated porcelain where the reduction of strength can be in the order of 80%. However, the same scratch in chemically treated porcelain will lead to a reduction of about 60%. Grinding the surface will do far less damage.

The porcelain–enamel complex

Surface flaws, voids and cracks are the greatest weakness in porcelain and tensile stress in their presence will lead to failure. However, if a porcelain surface can be bonded mechanically or chemically to a solid base support it will become more difficult to inflict tensile strain on the bonded surface. This means that a porcelain veneer bonded to enamel through a resin-based cement will have considerable strength. Care must be taken to preserve enamel so as not to sacrifice the stiff support and, conversely, gross enamel loss will severely compromise the prognosis. Both

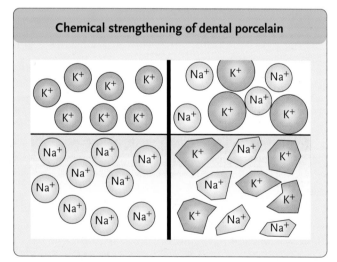

Chemical strengthening of dental porcelain

Fig. 12.8 Chemical strengthening of dental porcelain. A diagrammatic representation of the ion exchange that occurs in the surface layer of porcelain as a result of immersion in pure crystalline potassium nitrate at 500°C for 6 hours as described.

the enamel and the porcelain should be etched and a silane coupling agent applied to the clean, dry porcelain fitting surface to obtain the strongest bond possible.

METAL–CERAMICS

Combination of metal and porcelain

The metal–ceramic crown is the most widely used restoration in fixed prosthodontics, although the combination of the two materials places additional demands on the physical properties of both.

Porcelains and their properties

As discussed above there are very few modifications available which can be incorporated in porcelain, so variations must be found in the metal alloys.

Alloys and their properties

The alloys used in this work can be subject to great variation and they are very different from the traditional gold alloys discussed previously. These alloys must not only possess acceptable mechanical properties, such as high modulus of elasticity, high yield strength and hardness, but they must also show a high resistance to creep at elevated temperatures and a thermal expansion which matches the porcelain that is fused on to them.

They must be sufficiently rigid to retain form under stress. Young's modulus is a measure of rigidity; so, in a given framework design placed under a constant load, the higher the modulus the lower the degree of elastic deformation. Young's modulus is inversely proportional to the cube of the thickness. Therefore, the same degree of elastic deformation is produced when, on changing thickness, other parameters are kept constant. This means that if the thickness of metal is to be decreased by a factor of 2, the metal used should have a Young's modulus eight times greater to obtain the same degree of elastic deformation. Base metal alloys generally have a Young's modulus about twice that of noble alloys.

The bond between the two

The bond between porcelain and metal cannot contribute significantly to the strength of the crown so, to minimise stresses forming at the interface, the thermal expansion of both the metal and porcelain must be compatible. The primary function of the bond is to prevent the porcelain peeling from the metal sub-base after it fractures and, in fact, even low bonding strengths can be effective.

Metal–ceramic alloys

A large number of metal–ceramic alloys have been developed for dental applications and they can be classified in groups as follows.

- Noble metal alloys
    high gold
    gold–platinum–palladium
    gold–platinum–tantalum
- Low gold
    gold–palladium–silver
    gold–palladium
- Gold-free
    palladium–silver
    palladium–indium–tin–cobalt
    palladium–tin–gallium
- Base metal alloys
    nickel–chrome
    cobalt–chrome (rare).

The metal–ceramic bond

Several theories have been advanced to explain the adhesion of porcelain to the metal alloys used in dentistry.

- Chemical reaction theory proposes that primary valence bonds occur at the interface between alloy substrate oxides and the porcelain. Chemical reactions probably occur, but there is no proof that the products increase the mechanical strength of the bond.
- Van der Waals bond theory considers the development of adhesion through wetting to be the main source of bonding.
- Diffusion theory postulates the diffusion of metal ions across the interface. Elements such as indium, tin and iron in noble alloys and nickel and chromium in nickel alloys diffuse into the porcelain during firing.
- Mechanical bond theory suggests a micromechanical interlock between the two materials.

Failures in bonding are almost always cohesive inasmuch as failure takes place either in the adhesive, the adherent or in the weaker oxide layer. Microscopic study of the interfacial separation region following fracture is necessary to determine the weakest layer. Adhesive failure is normally only observed with pure noble metals.

Metal–ceramic porcelain

The ceramic used in the metal–ceramic crown can be modified to a very limited degree to assist in reducing the stresses imposed on the union of the two materials. Aluminosilicate glasses containing up to 11% potassium oxide have a firing temperature of about 1250°C and cannot be crystallised by prolonged heating. However, the softening temperature can be lowered by decreasing the alumina content and increasing the sodium oxide content as well as adding alkaline earth oxides and zinc oxide. The glass-forming oxide, B_2O_3, also has a pronounced effect on the softening point of silicate glasses. Typical compositions of materials firing at different temperatures are shown in **Figure 12.9**.

Low firing jacket crown porcelains have a thermal expansion coefficient in the range $5.5–7.5 \times 10^{-6}/°C$, thus making them compatible with platinum and iridio-platinum alloys. However, the metal–ceramic noble metal and base metal nickel–chromium alloys have a thermal expansion coefficient of about $13.5–15.5 \times 10^{-6}/°C$.

In 1962, Weinstein *et al.* described the production of metal–ceramic restorations on dental alloy frameworks using porcelain powders containing 11–15% potassium oxide. Thermal expansion was controlled by mixing feldspar-based compositions with high K_2O frits, resulting in the crystallisation of leucite ($K_2O.Al_2O_3.4SiO_2$), which has a coefficient of thermal expansion of about $27 \times 10^{-6}/°C$.

When soda–potash aluminosilicate glasses containing not less than 11% K_2O are subjected to heat treatment at temperatures from 700°C to 1200°C, leucite will crystallise out. To increase the base glass thermal expansion to the $13.5–15.5 \times 10^{-6}/°C$ range required for porcelain–metal bonding, 15–25% leucite is required. The proportion of leucite is governed by the K_2O content and the temperature and time of heat treatment. **Figure 12.10** shows an average composition for a dental metal–ceramic porcelain.

Leucite crystals form in the glassy matrix and if these inclusions reach a critical size they will reduce both the strength and thermal expansion. This can lead to crack formation in the matrix with a reduction in coupling between the phases.

The refractive index of leucite is 1.508–1.509 and that of the porcelain matrix is about 1.495, so the effect of the leucite crystals on the translucency of the porcelain is not significant.

Comparison: noble metal *versus* base metal alloys in metal–ceramics

Advantages of gold alloys

The gold–platinum–palladium alloys are very acceptable chemically. They are easy to cast and, since the addition of base metals such as indium and tin can be carefully controlled, oxide production is not excessive. The tin and indium oxides diffuse into the porcelain at the interface, bringing the metal into atomic contact with the porcelain. For most clinical situations the strength of gold alloys is adequate for coronal restoration. Gold–palladium alloys have higher melting temperatures and, therefore, a reduced risk of metal creep on firing. They also possess good mechanical properties

Disadvantages of gold alloys

High gold alloys are more expensive and they can undergo metal creep when the porcelain is fired onto them. The melting range for alloys containing 84–85% gold is close to the porcelain firing temperature of 900–950°C.

Advantages of base metal alloys

Base metal alloys are cheaper than noble metal alloys. They have a higher melting range and their modulus of elasticity is twice that of the noble metal alloys. They possess exceptional strength, especially at high temperatures, and are poor thermal conductors.

Disadvantages of base metal alloys

Base metal alloys have less than half the density of gold alloys and are more chemically reactive. When freezing from the molten state the shrinkage is 60% greater than that of noble alloys and the casting technique needs to be modified accordingly. They oxidise readily, even though they contain approximately 20% chromium to protect against corrosion and tarnish. At high temperatures a substantial layer of chromium oxide may form on the surfaces, allowing chromium or nickel to diffuse into the porcelain. Also the thermal expansion is lower leading to high residual stress at the interface.

Firing temperatures			
Material	1250–1300°C	1060–1100°C	900–980°C
SiO_2	70.6	63.7	67.3
Al_2O_3	17.2	19.5	10.8
CaO			2.2
Na_2O	2.8	2.2	4.6
K_2O	9.4	8.2	7.9
B_2O_3			6.8

Fig. 12.9 **Firing temperatures.** The typical composition of a series of dental porcelains and the firing temperatures, which vary according to content.

Composition of a typical metal–ceramic porcelain			
SiO_2	63.2%	Al_2O_3	17.5%
CaO	0.8%	Na_2O	5.7%
K_2O	11.7%	B_2O_3	1.0%

Fig. 12.10 **Composition of a typical metal–ceramic porcelain.**

FURTHER READING

Charles RJ. Static fatigue of glass; I, II. *J App Phys* 1958; **29**:1549–60.

Fishlock D. Towards tougher materials. *N Sci* 1966; **29**:283–5.

Jones DW. Statistical parameters for the strength of dental porcelain. *Dent Pract* 1971; **22**:55–7.

Jones PA, Wilson HJ. Modulus of elasticity of dental ceramics. *Dent Pract* 1972; **22**:170–3.

Lehman ML. Stability and durability of porcelain jacket crowns. *Br Dent J* 1967; **123**:419–26.

McLean JW, Hughes TH. The reinforcement of dental porcelain with ceramic oxides. *Br Dent J* 1965; **119**:251–67.

McLean JW. *The science and art of dental ceramics, Vol. I. The nature of dental ceramics and their clinical use.* London: Quintessence Books; 1979.

McLean JW. *The science and art of dental ceramics, Vol. II. Bridge design and laboratory procedures in dental ceramics.* London: Quintessence Books; 1980.

Phillips RW. *Skinner's science of dental materials, 9th ed.* Philadelphia: WB Saunders; 1991 Chap 20:359–384 & Chap 26:505–528.

Southan DE. Strengthening modern dental porcelain by ion exchange. *Aust Dent J* 1970; **15**:507–10.

Southan DE. The development and characteristics of dental porcelain. *Aust Dent J* 1970. **15**:103–7.

Southan DE. Defects in porcelain at the porcelain-to-metal interface. In: Yamada, HN ed. *Dental porcelain: the state of the art.* Los Angeles: University South California; 1977:143–7.

Southan DE. Factors affecting the translucency of dental porcelain. *Quintessence Int* 1987; **18**:197–202.

Southan DE. Optical density-strength relationships in dental porcelain. *Quintessence Int* 1987; **18**:261–3.

Southan DE, Jorgensen KD. Faulty porcelain jacket crowns. *Aust Dent J* 1972; **17**:436–40.

Southan DE, Jorgensen KD. Precise porcelain jacket crowns. *Aust Dent J* 1972; **17**:269–73.

Southan DE, Jorgensen KD. An explanation for the occurrence of internal faults in porcelain jacket crowns. *Aust Dent J* 1973; **18**:152–6

Southan DE, Jorgensen KD. The endurance limit of dental porcelain. *Aust Dent J* 1974; **19**:7–11.

Weinstein M, Katz S, Weinstein AB. *Fused porcelain-to-metal teeth.* US Patent 3 052 982.

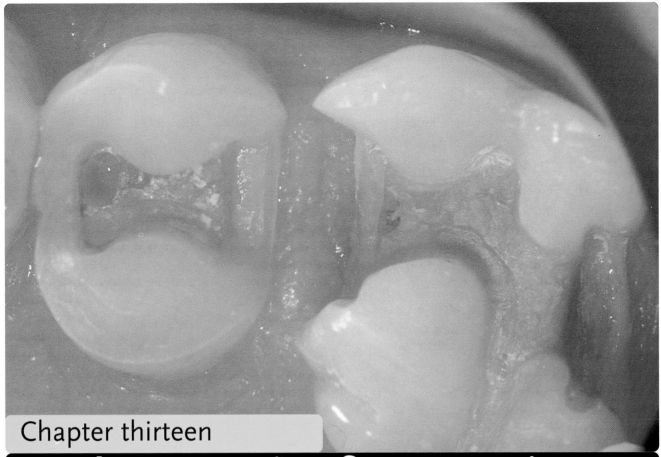

Chapter thirteen

Tooth preparation for restoration with rigid materials

G.J. Mount

The general principles for removal of tooth structure during preparation for restoration were described in Chapters 6, 7 and 11. The essential difference between a cavity designed for placement of a plastic material and for the acceptance of a rigid restorative material is that the restoration itself will be fabricated outside of the mouth rather than in the tooth. This has several implications for preparation design. Probably the most important is that it must be possible to take an impression without distortion, and then insert the restoration into the cavity without it binding or imposing stress on remaining tooth structure.

Preservation of remaining tooth structure is still of paramount importance because all restorations rely upon the strength and integrity of remaining tooth structure for their retention. To a limited extent, the restorative material can be used to protect and reinforce the remaining tooth, but in the long run the less dentine and enamel there is, the weaker the remaining tooth structure will be and the greater the risk of failure.

GENERAL PRINCIPLES

The placement of rigid materials requires preparation of a cavity with divergent lateral walls to allow a path of withdrawal and insertion of the completed restoration. This 'line of draw' is necessary so that a pattern or impression of the cavity can be withdrawn without distortion, and the finished restoration can be inserted into the tooth without generation of stress. At the same time, the design must include features to ensure retention, such as near-parallelism of major cavity walls. These restorations must be luted or cemented in place to prevent microleakage and, in most cases, to prevent removal along the line of draw by gravity or sticky food. The strength of retention of indirect restorations depends upon the area of the vertical walls of the cavity and their degree of divergence. Except in the case of resin-bonded veneer restorations, the luting agent is not a major contributor to retention.

Indirectly fabricated restorations can be either intracoronal or extracoronal.

- Intracoronal restoration is usually supported within the remaining tooth structure; it is known as an inlay or onlay (**Fig. 13.1**).
- Extracoronal restoration surrounds the circumference of the remaining tooth structure, either entirely, or to a substantial degree.

If the full circumference of the tooth is included, the restoration is called a full crown. However, there are many designs for less than full replacement of the external surface; these are called partial coverage crowns or partial veneers. Gold and porcelain are the materials most commonly used, but composite resin can also be polymerised, using an indirect technique, to construct a crown, veneer or inlay.

The following are the essential parameters for the design and preparation of teeth for restoration with rigid materials.

INTRACORONAL RESTORATIONS

Retention

Because the strength of retention is directly proportional to the area of the vertical walls of the cavity, care must be taken to preserve coronal height as far as possible. Where there is adequate tooth structure present, pins and grooves can be used to effectively increase wall length and area. The contraindications for the use of pins, particularly self-threading pins, were discussed in Chapter 7, page 47; however, under these circumstances, the pins are being placed to extend the area of the vertical walls and will not place stress on the dentine.

Both pins and grooves should be prepared using a tapered fissure bur (#168MS) (**Fig. 13.2**) at a low speed under air–water spray. Prefabricated systems are available for producing parallel sided or tapered pin holes, but a simple technique is to cut a pin hole with a tapered fissure bur; then, while holding the bur vertically, move it later-

ly to one side or the other to extend the pin hole laterally so that it becomes a groove or ditch. This will increase the area of the vertical walls still further, enhance the strength of the pin and simplify impression-taking procedures (because a groove is less likely than a pin hole to retain an air bubble when impression material is syringed into it).

Strength of walls

When an inlay is seated within a tooth, maintainance of retention under masticatory stress will depend upon the strength and integrity of both the buccal and lingual cusps. Under load, the point of rotation of an inlay out of a tooth will be around the most gingivally positioned buccal or lingual point angle, and, regardless of design, it is virtually impossible to gain strength and retention from the opposite remaining cusps. Therefore, if either side of remaining tooth structure is already very weak, or indeed split, an inlay is contraindicated and an extracoronal restoration should be designed instead.

Angle of divergence of the walls

The buccal and lingual walls should diverge from each other at an angle of between 5° and 10°. If the angle is less than 5° the remaining tooth structure will be subjected to undue stress during cementation procedures. If the angle is greater than 10°, retention will be compromised.

Modification of cavity to allow a line of withdrawal

If a tooth is deeply carious, or has been restored previously with a plastic restorative material, there may be undercuts in relation to the facial, lingual or axial walls that will compromise the line of withdrawal. The problem can be overcome by one of two techniques. If the problem is anticipated before commencement of cavity design, all existing caries and old restorative material should be

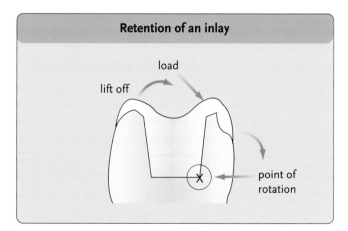

Fig. 13.1 Retention of an inlay. It is important to recognise that an inlay will be retained by one side only of a tooth at any one time so both cusps must be equally strong to withstand occlusal pressures. The point of rotation of the inlay out of the tooth will be the most buccogingival or linguogingival point angle of the cavity.

replaced first with a Type II.1 or a Type II.2 glass–ionomer (Chapter 8, page 75). Because these are strong cements, they can be regarded as dentine substitutes and the final cavity can be prepared ensuring that all margins are on sound enamel or dentine. Major retentive factors such as pins and grooves must be in sound dentine. Alternatively, if the problem is only minor and becomes apparent after completion of the cavity design, small defects can be eliminated using a Type III glass–ionomer lining cement providing it is entirely covered subsequently by the final restoration.

Modifications for specific materials
Gold
Because gold is strong as well as ductile and moderately flexible, it can be used in thin section to veneer and protect the remaining tooth structure. Wherever possible, margins should be placed in areas that will not be subject to direct vertical occlusal load, because of the potential for fracture of enamel rods leading to ditching at the margins. Very little protection is required over a nonworking cusp, and the margin should be taken just to the tip of the cusp and lightly bevelled outwards. Working cusps, however, should be covered with approximately 1.5 mm of gold for strength and protection, and the margin should be taken out to the extent that it can be burnished into place by the passage of the food bolus during mastication. All other margins should be provided with a long fine bevel to ensure minimum exposure of cement to the oral environment. Gold can be cast to a high degree of accuracy in very thin section and a type A or B gold can be burnished to virtually close a margin. However, if a type C gold is used, it will only be subject to burnishing if it is heat treated and subsequently quenched (Chapter 12, page 157), so accuracy of design and casting is of paramount importance.

Porcelain
As porcelain is essentially a brittle material, it cannot be used in thin sections to protect the remaining tooth structure. Wherever possible, the porcelain cavo–surface margin should be not less than 90° and, if possible, it should be placed on the tooth where it is free from direct vertical occlusal load. Gingival margins should have a flat butt joint with no bevel or chamfer.

Composite resin
Composite resin can be employed using an indirect poly-merisation technique for the fabrication of an inlay, although its physical properties are such that it cannot withstand heavy occlusal load. Nor is it strong enough to be used in thin section in an attempt to protect remaining tooth structure. The cavo–surface margins in resin should not be less than 90° and they should be placed on the tooth in a position where they are free of occlusal load. Gingival margins should be a flat butt joint with no bevel or chamfer.

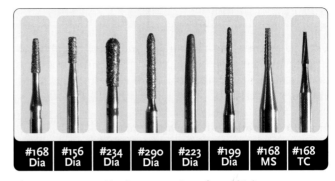

#168 Dia | #156 Dia | #234 Dia | #290 Dia | #223 Dia | #199 Dia | #168 MS | #168 TC

Fig. 13.2 Burs used in the preparation of a gold inlay.

Instrumentation for a gold inlay
Whether the inlay is being constructed to replace an existing restoration or to deal with an active carious lesion, the method of preparation will be similar.

Basic outline
Remove old metal restorations with a small tungsten carbide bur (#168TC) at ultra-high speed under copious air–water spray. Alternatively, enter a new cavity at ultra-high speed with a small tapered diamond (#156Dia). Open the cavity to a minimum outline form to identify the extent of the problem.

Use a small tapered diamond cylinder (#168Dia) with a 5° taper at intermediate high speed under air–water spray to extend the cavity far enough to define the entire outline. Maintain the diamond in a single vertical plane at all times so that the taper on the bur becomes the flair in the cavity.

Identify cusps which require coverage or protection and reduce these cautiously using a small pear-shaped diamond (#234). Reduce working cusps approximately 1.5 mm and nonworking cusps about 0.25 mm at this point.

Identify areas of sound dentine in which to enhance retention. Use a tapered fissure mild steel bur (#168MS) at low speed under air–water spray to cut pin holes and ditches whilst maintaining the bur in the same vertical plane. A ditch can be regarded as a lateral extension of a pin hole and is to be recommended as a method of enhancing retention. A ditch will enhance the area of the vertical walls and therefore improve retention. Also, it is easier to obtain an impression of a ditch than a pin hole, because it is less likely to incorporate an air bubble in the impression material.

Preparation of the margins
Refine the marginal finish around the full circumference of the inlay using very fine diamonds (#223) at intermediate high speed under air–water spray. Choose an appropriately shaped, very fine diamond to polish and lightly bevel margins on nonworking cusps.

Place a reverse bevel around working cusps with a chamfered margin of varied depth depending upon the load to be sustained. Use a long tapered (#199Dia) or flame-shaped diamond to prepare a long fine flair on proximal margins, particularly along the gingival margin.

Final finish

Polish all margins with very fine polishing diamonds (#223Dia). Smooth the floor and walls and eliminate all instrument marks as far as possible. Enhance retention areas and eliminate undercuts with glass–ionomer lining cement if necessary.

Instrumentation for porcelain or resin inlay

The basic instrumentation for these cavities is essentially the same as for gold. However, in view of their susceptibility to marginal fracture, it is necessary to provide a butt joint along all margins.

Basic outline

Follow the procedure outlined above for a gold inlay and develop a similar degree of taper on approximating walls. Do not reduce the cusps unless they need to be fully protected from occlusal load.

Preparation of margins

Using fine diamonds refine all margins to a smooth butt finish, particularly at the gingival floor and the proximal walls. If the cusps require protection from occlusal load they will need to be reduced in height by at least 2 mm at an angle to the vertical which is parallel to the original occlusal cuspal incline. This will ensure an even thickness of restorative material over the cusp and avoid acute angles within the restoration which may become stress points leading to initiation of fractures. Do not provide reverse bevels beyond the margins because a fine bevel will lead to fine fragile margins in porcelain or resin.

Fabrication of restorations

Fabrication of the restorations for these cavities is a laboratory procedure and will not be dealt with in depth in this text. Generally, gold inlays are cast as discussed in Chapter 12, pages 156–157, and porcelain inlays are constructed in much the same way as a porcelain crown using a pervious die. However, recent developments in the accuracy of computer-generated cutting machines means that there is now a possibility of forming an inlay from a block of porcelain to fit a cavity preparation that has been scanned *in situ* in the oral cavity. To date, accuracy of fit is less than ideal and resin cements are recommended for luting to compensate for this. No doubt, accuracy will improve and such restorations will be possible providing always that both sides of the tooth are equally strong as discussed above.

EXTRACORONAL RESTORATIONS

It is necessary to utilise extracoronal restorations in those situations where remaining tooth structure is sufficiently weakened to be unable to withstand the stresses to which it will be subjected in supporting an intracoronal restoration.

Construction of these restorations requires external fabrication after the tooth is prepared. A model of the final restoration is made on the die, usually in wax or nonbonded resin. The 'pattern' is then removed and used to make the final restoration, either by investment and casting replication or, in the case of some composite resin inlay techniques, by heat activation, light activation, or both, to enhance the degree of polymeric conversion.

The strength and retention for these restorations is best gained in the gingival one-third of the crown. The design need not necessarily encompass the entire circumference of the tooth providing it involves the bulk of the remaining sound tooth structure. Three-quarter crowns and seven-eighths crowns are desirable if it means that it is possible to retain the aesthetics and anatomy of natural enamel without compromising strength and retention of the restoration.

Retention

As retention is directly proportional to the area of the vertical walls, it is generally desirable to first build or rebuild the basic tooth structure to the full available occlusal height in a plastic restorative material, preferably amalgam, before carrying out the final preparation. The amalgam should be firmly interlocked with remaining dentine, utilising ditches and grooves (Chapter 7, page 60) and, for a nonvital tooth placement, of a post in each root canal is recommended (Chapter 19, page 219). Because the physical properties of amalgam are similar to those of dentine, amalgam can be regarded as a dentine substitute and the full length of the walls can be expected to provide retention. The alternative plastic restorative materials which could be used, such as composite resin and glass–ionomer, lack the required physical properties and should be used with caution in limited areas only (**Figs 13.3** and **13.4**).

Strength of remaining tooth structure

A number of materials can be used to replace remaining tooth structure prior to preparation for a crown. However, as it is the lateral stresses to which the tooth is subjected which are the most destructive, the tensile strength of the material used for the build-up may be the weakest link. Providing there is at least 2–3 mm of sound tooth structure

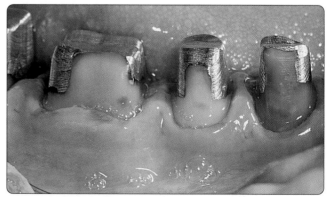

Fig. 13.3 Amalgam build-up. Three teeth which were restored with amalgam before preparation for full crowns.

remaining around the circumference at the gingival margin then the relatively more flexible and weaker materials, such as composite resin and glass–ionomer, can be used to make up the difference in the vertical height. Well-retained amalgam will provide more support but if there is virtually no tooth structure left above the gingival margin, it may be

necessary to devitalise the remaining roots and place either cast gold, stainless steel or titanium posts within each root canal. This will change the point of rotation of the crown off the root to a point approximately one-quarter of the distance up from the tip of the post and make maximum use of remaining tooth structure. However, there is then a risk of a split developing in the root that will bring about the ultimate demise of the tooth and the restoration.

Angle of convergence

All the walls of an extracoronal restoration should converge at an angle of approximately 5° and no greater than 10°. With a full crown, if the angle is 5° or less it will be necessary to put a vent hole in the crown to allow it to be seated fully without retaining excess cement on the occlusal surface. If the angle is greater than 10° the retention may be compromised, particularly if the preparation is short. In fact, a crown may rotate off the tooth because the point of rotation is always at the gingival margin opposite the side of lift-off (**Fig. 13.5**).

Modification to enhance retention

It is usually not necessary to provide additional enhancement for retention of a full crown because, unless the preparation is perfectly circular, it is impossible for the crown to rotate in a horizontal plane. Also, providing there is sufficient length and a fine taper, as described above, it cannot rotate in a vertical plane. However it may be necessary to place vertical grooves in one or more walls to compensate for an inability to minimise the convergence angle. These grooves should diverge no more than 10° from each other or from another wall and they will effectively increase the area of available vertical wall.

Retention for a three-quarter or seven-eighths crown is enhanced with grooves at the mesial and distal end of the preparation placed, if possible, in sound tooth structure. They should be cut with a tapered fissure bur or a diamond of a similar size and a further groove extended across the occlusal/incisal surface, in tooth structure, to join the two proximal grooves together. This will provide a reinforcing strut effect for the mesial and distal wings of the restoration to minimise flexure under load (**Figs 13.6** and **13.7**).

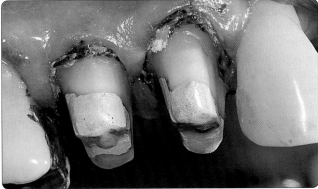

Fig. 13.4 Glass–ionomer cement build-up. Two bicuspids built with glass–ionomer cement before crown preparation. There is 3 mm of sound dentine all around the gingival margin.

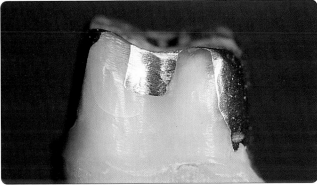

Fig. 13.5 Crown retention. A preparation for a full crown on a lower molar. Note the length of the preparation and the fine taper of less than 10°. The buccal cusp was split and an old amalgam was replaced before preparation. Note that there is still adequate natural tooth structure remaining for optimum retention.

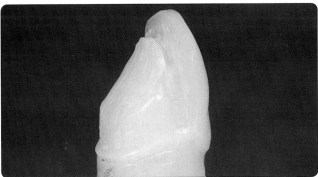

Fig. 13.6 The preparation for a three-quarter crown. Note proximal and incisal grooves.

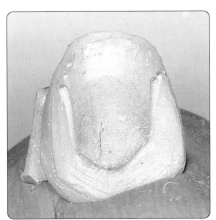

Fig. 13.7 Three-quarter casting before trimming. Note the strengthening effect of the proximal and incisal grooves.

Modification for specific materials

Extracoronal restorations can be fabricated using a variety of materials, and variations in cavity design may be required to provide adequate strength when using some materials (**Fig. 13.8**).

Gold

Because gold is strong as well as flexible and ductile it can be utilised in very thin section and cast with great accuracy. This means that conservative tooth reduction is possible. The thickness of gold can be in the range 0.5–1.0 mm in areas not under occlusal load but this should be increased to 1.5–2.0 mm when protecting working cusps or areas under heavy load. For preference the gingival margin should finish to a fine chamfer although, under some circumstances, it is acceptable to finish to a feather edge.

Porcelain bonded to metal

In view of the brittle nature of porcelain, and the need to build it in depth for aesthetics, it is necessary to remove more tooth structure than for gold alone. To enhance strength, full crowns are often constructed as a gold or alloy thimble and the porcelain is fused to the metal. The metal coping will need to be at least 0.75 mm thick in all areas. In those areas where porcelain will be added an additional 1.0 mm of tooth reduction is necessary. Whilst it is possible to develop a margin in porcelain to fit directly to tooth structure it is desirable, in all areas where aesthetics is of no concern, that the margins should be in metal. The finish line for the metal casting should be as described above. However, if the margin is to be in porcelain there will need to be a shoulder at least 1.3 mm wide. In addition there will need to be an occlusal clearance of at least 1.75 mm to allow for a thickness of metal as well as porcelain.

As unsupported porcelain is liable to shear under occlusal load it is desirable to provide a substantial shoulder of gold interproximally to support the marginal ridge if it is to be built in porcelain.

Porcelain alone

Optimal aesthetic restoration of tooth structure can only be achieved using ceramics. However, in view of its relatively brittle nature, porcelain requires substantial bulk in all dimensions. As far as possible, the thickness should be even overall, with a minimum clearance of 2 mm in areas subject to heavy load. The margins should always be finished as a butt joint at right angles to the long axis of the tooth. All external angles of the preparation, other than the gingival margin, should be lightly rounded over because sharp angles tend to provide areas of stress concentration, which may lead to subsequent fracture.

Rubber dam

As discussed in Chapter 7, page 66, the use of rubber dam as a routine, for protection of the patient as well as the operator, is strongly encouraged. Place an anchor clamp on a tooth distal to the one to be prepared and use an additional clamp, if required, on the appropriate tooth. There are distal extension clamps available if the anchor tooth is involved. Specially designed hand instruments are available to act as retractors and protection for both the dam and the gingival tissues.

Instrumentation

As strength of retention is related to the area of the vertical walls it is desirable to prepare those walls first before modifying other surfaces, such as the occlusal, to make room for the restorative material. As a large part of the external anatomy of the original tooth is to be removed and altered, the maintenance of visual orientation with remaining tooth structure may be difficult. Each step of the preparation should be undertaken to maintain the relationship of the preparation to the original anatomy of the crown of the tooth.

Basic preparation

Begin the preparation with a long, parallel-sided diamond (#290) (**Fig. 13.9**) at ultra-high speed under air–water spray to produce a depth cut through the enamel to the dentine on the buccal surface. This can then be used as a guide for the removal of remaining tooth structure as well as the development of the retentive design. Make a similar groove, parallel to the first, on the lingual of the tooth and then prepare one-half of the tooth only, interproximally, to unite the buccal with the lingual groove. Maintain the vertical plane at all times. It will generally be necessary to use a long, fine, tapered diamond (#199) to open interproximally without damaging the adjacent tooth.

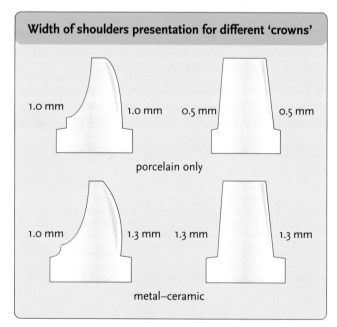

Width of shoulders presentation for different 'crowns'

1.0 mm   1.0 mm   0.5 mm   0.5 mm

porcelain only

1.0 mm   1.3 mm   1.3 mm   1.3 mm

metal–ceramic

Fig. 13.8 Anterior crown design. Diagrammatic representation of the minimum depth of preparation for a porcelain and metal–ceramic crown. Note that additional tooth structure is removed to allow for the metal thimble required for the metal–ceramic crown.

Develop the gingival margin in approximately its correct position just above the gingival tissue.

After the preparation of one end of the tooth, prepare the other end in a similar fashion. Now, reduce the occlusal surface of a posterior tooth, or the incisal edge of an anterior, allowing sufficient room for the selected restorative material. Use a pear shaped diamond stone (#234) at ultra-high speed under air–water spray.

Finally, reduce the remaining lingual or buccal surface of the tooth to conform to the original tooth anatomy but without compromising the gingival retentive areas. Retentive elements, such as grooves, can be developed using the #168 tapered diamond.

Refine the cavity outline

The gingival margins and the final surface of the preparation should now be refined using a very fine, tapered diamond (#223) with a 5° taper. Keep the bur vertical at all times when preparing the gingival margin and the retentive walls. If restoring with gold the diamond stone should have a rounded end to prepare a chamfer margin at the appropriate level. To prepare the butt joint for porcelain use a diamond with a flat end and tapered sides (#168).

Polish the entire preparation using very fine diamonds

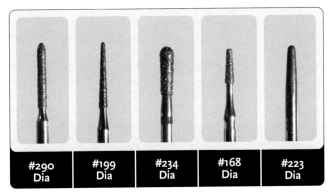

#290 Dia   #199 Dia   #234 Dia   #168 Dia   #223 Dia

Fig. 13.9 Burs used in the preparation of an extracoronal restoration.

under air–water spray at intermediate high speed and round over all sharp angles which may become stress points.

The position of the gingival margin will be dictated by several factors and these are discussed in detail in Chapter 14, page 176, in relation to gingival retraction.

FURTHER READING

Behrend DA. Ceramometal restorations with supra gingival margins. *J Prosthet Dent* 1982; **47**:625.

Gardiner FM. Margins of complete crowns [Review]. *J Prosthet Dent* 1982; **48**:396–400.

McLean JW. *The science and art of dental ceramics. Vol. 1. The nature of dental ceramics and their clinical use.* Chicago: Quintessence Publishing Company; 1979.

Rosner D. Function, placement and reproduction of bevels for gold castings. *J Prosthet Dent* 1963; **13**:1160–6.

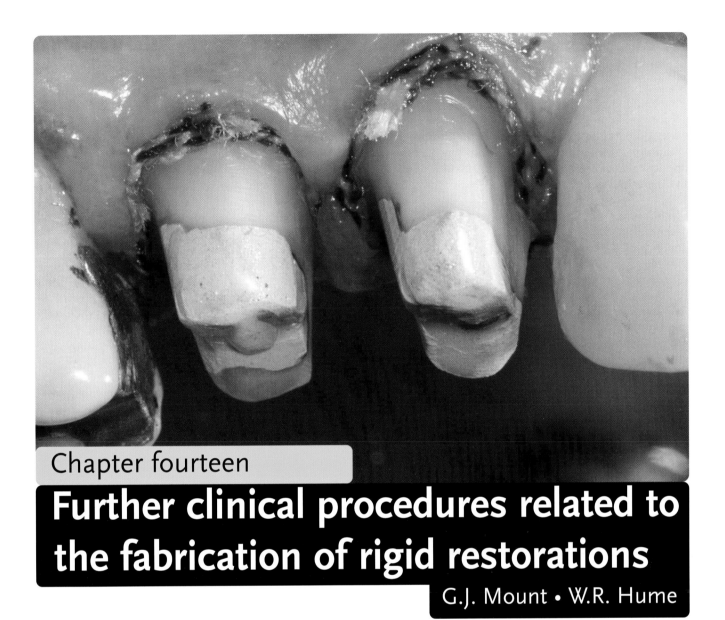

Chapter fourteen

Further clinical procedures related to the fabrication of rigid restorations

G.J. Mount • W.R. Hume

After preparation of a tooth for the fabrication of a restoration using an indirect technique, it is essential to ensure that neither errors nor distortions occur during the successive stages of production. All members of the dental team are involved in these routines and care and attention to detail is essential at all times.

GINGIVAL RETRACTION

The gingival tissue in health

Normal healthy gingival anatomy is discussed in detail in Chapter 20, page 227; as far as possible, the gingival tissue should be in complete health before commencement of cavity preparation for an indirect restoration. Any pre-existing gingival disease should be treated and eliminated and active caries removed and restored with plastic restorative materials, at least on a temporary basis.

Significance of the emergence profile

The integrity of the gingival margin of a restoration and the anatomy of the emergence profile are also discussed in Chapter 20, page 228. One of the great challenges in restorative dentistry is to reproduce natural anatomy in the area of the gingival crevice and, in fabricating an indirect restoration, the responsibility is generally left in the hands of the dental technician. Unless the technician is offered an accurate reproduction of the tooth anatomy for about 1 mm beyond the final cavity outline, the potential for development of a margin free of over-contour or under-contour, and with the correct emergence profile, is severely compromised.

Significance of healthy gingival tissue

The gingival crevice cannot be regarded as a caries-free zone because it is not naturally plaque free. The presence of any foreign material or alteration to the anatomy of the tooth within the crevice, which is likely to encourage the growth and retention of plaque, will inevitably lead to gingival inflammation and, possibly, the generation of caries, periodontal disease, or both.

It is not always possible to obtain perfect health and contour in the gingival tissues beforehand and compromises may be necessary to overcome any problems arising. In the presence of restorations that are over-contoured or do not have a desirable emergence profile, the gingival tissue may become hypertrophied and fibrous. Also the gingival tissue will adapt very rapidly to the development of any negative contour around the gingival margin and will quickly cover over remaining tooth structure following a subgingival fracture. However, it is necessary to obtain an accurate reproduction of the anatomy of the tooth to a point beyond the finish line of the preparation, without contamination and distortion, using the impression material of choice. This objective will be made more difficult in the presence of gingival haemorrhage or excess gingival tissue. Hence the value of achieving a normal healthy state beforehand.

If the final margin of the preparation is outside the gingival crevice by a minimum of 1.0 mm around the entire circumference of the tooth then it will be unnecessary to disturb the gingival tissue. However, there are a variety of reasons for taking the margin into the gingival crevice even though this may complicate the impression-taking procedures.

Reasons for gingival retraction

Subgingival margins

Very often, following preparation for an extracoronal restoration, there will be at least one section of the margin that will be subgingival because the margin of the original restoration was in this position. Other causes include active caries, recurrent caries beyond the margin of a previous restoration or fracture of a cusp. Treatment of any defect beforehand, at least on a temporary basis, will often assist the recovery of the gingival tissue to the point where the problem is reduced, and at least part of the margin may become supragingival.

Aesthetics

Particularly in the construction of aesthetic ceramic restorations it is necessary to place the labial or facial gingival margin about 0.5 mm into the gingival crevice to disguise the transition from restoration to tooth. Preparation of the tooth beyond this point is both unnecessary and undesirable.

Bulk fracture of tooth structure

On occasion, the construction of an indirect restoration is undertaken to compensate for the loss of a cusp from a tooth that had been restored previously or been subject to major trauma. The position of the fracture line may be well subgingival.

Enhance retention

For an indirect restoration the strength of retention is directly proportional to the area of the vertical walls (Chapter 7, page 61). There will therefore be occasions when it is necessary to extend the tooth preparation below the gingival margin to enhance retention. There may even be a need for minor gingival surgery and, possibly, re-contouring of the alveolar bone crest.

Retraction before preparation

To enhance access and to prevent damage to the soft tissue during cavity preparation procedures, it may be desirable to carry out some degree of gingival retraction prior to commencement of preparation. It is easy to abrade the soft tissue with rotary cutting instruments and this will both complicate impression taking and may also result in migration of the gingival tissue during healing, to the extent that, a margin that was designed to be subgingival, is subsequently exposed, thus downgrading aesthetics.

Placement of one, or possibly two, lengths of retraction cord within the gingival crevice, before commencement of preparation, will move the tissue outwards and apically away from the area of operation and will lessen the risk of damage. When dealing with an aesthetic problem, such as a ceramic crown on an anterior tooth, it may be desirable to define the outline of the gingival tissue first, with a marking pen or pencil, before placing retraction cord and then take the final marginal preparation up into the gingival crevice to the desired depth, beyond the pencil mark.

Simple gingival retraction

The object of gingival retraction is to open the gingival crevice to a limited extent to allow the ingress of impression material in sufficient bulk to record the anatomy of the surface of the tooth within the crevice. Upon withdrawal, the impression material must have sufficient bulk that it does not tear. It must also withstand the stresses of construction of a model without distortion. This can be achieved by gentle placement of a length of cord into the base of the crevice in such a way as to displace the gingival cuff laterally without disturbing the integrity of the epithelial attachment. A second cord of slightly greater diameter can be placed over the first so that the crevice is opened a little wider at the entry than at the base. If the tissue is in complete health it should be sufficient to leave these cords in place for approximately 3 minutes and, upon removal of one or both cords, the crevice will remain open long enough for the placement of the impression material.

Haemostasis

In the presence of minor haemorrhage, it may be necessary to use a styptic or haemostatic agent, either on or in conjunction with the cord, to ensure the crevice remains dry during the impression procedures. Low-concentration epinephrine (adrenaline), aluminium trichloride or zinc chloride are useful, particularly when the cord has been soaked in the chemical and allowed to dry first. The use of epinephrine carries the risk of increasing the pulse rate and blood pressure of some patients and it must therefore be used with caution; zinc chloride is strongly caustic.

Complex retraction
Chemical retraction

Chemical cautery of the gingival tissue can be carried out simply and effectively using concentrated trichloroacetic acid. The material is available in crystalline form and will readily deliquesce in air, producing a super-saturated solution of the acid. Application of a very small quantity to the surface of the tissue will bring about immediate haemostasis and control of gingival fluid flow. Place a single drop of the acid solution into a Dappen's dish. Wet the tip of the blade of a small flat plastic instrument in the liquid and touch it to the soft tissue which is to be cauterised. Leave alone for 1 minute and wash thoroughly. Care should be taken in its application but it is self-limiting in penetration into the tissue and the cauterised wound will heal rapidly without any inflammatory response. An impression can be obtained immediately, free of interference and contamination, and within 1 week there will be complete healing of the soft tissue.

Surgical retraction

In circumstances where there is an excess of hypertrophied tissue or where the gingival margin is well subgingival as a result of traumatic fracture, it may be necessary to use standard surgical procedures to remove tissue. This can be carried out at the time of impression taking and

supplemented with trichloroacetic acid to achieve a dry field. However, it is generally recommended that the surgery be completed at least 2 weeks before cavity preparation and impression taking to allow healing in the soft tissue. Any deficiency in the anatomy of the remaining tooth will need to be made good with an adequate temporary restoration to ensure satisfactory healing to the required shape.

Electrosurgery

Summary

Electrosurgery

To cut + haemostasis:
- use fully rectified current (RF)
- cut for 3 seconds
- pause for 5 seconds

To cut only:
- use fully rectified filtered continuous wavelength current (CWRF)

Soft tissue reduction with electrosurgery is relatively straightforward and, possibly in conjunction with trichloroacetic acid, may be very effective. Electrosurgery provides rapid, atraumatic cutting of soft tissue and sterilises the wound at the same time, leaving a dry field free of haemorrhage. There should be healing by primary intention without pain, swelling or scar formation.

When using this technique it is necessary to have a full understanding of the method and instrumentation because there is a potential for tissue damage beyond the area of operation. To cut gingival tissue and provide haemostasis at the same time a fully rectified (RF) current is used; the length of time of contact with the tissue is important. Considerable heat can be generated in the tissue in a very short period, so a pause of 5–10 seconds must be allowed between applications of the cutting tip. Cutting without haemostasis can be achieved using a fully rectified filtered continuous wavelength current (CWRF), following which haemostasis can be achieved with trichloroacetic acid.

The technique is probably of greatest use for the removal of hypertrophied fibrous tissue of long standing which is not responding to conservative periodontal treatment. For this purpose it is best to carry out the surgery at least 2 weeks before cavity preparation and impression taking.

Laser surgery

Soft tissue reduction with lasers in the field of dentistry has been subjected to intense scrutiny in recent years. Some of the hard lasers such as CO_2 lasers (CO_2 gas), Nd–YAG lasers and Ar lasers (Argon ions) have been used for soft tissue surgery in medicine and oral surgery, for some time with success. Lasers work through photoablation and produce completely blood-free incisions followed by rapid, pain-free healing with no underlying inflammation. The Nd–YAG laser is preferred for re-section of oral soft tissues and can be used successfully without local anaesthesia for gingival retraction prior to impression taking, particularly in the presence of hyper-trophied tissue.

The pulsed Nd–YAG laser beam is directed to the operative site through a flexible quartz optical fibre. As this beam is invisible at the correct operating wavelength, a red helium–neon laser is used to provide a visible aiming beam coaxial with the YAG laser. The tip of the fibre extends approximately 1 mm from the handpiece and provides accuracy for positioning and directing the beam. The tip of the fibre is kept in touch with the soft tissue and is moved and directed in much the same way as a conventional scalpel. The laser technique is a little slower than using a scalpel but produces very controlled tissue removal free of haemorrhage and pain. Healing is rapid and uneventful.

IMPRESSIONS

Successful construction of an indirect restoration requires an accurate model of the prepared tooth. A full description of the steps involved in fabrication of restorations is beyond the scope of this book, principally because of the wide variation of techniques for the various materials used. However, the first step in impression taking is common to all materials and methods of manufacture. The main groups of impression materials now available are listed below and the techniques used with each briefly described.

Summary

'Reversible' hydrocolloid
- Boil for 15 minutes
- Store at 61°C until ready to use
- Temper at 43°C for 3 minutes
- Hold water-cooled tray for 3 minutes
- Remove with a 'snap'
- Cast model quickly

Agar hydrocolloid ('reversible' hydrocolloid)
This water-based material undergoes a temperature-dependent, sol–gel phase change. It gives high-precision results, is of relatively low cost, and is more tolerant of undercuts, in terms of ease of removal without tearing, than the other materials described below. It is prepared for use by converting to a sol in boiling water and subsequent gelation will occur following cooling. The impression is taken in a water cooled tray, so gelation will proceed from the cooled metal surface of the impression tray towards the tooth, with the hydrocolloid at the tooth surface being the last to change to a gel. This provides excellent conditions for very high precision. As

the agar hydrocolloid is water based it is tolerant of moisture on the tooth surface; the dentine should be subjected to a very fine water spray immediately before impression taking.

Time and temperature cycle
The successful use of agar hydrocolloid requires careful attention to procedural detail, particularly in regard to temperature control. A temperature-controlled water bath is required in which the material can be immersed in boiling water for 15 minutes. The material is then moved to a storage bath and held at 61°C until it is required for use. Final preparation involves loading the water-cooled tray with the material and immersing it in a tempering bath at 43°C for 3 minutes. The tray is then placed in the mouth and cold water is circulated through the tray for a further 3 minutes, by which time it is set and the impression is removed.

Clinical routine
Agar hydrocolloid is also available in a light body form in glass Carpules and is passed through only the first two stages of softening before use. The Carpules can then be placed into a fine tip syringe and the material syringed directly onto the prepared tooth surfaces and into the gingival crevice, to ensure that air bubbles are not entrapped. After tray placement the material is cooled over a period of about 3 minutes so that, when gelation is complete, the impression can be removed with a sharp 'snap' movement to reduce the chance of tearing or distortion. The impression can be stored in potassium sulphate for a few minutes but the modelling stone must be poured into the impression very shortly thereafter. If there is to be a delay before pouring, the impression must be stored in high-humidity air to reduce the risk of dimensional change through water loss. (Alginate hydrocolloid [irreversible] is not sufficiently accurate for use in indirect restorative work and will not, therefore, be discussed here.)

Polysulphide rubber (mercaptan)

Summary

'Rubber base'
- Always use custom tray
- Dispense equal lengths
- Mix thoroughly
- Use light body form in syringe to avoid air bubbles
- Hold 5–8 minutes
- Pour model within 30–60 minutes

This material, commonly called 'rubber-base', must be used with a well fitting, rigid, custom-made tray for each patient, to ensure a relatively even layer of material of 1–2 mm thickness throughout the impression. In these circumstances very accurate impressions can be obtained.

Clinical routine

The material is prepared for use by mixing the two components, in correct proportions, for a defined period of time. It is generally marketed in three consistencies, light, medium and heavy bodied, and these can be used in combination. The light-bodied or medium-bodied material is placed, using a syringe, into the gingival crevice and around the prepared teeth to minimise the inclusion of air bubbles, while a heavier consistency is loaded into the impression tray. Upon seating the impression tray into the mouth, the heavy body material applies pressure to the light body material which in turn leads the heavy body into the fine details of the prepared tooth, thus producing great accuracy with a minimum of voids. After setting there is a chemical shrinkage over time of about 0.25% over the first 24 hours. In addition there may be minor distortions of the impression during removal from the mouth which will take a few minutes to recover. Because of these two factors impressions should not be poured until approximately 30–60 minutes after mixing.

Polysulphide rubber is considered difficult to mix, relatively slow to set, and is hydrophobic compared with agar hydrocolloid. It also has an unpleasant smell and taste from the patient's point of view. However, it is not expensive and, if properly used in a custom tray and the teeth are carefully dried before placement of the impression, it is possible to achieve excellent results.

Condensation silicone rubber

This material is handled in the same manner as are the polysulphide rubber materials and is considered an attractive alternative because of its relative ease of mixing, rapid set and lack of odour and taste. However, it is very hydrophobic and has a high shrinkage after setting. It can be used in combination with a more dimensionally stable putty phase to decrease the thickness of the silicone material but even so, the impression should be poured as soon as possible after removal from the mouth before the shrinkage becomes significant.

The clinical handling routines are similar for each of these materials and the ones that follow.

Addition-cured silicones (vinyl silicones)

Summary

Addition-cured silicones
- Always use custom tray
- Dispense equal lengths
- Mix thoroughly
- Use light body form in syringe to avoid air bubbles
- Rigid when set
- May be difficult to remove from the mouth and/or model
- Dimensionally very stable – model need not be poured for days

These materials give more detailed results, with very low shrinkage on setting and excellent recovery from deformation. They are also less hydrophobic and are more stable after removal from the mouth than the condensation silicones. Because of their good dimensional stability they can be used satisfactorily in stock impression trays, although construction of a custom tray is a far more economical use of impression material and offers a more directional impetus to the material during placement.

The addition silicones are relatively expensive and are rather rigid after setting, which may make removal from undercut areas in the mouth difficult. Also, removal of the model from the impression can pose problems because of the possibility of breakage of fine sections of the model. Some products that do not contain finely divided palladium as a hydrogen scavenger may release hydrogen gas on setting. With these materials it is advisable to wait for at least 1 hour after removal of the impression from the mouth before pouring the model to avoid surface bubble defects on the cast. Multiple models can be made from a single impression, and the material is so dimensionally stable that impressions need not be poured for several days. This is an asset if the laboratory is situated at a distance from the dental office.

Polyether rubbers

These materials are similar in accuracy and working characteristics to the addition silicones. Because of their short working time and rapid setting time they are most useful for taking an impression of a small number of prepared teeth using a sectional tray. Like the addition silicones they set very hard and difficulties may arise if the model is at all fine and fragile.

Visible light cured materials

A polyether urethane dimethacrylate elastomer resin material which is photoinitiated is available. The material requires no mixing and is relatively rigid when cured but it requires a transparent impression tray and may pose problems in achieving an even and complete setting reaction.

TEMPORARY RESTORATIONS

After preparation of a tooth for an indirectly fabricated restoration it is necessary to construct a temporary or provisional restoration for the tooth. This is necessary if there is to be a delay greater than 1–2 hours between taking

Notes

Temporary restorations

These must:
- Protect prepared dentine from contamination
- Maintain aesthetics
- Protect all teeth against migration

the impression and cementation of the permanent restoration. Temporary restorations have several functions, as listed below.

- Protection of dentine and pulp from oral bacteria, osmotic change and temperature change.

  As a preparation generally involves dentine there will be some degree of immediate pulpal inflammation, rendering the dentine and pulp hypersensitive to normal intra-oral fluctuations in osmolality and temperature. It is also desirable to minimise bacterial access to freshly cut dentine. A temporary restoration, luted with a relatively soft cement to facilitate subsequent removal, will help protect the pulp, and reduce dentinal sensitivity.

- Maintenance of aesthetics.

  It is often an important service to the patient to provide an aesthetically acceptable interim restoration. Most of the materials used for temporary restorations are tooth coloured and it is possible to colour match to a reasonably satisfactory degree.

- Maintenance of stable tooth-to-tooth relationships.

  If a tooth is disarticulated through a cavity preparation there is a physiological tendency for it to erupt until occlusal contact is regained. Mesial tilting may also occur until approximal contact is re-established. Less commonly, distal migration can occur after surgical loss of distal contact. A tooth may move as much as 1 mm in a week in the initial period after it has been relieved of occlusal load. A well fabricated temporary restoration is designed to replace hard tissue lost in cavity preparation and prevent this movement. Maintenance of both occlusal and approximal relationships during fabrication of the final restoration will minimise problems at the time of insertion and cementation.

  Conversely, a tooth which did not originally have an occlusal or proximal contact will not move following cavity preparation and disarticulation.

- An accurate temporary restoration may also serve as an immediate model of the form of the final restoration. Therefore the temporary restoration is of value to check that tooth reduction during the preparation of the cavity was sufficient, at a time when modifications to design can be made readily.

Long-term temporaries

When there is an immediate need to replace missing tooth structure, but there is a reason to delay final restoration for an extended period, long-term provisional restorations may need to be made using more durable materials. There may be a delay whilst awaiting the outcome of periodontal therapy or the occlusal pattern may need to stabilise as part of a complex reconstruction. In these cases it may be necessary to use longer-term provisional restorations. Fully polymerised methyl methacrylate materials are preferred in these instances rather than the self-cure materials used for simpler cases. An alternative is to construct provisional restorations using permanent materials, such as gold, and place them using a temporary cement.

Materials used and fabrication techniques
Methyl methacrylate

Tooth-coloured methyl methacrylates, similar to those used in the fabrication of removable denture bases, are commonly used. The self-cure variety contains a chemical activator and initiator as separate components to initiate the setting reaction. They can also be heat cured. Heat-cured resin temporary restorations can have sufficient strength, wear resistance and colour stability to serve as provisional restorations for long periods of time.

External coronal form for the temporary restoration can be determined by taking an impression of the tooth shape before reduction, either directly in the mouth or from a model using, for example, an irreversible hydrocolloid impression material. The tooth form should be modified, if necessary, before taking the impression.

Fabricaton of a self-cure temporary restoration

With a self-cure resin, the temporary restoration can be fabricated directly on or in the prepared tooth by putting the freshly mixed resin into the impression and then placing the impression onto the model or into the mouth and retaining until initial cure is complete.

Fabrication of a heat-cure temporary restoration

When using heat-activated resin it is necessary to make a plaster model of the prepared tooth and build the temporary restoration on the model before heat curing under pressure. The technique is more time consuming but the result is a harder, more durable restoration which may well justify the additional work.

Epimine resins

These are self-cure epimine resin polymers that are tooth coloured and are useful for short-term provisional restorations. They are dimensionally very stable and relatively simple to fabricate using the approach described above for self-cure acrylic resins. The original shape of the tooth is recorded with an alginate impression before commencing tooth reduction. After preparation, the resin is placed into the impression and the impression is replaced in the mouth and retained while the resin sets. Use for longer-term temporary restorations is limited by colour instability, relatively poor resistance to wear and lack of fracture strength.

Preformed crowns

Shells of rigid or semirigid materials such as tooth-coloured polycarbonate, stainless steel, aluminium or tin are available for temporary restoration of a single tooth. The shell form can be modified to an appropriate external form by grinding, cutting or bending, then filled with one of the cold-cured resins described above or with a soft cement (see below). The shell is then seated on the prepared tooth and held in position until initial cure occurs. It can then be removed from the tooth for adjustment of the shape and polishing, before cementation with a temporary cement.

Although this technique may be quicker with preformed crowns it is not as accurate as the fully customised approach in either fit or external form. Their use may well result in movement during the temporary restoration phase.

Plastic restorative materials

Providing the principal occlusal contact of a tooth has not been removed during preparation for a rigid restoration, relatively soft materials such as zinc-oxide–eugenol or poly-carboxylate cement may be used as a temporary restoration. If, however, the full occlusal surface has been reduced a resin material is necessary to maintain stability of tooth position. Partially bonded, directly formed composite resin may be used as a provisional restoration for teeth prepared for enamel-bonded veneers on the labial surface of anterior teeth. However, if approximal contacts, occlusal contacts or dentine are not involved or exposed it may be unnecessary to place a temporary at all.

Temporary cementation

Zinc-oxide–eugenol cements are useful as temporary luting agents, not only because of their relative softness but also because of their antibacterial and sedative effects. There is a wide range of temporary cements available in this category. Note, however, that the 'reinforced' versions of these cements are not suitable for temporary cementation.

It is necessary to find a balance between retention of the provisional restoration for the desired period with ease of removal, without damage to the cavity design, at the time of final cementation. As a general principle, a retentive preparation with a well fitting temporary crown retained by a relatively soft luting agent is the best combination. Softness of the lute also aids in removal of excess cement after placement because retention of debris may compromise gingival health or seating of the crown.

Note that eugenol-containing materials must not be used if addition-cured silicone impressions have yet to be taken or if it is intended to use a resin luting cement. The setting reaction of both these groups of materials is inhibited by eugenol, even in very small quantities.

LUTING CEMENTS

When a rigid restoration is finally installed into a prepared tooth it is necessary to lute the space between the tooth and the restoration to prevent the ingress of bacteria and to unite the restoration to the tooth. The cement must not be regarded as the primary means of retaining the restoration because of the limitations of physical properties in the cements available and the difficulty of developing true long-term adhesion in the oral environment. The restoration should rely mainly on resistance and retention design in the cavity preparation to remain in place, and the accuracy of fit of the restoration will limit the quantity of cement required to lute the space. The only contribution

to retention that the cement can achieve is to limit the possibility of the restoration being removed back down the original path of insertion.

Properties of a luting cement

The important requirements of a luting cement can be listed as follows.
- Biocompatibility
- Fine ultimate film thickness
- Low solubility
- High ultimate compressive strength
- High ultimate tensile strength
- Radiopacity (is desirable).

Zinc phosphate cement

! Be aware

Zinc phosphate
- May cause post-insertion sensitivity
- Do not remove smear layer
- Apply two coats of copal varnish first
- Always vent a full crown to allow complete seating

Zinc phosphate cement has been available for many years and has proved to be a very useful material. Although it has a low pH immediately after mixing and is subject to filtration – separation of the powder and liquid during the application of high pressure in seating a restoration – it is relatively biocompatible. Dentine is an effective buffer and can counter the initial low pH, particularly as it rises quite rapidly over the first 2 hours after placement. Postinsertion sensitivity can be controlled by the application of either two layers of copal varnish or a mineralising solution over exposed dentine before cementation.

Seating

Mixed at a low powder : liquid ratio it is possible to achieve an ultimate film thickness of approximately $25\,\mu m$, but care must be taken to maintain pressure on the newly placed restoration until the initial set has taken place because the restoration tends to rebound off the tooth before setting is complete.

Venting

Alternatively, a full crown can be vented through the occlusal surface to allow escape of excess cement; this will minimise the problems associated with rebound.

Properties

Solubility is low and the compressive and tensile properties are adequate providing the powder content is maintained at the recommended level. Working time can be extended by mixing on a glass slab which has been chilled to just above the dew point or else by adding the powder to the liquid in small increments and spatulating widely over the slab to dissipate the heat of reaction. Care must be taken to maintain the prescribed powder : liquid ratio or the physical properties will be downgraded.

Adhesion

The zinc phosphate cements do not adhere chemically to tooth structure so they rely entirely on mechanical interlocking for retention. It is therefore undesirable to polish the prepared tooth surface. Sandblasting the interior of the restoration immediately before cementation is recommended because this will slightly roughen the surface.

Glass–ionomer cements

Be aware

Glass–ionomer
- Do not rely on the ion-exchange adhesion to retain a restoration
- Do not remove smear layer at time of insertion
- Apply mineralising solution at time of preparation
- No need to vent full crown

A relatively new group of cements, these materials have had an excellent record over recent years. They have a high biocompatibility, in part because of the high fluoride content, and a continuing release of fluoride over many years. The liquid is a polyalkenoic acid with a relatively high molecular weight and complex chain formation and, in view of the excellent buffering capacity of the dentine, it has no untoward effect on the pulp. The initial pH immediately after mixing is in the vicinity of pH 1.5–2.0, but this rises to pH 3.5 within the first 20 minutes and does not appear to cause problems (see Figure 8.19, page 81).

Seating

The flow is thixotropic in nature so it is simple to place a restoration completely into or onto a preparation without risk of rebound. An ultimate film thickness of $20\,\mu$m can be achieved quite readily and the need to vent a crown is rendered less likely.

Properties

The cement shows the lowest solubility rate of the luting cements and acts as a fluoride reservoir, probably for the life of the restoration. Working time cannot be varied to any significant degree although mixing on a cooled slab will add up to 25% to the available time. Care must be taken not to cool the slab below the dew point because of the risk of adding water to the mix. The powder to liquid ratio will dictate the physical properties and, within limits, the higher the powder content the higher the physical properties.

Adhesion

The glass–ionomer cements are noted for their ability to adhere to tooth structure through ion exchange and, when used as restorative cements, they do not require a retentive design in the cavity. However, as a luting cement mixed at the prescribed ratio of 1.5 parts of powder to 1 part liquid, the physical properties are not as great as those of the high powder : liquid ratio restorative cements. Although the ultimate compressive strength is adequate, the tensile strength is only about 2–3 MPa, so glass–ionomer cement cannot be relied upon with its adhesive properties to retain a poorly fitting restoration. Although it is possible to achieve adhesion to tooth structure, it is probably unwise to attempt it under these circumstances, but rather to rely on the retentive design of the restoration itself. To gain adhesion the dentine would need to be conditioned and the smear layer removed to allow development of the ion exchange and, particularly when cementing a full crown, the hydraulic pressure that can be developed may force the cement liquid through open dentine tubules to the pulp, leading to post-insertion sensitivity. It is therefore recommended that the dentine surface be remineralised instead with an oxalate-containing solution immediately after completion of the preparation. Alternatively, it can be sealed with a resin–dentine bonding agent that contains a polyalkenoic acid.

Adhesion to noble metals

It is possible to gain adhesion to a gold casting or platinum foil by laying down a fine layer of tin oxide on the fitting surface of the restoration immediately after try-in and occlusal adjustment, and just before cementation.

Polycarboxylate cements

These were the first of the cements to be regarded as adhesive to tooth structure. The liquid is a polyacrylic acid that can develop an ion exchange adhesion with dentine or enamel. The powder is essentially zinc oxide with a small quantity of manganese; biocompatibility is high. The buffering capacity of the dentine is enhanced by the presence of zinc oxide; these cements have an excellent record for cementation free of postinsertion sensitivity.

Seating

From a clinical point of view these cements are a little difficult to handle because, at the prescribed powder : liquid ratio, the mix is initially very thick and it does not achieve a workable consistency until late in the mixing process. There is therefore a tendency to reduce the powder content to make the mixing easier but this will downgrade the ultimate physical properties and should be avoided. Properly handled, the ultimate film thickness is satisfactory because of the thixotropic flow properties but it is generally not possible to reduce the cement to an ultimate film thickness of less than $30\,\mu$m.

Properties

The physical properties are generally lower than for the

first two groups so, even though adhesion to tooth structure is possible, it is not advisable to rely on the ion exchange to enhance retention of the restoration. Also, the solubility is higher than for the other cements and it seems there is a tendency for the cement to hydrolyse over time and wash out. This cement is recommended for cementation of full crowns where an ongoing pulpitis is suspected and where, therefore, other cements may cause postinsertion sensitivity. However, the retention form for the restoration should be of a high standard.

Reinforced zinc oxide cements

There is a group of cements in this category which essentially consists of zinc oxide and eugenol, with additives to increase the physical properties. They have been noted for their biocompatibility and obtundant properties but their remaining properties do not match up to those of the other materials listed in this group. There is a tendency for them to hydrolyse over time and break down to a zinc eugenolate washing out around the margins.

Their greatest value lies in the field of temporary cementation where their obtundant properties are of great value to sedate a relatively traumatised pulp following cavity preparation.

Seating
It is relatively difficult to develop a fine film thickness when using the prescribed powder:liquid ratio; these cements will almost invariably hydrolyse over time, revert to a zinc eugenolate and break down.

Properties
Their relatively low physical properties make it easier to remove the temporary restoration without doing any damage to the cavity preparation. Their strength can be reduced still further, if necessary, by the incorporation of a small quantity of petroleum jelly during mixing procedures.

Resin cements
This is a relatively new group of cements that are gaining popularity because of their high physical strength and translucency. Their biocompatibility is acceptable, inasmuch as any toxic by-products are buffered by the dentine or dissipated in the pulp over a period of a few days. They are essentially methacrylates with a variable quantity of HEMA and they contain small quantities of fine filler particles. Their use is strictly contraindicated if any eugenol-containing cement has been placed on the tooth previously.

Seating
Seating a restoration with these cements is not easy because of limited flow properties. The ultimate film thickness will vary depending on the quantity and size of the filler particles; a film thickness of less than $100\,\mu m$ is difficult to achieve.

Properties
Their main advantages include low solubility and high strength. However, their strength and retention may, in the long run, be a disadvantage inasmuch it can be very difficult to remove a restoration which has been seated with a resin cement, has subsequently failed, and which requires replacement.

Adhesion
These cements do not develop a long-term chemical adhesion to tooth structure but show a high degree of mechanical interlock, with enamel in particular, and possibly to acid-treated dentine also. They may also adhere mechanically to the restoration, particularly to an etched ceramic crown or inlay.

Resin cements are recommended for cementation of porcelain crowns, laminate veneers and porcelain inlays in particular, because they can be useful for varying or modifying colour matching and translucency. They may also compensate, to a degree, for the relative lack of fit of this type of restoration. They can compensate for marginal discrepancies of up to $100\,\mu m$ and, owing to their relatively low solubility, they wash out very slowly but, over time, they may wear out leaving a ditch at the margin.

CLINICAL PLACEMENT OF RESTORATIONS

The essential requirements for successful clinical placement of a rigid restoration are quite straightforward keeping in mind that dentine is a vital tissue and the surrounding gingival tissue may be subject to damage.

Removal of temporary restoration
Remove the temporary restoration without damaging the surrounding soft tissue and gently clean off the residue of the temporary cement. At this point do not scrub the exposed dentine or condition it with polyacrylic acid because this will remove the smear layer and open the dentine tubules. This may lead to a positive dentine fluid flow with the potential for reducing the physical properties of the final cement.

Dentine protection
It is better to protect the dentine with a 1 minute application of an oxalate solution or 25% tannic acid to seal the tubules and inhibit a positive dentine fluid flow. Alternatively, apply a very low viscosity resin dentine bonding agent containing a polyalkenoic acid. Such a seal will reduce the possibility of postinsertion sensitivity, which may arise through the ingress of toxins from the cement into the pulp under hydraulic pressure. It will also enhance the mechanical interlock between the cement and the relatively 'rough' tooth surface.

Control of gingival tissue
Reduce the potential for a positive fluid flow from the gingival crevice before mixing the cement. A light

application of trichloroacetic acid will cauterise the tissue, without the need for local anaesthesia, sufficient to maintain complete dryness for the required time. A short length of a thin gingival retraction cord may be equally successful. Placement of a rubber dam may be required on occasion although keeping the dam away from the prepared margins may then be a problem.

Venting

Venting of full crowns is desirable when using a cement with limited flow properties such as zinc phosphate or resin cement. The vent hole should be small and placed in such a position that it will lead from the inner occlusal surface of the preparation out to either the occlusal or the lingual surface of the crown. If it opens on to the occlusal it should be placed within a fissure rather than on a cuspal incline. It can be sealed immediately after the successful positioning of the crown with either a threaded or a cast pin. Alternatively it can be sealed, on a later occasion, with amalgam.

Mixing cement

Mix the cement at the correct powder:liquid ratio. Mechanical trituration in a capsule is the preferred technique because it is rapid and will lead to a consistently standard result. However, the only way to extend the working time to any significant degree is to mix by hand on a chilled glass slab.

Placement

Apply a generous layer of cement to the tooth surface using a small stiff bristle brush making sure to cover all the walls. Wind cement up into pin holes using a lentulo spiral or similar. Paint a generous layer of cement with the brush over or into the restoration and marry the two together. Apply sufficient pressure to ensure the expression of all excess cement, leaving the finest possible film behind. When using glass–ionomer cement the pressure can be released at this point but with zinc phosphate or resin cements it is advisable to maintain pressure until the first stage of the setting chemistry has been achieved.

Clean-up

When using resin cements remove all excess cement immediately after placement because of the difficulty of detecting and removing the residue once it has set. With other cements allow the cement to set sufficiently hard that it cannot be indented with a sharp probe, and then clean out the residue before it sets too hard. Further delay complicates the task, and it is essential that all residue be removed or it will become a plaque trap and lead subsequently to gingival irritation.

Review

Always review rigid restorations within 1 week after placement to ensure that the occlusion is correct and that all cement residue has been removed.

FURTHER READING

Bebermeyer RD, Berg JH. Comparison of patient-perceived post-cementation sensitivity with glass–ionomer and zinc phosphate cements. *Quintessence Int* 1994; **25**:209–14.

Brackett WW, Vickery JM. The influence of mixing temperature and powder:liquid ratio on the film thickness of three glass–ionomer cements. *Int J Prosthodont* 1994; **7**:13–16.

Brannstrom M. Reducing the risk of sensitivity and pulpal complications after the placement of crowns and fixed partial dentures. *Quintessence Int* 1996; **27**:673–8.

Johnson GH, Powell LV, Derouen TA. Evaluation and control of post-operative cementation pulpal sensitivity: zinc phosphate and glass–ionomer cements. *J Am Dent Assoc* 1993; **124**:39–46.

McLean JW. *The science and art of dental ceramics. Vol. 1. The nature of dental ceramics and their clinical use.* Chicago: Quintessence Publishing Company; 1979.

Metz JE, Brackett WW. Performance of a glass–ionomer luting cement over 8 years in a general practice. *J Prosthet Dent* 1994; **71**:13–15.

Phillips RW. *Skinner's science of dental materials, 9th ed.* Philadelphia: WB Saunders; 1991, [Chaps 7–9:107–56 & Chap 25:479–504].

Schweikert EO. Feather-edged or knife-edged preparation and impression technique. *J Prosthet Dent* 1984; **52**:243–6.

Tjan AHL, Miller GD, Sarkission R. Internal escape channel to improve the seating of full crowns with various marginal configurations; a follow-up study. *J Prosthet Dent* 1985; **53**:759–62.

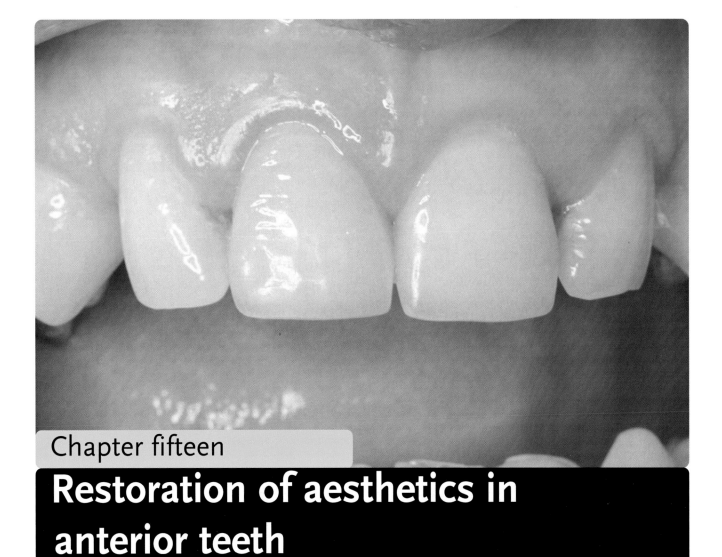

Chapter fifteen

Restoration of aesthetics in anterior teeth

D. Southan

Restoration of the single anterior tooth is a difficult aesthetic challenge and the single maxillary central incisor is the most difficult of all to deal with. Dentine is the prime source of colour in a tooth and enamel envelops the dentine with a translucent, prismatic mantle. The highest light transmission occurs at the incisal one-third and in the proximal regions. A section of enamel 1.0 mm thick can transmit up to 70% light. A section of dentine of the same thickness transmits only about 30% light. Unopacified porcelain is the best material available to simulate these optical properties of teeth.

Both the colour and shape of natural teeth are constantly changing throughout life but porcelain restorations show little change in service. Therefore, at present, it is not possible to guarantee to provide a single anterior restoration that remains permanently, aesthetically undetectable. There are a number of problems which occur that alter the aesthetics of teeth, and a number of methods are available that can be employed to modify or improve the situation. Not all these methods are perfect or permanent in their effect but the alternatives should be offered and discussed with the patient.

PROBLEMS AND POSSIBLE TREATMENTS

There are a number of problems encountered in clinical practice which will compromise the aesthetics of anterior teeth and require a solution. The principal ones can be listed as follows.

- active caries
- discoloration from pulp loss, hypoplasia or iatrogenic causes
- fracture
- malformation such as a peg lateral incisor
- ectopic eruption – canine transposed to the lateral incisor position
- a diastema between teeth
- misalignment of teeth
- erosion and abrasion.

There are a number of approaches available for overcoming these conditions and one or more may be indicated to deal with a particular situation.

- ameloplasty
- bleaching, both vital and nonvital
- orthodontic treatment
- restoration with: composite resin restoration; composite resin veneering; porcelain laminate veneering; porcelain veneer crown or a metal–ceramic veneer crown.

Ameloplasty

Ameloplasty involves importing subtle changes to the contour of a tooth by removing enamel. It is a limited form of treatment which applies principally to anterior teeth and it can be used successfully to soften incisoproximal angles and ridges or to smooth roughened and chipped incisal edges. Tooth form and shape can be delicately modified with fine diamonds to great effect. Care must be taken to polish afterwards to a fine sheen and it is important to note that the occlusal relationships and anterior guidance, particularly in centric occlusion and lateral excursions, must remain unchanged.

Bleaching of vital and nonvital teeth

Bleaching techniques can be effective for lightening the colour of teeth stained by fluorosis, tetracycline administration and acquired superficial discoloration. Bleaching or chemical alteration is the preferred primary aesthetic treatment, to be followed up later, as required, with composite resin bonding, labial resin veneers or porcelain laminate veneers.

Preparation

The tooth or teeth to be bleached should be isolated under rubber dam and cleaned with pumice and water. As the materials used are very irritating the operator and the patient must be protected with eye glasses and drapes; gloves should be worn at all times. The treatment should be performed without anaesthesia so that the patient can be constantly monitored for pain or discomfort. The pulp chamber in a nonvital tooth must be thoroughly cleaned of

all restorative material and the entry to the root canal completely sealed just apical to the gingival tissue margin with a glass–ionomer cement. Allowing bleaching chemicals to penetrate through subgingival dentine tubules may possibly lead to idiopathic external resorption of the root surface.

Summary

Bleaching with heat and light
- Hydrogen peroxide: 30–35%
- Heat: 40–57°C
- Time: 20 minutes maximum
- Vital teeth: monitor for pulp damage
- Nonvital teeth: apply within pulp chamber

Heat and light techniques

Techniques involving the application of heat or light can be used for both vital and nonvital bleaching. All the methods involve the release of oxygen from hydrogen peroxide using heat or light or a combination of both. A solution of 30–35% hydrogen peroxide is applied to the tooth and subjected to a low heat of 40–57°C for about 20 minutes at a maximum. Pulpal damage is possible but will be rare as long as the patient is carefully monitored for any sign of discomfort. A minimum of at least three treatments are generally required in the first place with a careful periodical review for some time thereafter.

Vital techniques involve labial applications only, but, for nonvital teeth, bleaching is carried out via the pulp chamber after completion of the endodontic therapy. Careful colour checks should be used to monitor the progress of bleaching and if there is no real improvement after two sessions another form of restorative therapy should be considered, such as bonding, laminating or crowning. Generally, if the initial bleaching was only partially successful, the alternative treatments are more likely to succeed for the long term.

There have been suggestions that bleaching may be related to idiopathic external resorption but there is little evidence to substantiate this.

Bleaching gel techniques

All other methods are designed to deliver oxygen to the tooth surface, in the absence of heat or light, in sufficient concentration to cause a colour modification. These are essentially patient moderated and are therefore more time consuming and less effective.

- Fine silicon dioxide powder is mixed with 35% hydrogen peroxide to form a gel that is spread in a layer about 2 mm thick on the enamel of a vital or nonvital tooth; the gel is left for 10–20 minutes. It is then removed and the teeth washed well with water.
- Nonaqueous 10% carbamide peroxide solution at pH

Summary

Bleaching gel
- Silicon dioxide powder with 35% hydrogen peroxide
- Apply 2 mm layer on vital or nonvital teeth
- Leave for 20 minutes
- Repeat as required

Alternatively...
- Carbamide peroxide 10% at pH 6.8
- Apply in custom tray
- Leave 30 minutes
- Repeat as required

6.8 is applied to the teeth using a vacuum-formed tray custom-made for the particular patient. A small amount is placed in the tray and applied to the teeth for about 30 minutes, by which time the material has become sufficiently diluted to be ineffective. The treatment can be safely repeated three or four times a day.

With each of these systems the effectiveness of the bleach depends on:
- the type and intensity of the original stain
- the contact time
- the amount of available active ingredient in the bleach.

Orange–brown stains on ageing teeth, fluorosis, smokers' stains and tetracycline stains respond quite readily to bleaching, and perceptible colour change will occur between 1 and 10 days, depending on the type and intensity of the stain. However, success is not guaranteed and an improvement may not last for long.

Microabrasion techniques

Teeth may be discoloured by hypocalcification or hypoplastic defects and the defect may not penetrate the full depth of the enamel. Such lesions may respond well to techniques which gently abrade away the stained enamel, with a low-pH vehicle containing an abrasive, leaving sound enamel beneath. Use dilute hydrochloric acid with fine flowers of pumice in a water-soluble paste. Apply the mix under firm pressure with a soft rubber cup and polish and abrade away small amounts of enamel with a slow-speed handpiece until sound enamel is exposed. An application of a topical fluoride should follow immediately to compensate for the lost enamel and remineralise the remainder. However, if the discoloration penetrates deeply into, or through, the enamel the result may be less than ideal and it may be necessary to utilise other techniques such as composite resin bonding or a porcelain laminate veneer.

Orthodontic treatment

The two main reasons for the introduction of orthodontic therapy for a patient are to improve the functional relationship of the two arches and to upgrade the aesthetic arrangement of the teeth – in particular the anteriors. It is often the responsibility of the dentist to recognise the former because the patient may not be aware of the problem but on many occasions it will be the patient who will insist on treatment for the latter situation. Discrepancies which appear minor to the dentist may be major to the patient and a sympathetic and understanding approach is required. There may, however, be problems which are only obvious to the dentist and timely advice is required to alert the patient to the problem.

Orthodontic treatment should always be considered in cases involving ectopic teeth, diastemata and misaligned teeth, particularly while the patient is young and the dentition is more subject to rearrangement. Timely diagnosis and effective treatment can obviate an insoluble functional and aesthetic problem in the future.

It is important to note if the canines have failed to erupt on time so that, if they are impacted, they can be assisted down into their correct position by appropriate surgical exposure and orthodontic treatment. It is very important that the canines be correctly positioned so that they can play their part in anterior guidance during the masticatory cycle.

The problem of missing or peg lateral incisors should be diagnosed early so that development can be monitored and guided rather than wait for complex treatment at a later stage. Orthodontic treatment is generally required to either open or close the spaces. Whilst it is possible to move a canine into the lateral position and disguise it using ameloplasty and composite resin it is generally far better to position the canine for proper function and to use other methods to replace the lateral.

Composite resin restoration

Composite resin is the material of choice for restoration of relatively minor defects on anterior teeth involving the incisal edge or labial enamel deficiencies, such as:
- damage from caries
- traumatic fracture
- modification of anatomy; for example, peg laterals, canine in lateral position, diastemata.

The advantages are that the technique is relatively non-invasive, prompt and inexpensive. Although the resin tends to wear and stain over time it can be repaired or replaced readily and atraumatically with minimum further loss of tooth structure.

The attachment of composite resin to enamel through the acid-etch technique is sufficiently effective to allow its use for the improvement of the aesthetic form of a malformed tooth such as a peg lateral incisor. Upper canines which have been moved to compensate for a missing lateral incisor can have their outline form softened so the change is less noticeable. Diastemata can be reduced or closed up, and misaligned, abraded, eroded teeth treated effectively. The limitations of these techniques include the relatively low physical properties of the composite resins, their poor covering power and low resistance to staining and abrasion.

507–508

Porcelain laminate veneers

The porcelain laminate veneer technique is irreversible but reasonably conservative. Porcelain is more resistant to stain uptake and colour change than resin composite veneers and it does not wear away. However, it is generally necessary to remove a greater amount of enamel to make room for the veneer, otherwise there is a risk of altering the emergence profile of the crown with subsequent periodontal problems. The porcelain laminate veneer is indicated in any situation where the enamel is severely defective, stained, malformed or fractured. However, in view of the fact that attachment to the tooth is dependent upon the presence of some remaining enamel it is contraindicated where the enamel has been lost or where there is a heavy occlusal load on the anterior teeth (**Figs 15.1** and **15.2**).

Great care must be taken in the preparation phase because it is necessary to retain some enamel to which to develop adhesion with the resin cement which is used for attachment. If dentine is exposed adhesion cannot be assured for longer than 3–4 years and leakage, particularly at the gingival margin, will destroy the aesthetic result and may lead to recurrent caries. There can be no certainty as to the thickness of remaining enamel because the patient may well have abraded some away already. Although the average thickness of the labial enamel on an upper central

incisor tooth is approximately 1.75 mm. there may be considerably less than this on a tooth which has changed colour to the extent that it requires a veneer.

Also, because a porcelain veneer is necessarily quite thin, there are limitations to the covering power that can be provided and the extent to which the veneer can be characterised to blend in with remaining natural teeth. From a cosmetic point of view it is much simpler to improve aesthetics by covering four to six anterior teeth than to replace a single tooth, particularly a single upper central incisor.

Porcelain jacket crown

The porcelain jacket crown is still the best method available to restore a single central incisor with optimal aesthetics. It can be made highly translucent and it can be characterised with lateral segmental build-up of porcelain to provide a depth of shade and character unmatched by any other system. Although aluminous porcelain itself is stronger than metal–ceramic porcelain it lacks the support provided by a strong metal framework and is therefore somewhat limited in its application. This means the porcelain jacket crown should be applied to the aesthetically demanding situation where no more than moderate occlusal stress is expected. Parafunction or thegotic activity is a contraindication (see Chapter 4). Porcelain jacket crowns built on pervious refractory dies can exhibit marginal adaptation of a very high order.

Metal–ceramic crown

Generally, metal–ceramic crown aesthetics suffer by comparison with the porcelain jacket crown because they cannot provide the depth of translucency of an all-porcelain restoration. It is necessary to provide covering power in the porcelain to mask the metal background and this gives an optical flatness to the restoration (**Fig. 15.3**).

CD
509

There are times where this optical effect can be utilised to aesthetic advantage but, generally, the metal–ceramic crown should only be used in the single anterior tooth when functional demands are excessive. That is, the aesthetic effect may have to give way to functional demands.

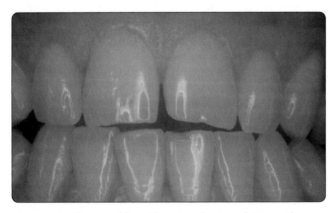

Fig. 15.1 Aesthetic problem. There is a diastema between the central incisors and a lack of regularity in the anteriors.

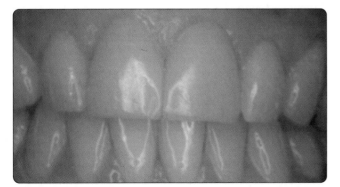

Fig. 15.2 Porcelain laminates. Porcelain laminate veneers were placed to improve aesthetics.

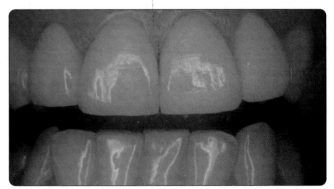

Fig. 15.3 Porcelain bonded to metal crowns. The upper anteriors are all porcelain bonded to metal crowns. Note excellent emergence profile and gingival contour as well as colour match.

PRINCIPLES OF AESTHETIC COLOUR MATCHING

Successful restoration of aesthetics in restorative dentistry can best be realised through an understanding of natural tooth form, texture, shade and anatomy.

Form and surface texture

Form and surface texture of a tooth are more important than shade in the provision of an aesthetic restoration. When preparing for and making a porcelain crown it is essential to develop the proper emergence profile and axial form in the cervical region so as to avoid compromising periodontal health. Careful preparation of the tooth is essential to allow sufficient space for the porcelain without compromising aesthetics. The gingival shoulder preparation should be at least 1.0 mm wide and there should be 1.5 mm of tooth removed in the midlabial region and at least 2.0 mm from the incisal edge.

The way in which light is reflected from the labial surface of a crown will also contribute greatly to the appearance of vitality so surface striae, notches, fissures and grooves should be included on the labial surface as required to control reflectance. A smooth, glossy surface will look brighter than a textured or matt surface because it reflects more light back to the observer. Therefore, careful observation of the tooth form will allow it to be texture matched as well as colour matched.

Shade selection

Commercial shade guides are not based on measured tooth colour so they are more appropriate for selecting teeth for complete dentures rather than colour matching for natural teeth. When a shade is selected it will not necessarily be a perfect match to the original tooth colour and modifications to the shade will often need to be made to achieve a complete colour match. This means that some understanding of the theory of colour is essential to consistently achieve a close shade match, especially for single restorations. Multiple restorations are far less demanding.

To perceive colour or shade there must be light falling on to, and reflected from, an object. The reflected light is perceived by the eye and brain. Some aspects of colour perception are subjective. It is necessary in dentistry, however, to derive an objective statement of the nature of colour so that effective communication can occur between manufacturer and dentist and between dentist and dental technician.

The dimensions of colour

Colour can be described as having three dimensions – hue, value and chroma.

Hue

Visible light resides in the electromagnetic spectrum of energy between wavelengths of 380 nm and 760 nm, that is, it lies above the ultraviolet and below the infrared regions.

Notes

Dimensions of colour
- Hue
  the family name of a colour
- Value
  relative whiteness or blackness of a colour
- Chroma
  intensity or saturation of the hue

Hue is a stimulus of radiant energy of a given wavelength or group of wavelengths and provides the 'family name' of the colour. The order of the physical hue is violet, indigo, blue, green, yellow, orange and red but within the visible spectrum there is no clear demarcation between discrete hues. They merge into one another so hue names such as red or blue define a hue range rather than a specific entity.

Value

Value is the relative whiteness or blackness or, alternatively, the lightness or brightness of a colour. The value of a colour is defined by comparing it with a grey of similar brightness. Therefore colours of low value are more like black and colours of high value are more like white. Coloured scenes or objects can be reduced to one-dimensional values as in, for example, black and white photography and television.

Value is extremely important in shade selection for teeth and it must be correct. Small differences in hue and chroma are relatively unimportant if the value is very close to correct.

Chroma

Chroma is the saturation of the hue and is only present when there is hue – unlike value, which occurs independently of hue. Intense colour denotes a higher chroma; for example, canine teeth usually have a higher chroma than incisors in the same mouth. Normal blood exhibits a given chroma but if it is centrifuged it will exhibit a higher chroma simply because of the compaction of the red blood cells.

Colour vision

The eye receives visual images through the reception of light, which it directs to receptor cells that convert this information and transmit it to the brain for interpretation and reaction (**Fig. 15.4**).

Light enters the eye through the cornea, which is a clear, lamellar structure of submicroscopic collagen fibrils. A protein-free plasma, the aqueous humour, lies behind the cornea and the iris controls the quantity of light admitted to the eye which then passes to the avascular lens. Light then passes through the jelly-like vitreous humor and is focused onto the cellular retinal layer lining the posterior surface of the eye. It travels through layers of blood vessels, nerve fibres and supporting cells to the rods and cones, which are the sensitive receptors lying at the back of the retina. Light reaching the photoreceptors is converted to nerve impulses that are sent through the optic nerve and tract to the lateral geniculate body in the brain. Here a synapse with another set of neurones is made and the impulses are directed to the occipital lobe of the cerebral cortex where the information is interpreted.

Cones and rods
The cones function in daylight conditions, and give colour vision while the rods function under low illumination, and give vision only in shades of grey. Cones are packed tightly in the foveal region, which is the centre of most acute vision but the rods are found away from the fovea and increase in numbers towards the periphery of the retina (**Fig. 15.5**).

Photosensitive pigments
There are three types of cones, with each type of cone containing a photosensitive pigment with a range of sensitivity to which it will respond. The pigments respond selectively to the additive primary colours of blue (445 nm), green (535 nm) and red (570 nm), so the human visual system is able to receive colour through the additive colour system because the pigments convert light to colour sensation. On the other hand, achromatic vision is mediated by the rods. Value can best be appraised by 'looking off' the fovea and squinting. When the eyes are narrowed, the light admitted is diminished and the focus becomes less acute. This favours rod function and judgements of value are enhanced.

Defective colour vision
Total colour blindness (monochromatism) is extremely rare; other less serious defects in colour vision are sex linked and affect about 8% of the male population. Normal colour vision is called trichromatic vision because it is derived from the three photosensitive pigments.

The most common defects in colour vision occur when the person can see all three primary colours but has a weakness or confusion in some area, usually the red or green area. There are also types of defect where the person can only see two of the primary colours.

Colour vision can be tested using numbers camouflaged by a series of dots and asking the person to perceive and identify the numbers. Inability to succeed in one group or another demonstrates either colour confusion or over-compensation of one or more of the primary photosensitive pigments rather than an inability to see colour. It is clear that colour defects should be identified in dentists so that compensatory steps can be taken.

Negative after-image
The colour vision phenomenon called negative after-image can influence shade selection. The ability to perceive the correct hue is progressively diminished with time. As light of a particular wavelength strikes the cones sensitive to that stimulus, the photosensitive pigments involved are depleted at a rate faster than regeneration can occur so the eye becomes progressively less sensitive to the hue range of that stimulus. The accuracy of shade judgements becomes rapidly less reliable through this phenomenon, which is termed 'hue adaptation'. Along with the waning ability to perceive a given hue the eye becomes more responsive to complementary hues of the adapted range. This means for example that intense red lipstick can make teeth appear greenish by reducing red perception.

To overcome the problem in the clinical situation, comparisons in shade selection should not exceed 5 seconds duration. The gaze should then be diverted to a card of a medium blue colour to adapt the vision to blue and sensitise it to yellow. The eye can then continue to be an accurate receptor.

Simultaneous contrast
The phenomenon of simultaneous contrast is an intensification of the difference perceived between two

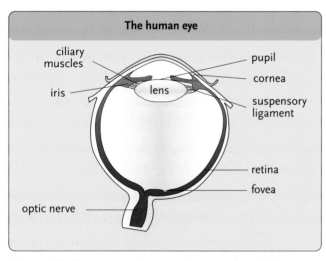

Fig. 15.4 The human eye. A horizontal section through the human eye showing the essential parts related to vision.

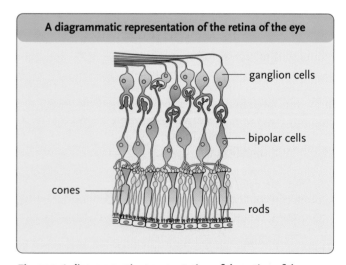

Fig. 15.5 A diagrammatic representation of the retina of the eye. The retina is the functional area of the eye essential to the discrimination of colour.

adjacent contrasting colours. When a yellow object is placed alongside a blue field, both appear brighter and more saturated. Colours can appear brighter against a dark background and darker against a bright background. Hues can appear more colourful against a neutral background or less colourful against a coloured background. All these situations can be encountered and affect shade matching.

Light source and shade selection

Colour is characteristic of the reflected light that enters the eye from an object. A change in the light source can change the object's appearance. If light of certain wavelengths is absent or deficient in the source of light, it cannot be reflected to the observer, even though the object might be capable of reflecting such light. Therefore it is essential to illuminate an object with full spectral lighting in order to assess its colour correctly.

As there is no perfect light source for shade selection there must, of necessity, be a compromise. A source of illumination can be evaluated by its apparent colour temperature, its spectral curve and its colour rendering index and, whichever source is chosen, its limitations must be recognised (**Fig. 15.6**).

Colour temperature

A light source suitable for shade selection should have an apparent colour temperature of about 5500 Kelvin and little or no hue dominance. The specifications of operating lights and fluorescent tubes that are colour corrected are available from their suppliers.

Level of illumination

Brightness contrast can also influence shade matching because the eye is more easily fatigued where ambient lighting is uneven. This means the dental clinic should always be evenly and adequately illuminated and there should not be a great contrast between the intra-oral

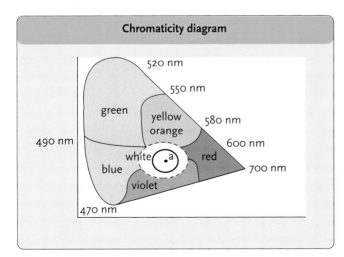

Fig. 15.6 Chromaticity diagram. A chromaticity diagram showing the equal energy point (a). The circle around this central point depicts the light sources with colour rendering indices of 92.

illumination and the surrounding work environment. Ideally, the walls of the dental surgery should be a neutral grey or pastel blue.

Metamerism

Two objects with identical spectral distribution curves will always match regardless of the nature of the illumination. When attempting to create different materials with the same colour, however, identical spectral distribution is very difficult to achieve. The usual outcome is that the two objects appear to be of the same colour under some lighting conditions but not others. Such objects are called metamers.

Tooth structure, porcelain and other tooth-coloured restorative materials have different spectral distribution curves. It is therefore necessary to test shades under various light sources such as:
- daylight
- a cool white fluorescent light
- an incandescent lamp.

The shade of the restorative material should be tested under each of the above and the colour that best matches adjacent tooth structure under these various conditions should be selected.

Shade matching routine

Every attempt should be made to match shades by using intrinsic rather than extrinsic colouring. Shade must necessarily have depth, and surface staining ought to be used only to simulate similar stains on adjacent teeth. Surface staining should never be employed to correct mismatches although this is an ideal that is not always possible to accomplish.

Variables to take into account

The variables of tooth colour are the value (lighter or darker), hue (more yellow or more red) and chroma (weaker or stronger), and the various porcelain systems available should be used with their own specific shade guide because different porcelains possess different optical properties. However, the usual dental shade guides lack a systematic arrangement or orderly relationship between tabs and they do not represent the range of colours encountered in natural teeth. This means that shade selection must acknowledge and allow for these limitations and proper communication with the ceramic technician is very important.

Check value first

Value is the most important property to be achieved because if value, translucency, and blue–grey effect are correctly matched there is a far greater chance of developing an undetectable restoration for an anterior tooth.

Range of shade guides

Within a controlled environment, as described above, shade selection should be a logical process. Have on hand three sets of shade guides for the particular ceramic system being used. The first guide should be left just as it is received. With the second shade guide remove the ridge lap portion of each tooth. For the third remove the glaze from the labial surface. The tab with the glaze removed can be used when modifications are needed to match natural teeth.

- Step 1: Clean the teeth with pumice and water.
- Step 2: Ask the patient to remove lipstick or dominant colour make-up.
- Step 3: Hold a moistened shade tab to the tooth being matched and compare the value. Increase the ratio of rod to cone vision by reducing the environmental lighting intensity and by squinting the eyes. Select the shade that most closely matches the value of the tooth. Note whether it is higher or lower in value.
- Step 4: Increase the background lighting intensity and assess the hue. View from directly in front of the teeth with the guide tab held in the same plane as the tooth being matched and use multiple light sources to choose the best compromise. Do not look at the teeth for longer than 5 seconds before relaxing the eyes by gazing at a blue card. Compare with the shade guide and the tooth both wet and dry.

Decide whether the shade guide tab is the same, more yellow than or more red than the natural tooth. Comparison with the canine can help in this decision as these teeth usually have denser hues than the others.

- Step 5: Assess the relative saturation of the adjacent teeth.
- Step 6: View again with the lips relaxed and reflected, and with the lipstick replaced. If no close match is achievable, always select a shade higher in value and lower in chroma, and modify the third shade guide using metal oxide stains. It is much easier to lower the value using the principles of subtractive colour than to raise it. If possible reassess the shade at two or three different appointments and compare the results.

The decision to select a shade that is higher in value and lower in chroma should be made only when modification of the restoration is possible. If no modification is to be made a restoration with a slightly lower value will be more acceptable.

Shade prescription

The objective in writing a shade prescription is to provide the ceramist with a detailed chart which will incorporate as much information as possible on the intrinsic translucency and coloration of the tooth to be matched. Localised effects and hairline checks should be included to be incorporated within the body of the crown using a lateral segmentation technique in the porcelain build-up.

Two diagrams for the restoration are generally required, the first depicting the outline of the tooth from the labial or buccal aspect and the other representing a sagittal cross-section of the crown (**Fig. 15.7**).

The shade tabs on the Lumin Vacuum Guide can be

arranged in descending order of relative value, or degree of brightness, as follows:

B1; A1; B2; D2; A2; C1; C2; D4; A3; D3; B3; A3.5; B4; C3; A4; C4.

Based on these tabs, the value can be determined relative to the value of surrounding teeth.

- If the shade varies more to the red side prescribe an A range.
- If the shade varies more to yellow prescribe a B shade.

Note the usefulness of the effect porcelains and append the requirements to the 'tooth map', which is the technician's guide to the ultimate crown.

The use of stains and coloured porcelains

Often, existing porcelain shades need to be modified and manufacturers of porcelains supply intensely coloured porcelain powders for this purpose. The problem is that the palette of pigments for ceramics is limited, especially the reds, and it is the red–yellow range which is required for teeth. Consequently, a modified colour wheel has been developed for dental shades in which cyan is removed and orange (yellow–red) inserted and in which the red used is, in reality, a pink.

Intrinsic colour

Colour and characterisation which is intrinsic or built-in is preferred but it is impossible to correct a poor colour match without repeating the restoration. Whilst it is less effective, extrinsic characterisation is reversible. The final colour match must be achieved early because repeated firing is very undesirable. The existing pigments tend to dissolve in the glassy matrix and decompose, and metal–ceramic porcelains will devitrify and opacify with over-firing.

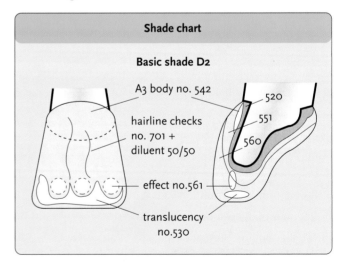

Shade chart

Basic shade D2

A3 body no. 542

520

551

560

hairline checks no. 701 + diluent 50/50

effect no.561

translucency no.530

Fig. 15.7 Shade chart. This is the basic type of shade chart that would be hand-drawn at the chairside and used for proper communication between the operator and the ceramist. Note that it is necessary to provide both a labial aspect as well as a proximal view to impart full detail. The more detail the better, and direct discussion may still be desirable if there are unusual modifications to be incorporated.

Extrinsic colour

Extrinsic modification can be carried out after all surface shaping and texture has been established and the glaze removed. Thoroughly clean the surface and replace the crown in the mouth. Surface stains can now be applied with a clean sable hair brush and the modifications carefully charted. Remove the crown from the mouth and clean off the stains. The modifications are then repeated in the laboratory and the crown fired at atmospheric pressure (no vacuum).

No more than three firings should be carried out for any one crown.

Age changes in the natural dentition

Tooth form and shade are constantly changing because of attrition, abrasion, erosion and biological changes in dentine and enamel. Teeth wear occlusally, incisally and approximally under normal function and they can also be abraded by brushing or eroded by dietary or gastric acid. Changes in the shade of natural teeth with ageing are due to an increase in translucency of the enamel, increasing mineralisation of the dentine, stain uptake and discoloration. Any restoration of a tooth must be recognised as a static remedy for a dynamic situation.

In young people, incident light passing through teeth is diffused and scattered by hydroxyapatite crystals and inter-crystalline defects of different refractive index. The teeth appear relatively white and opaque. With ageing hydroxy-apatite crystals in enamel become denser and inter-crystalline defects are gradually filled. The enamel tends to become more translucent. At the same time the density of mineralisation of dentine increases, and the body of the tooth therefore appears to become more yellow. The shade change will first appear in the cervical region of teeth because of the relatively thin enamel in this area.

Considerable variations may occur in this pattern of change. Incisal attrition will often change the dentine into a harder, more translucent tissue. The incisal dentine may appear opaque and stained in contrast to the more translucent enamel. Staining and discoloration may occur in the enamel, particularly in the cervical and proximal regions and in pits and fissures. Stains permeating into the superficial enamel layers from firmly attached foodstuffs, nicotine stain, bacteria and various metal ions can cause yellowish-brown discoloration and various pigments may permeate enamel cracks, making them more apparent as orange or brown lines.

Obviously the cosmetic life of a coronal restoration for a single anterior tooth in a young person is limited. Shade changes occur at varied rates in different individuals and a prudent clinician will always alert a patient to these facts before embarking on the coronal restoration of an anterior tooth.

FURTHER READING

Horn HR. Porcelain laminate veneers bonded to etched enamel. *Dent Clin North Am* 1983; **27**:671–84.

McLean JW. *The art and science of dental ceramics. Volume II. Bridge design and laboratory procedures in dental ceramics.* Chicago: Quintessence Publishing Company; 1980.

Nakagawa Y *et al.* Analysis of natural tooth colour. *Shikai Tenbo* 1975; **46**:527–37.

Rushton JD. Visual pigments and colour blindness. *Sci Am* 1975; 64.

Simonsen RJ, Calamia JR. Tensile bond strength of etched porcelain [Abstract]. *J Dent Res* 1983; **62**:297.

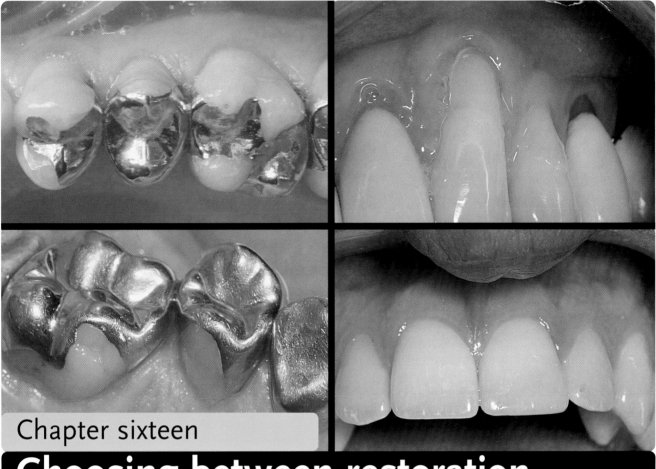

Chapter sixteen

Choosing between restoration modalities

G.J. Mount

It is necessary to take a number of factors into account in selecting the restorative material to be utilised in the restoration of any tooth. There are both advantages and disadvantages with each of the materials currently available and therefore none of them is ideal.

Maintenance of the original tooth structure should be the primary aim in treatment of the carious lesion, but as the lesion progresses and the cavity becomes larger there comes a stage where sacrifice of further tooth structure is required to provide protection from occlusal load to ensure maintenance of the remainder.

Because no restorative material is ideal and all materials display a potential life span of no more than 20 years, a considerable amount of the restorative work undertaken consists of replacement of old restorations.

Generally, replacement is indicated because of recurrent caries, failure of the previous restorative material or fracture of remaining tooth structure. Inevitably, there will be further loss and weakening of the remaining tooth structure. These factors will dictate the choice of the replacement material and this material must always offer the greatest longevity possible.

GLASS–IONOMER

Advantages

Summary

Glass–ionomer

Advantages
- Ion-exchange adhesion with dentine and enamel
- Continuing fluoride release
- Acceptable aesthetics
- Good wear factor
- Low solubility

Disadvantages
- Low fracture resistance
- Needs to be laminated if subject to load

Glass–ionomer is the only material currently available capable of true diffusion-based chemical adhesion to both enamel and dentine through an ionic exchange. It is a water-based cement and therefore stable in the oral environment and it has been shown that it is a dynamic material, inasmuch as the chemistry of the setting reaction will continue for a long period of time after placement. As a result of the method of manufacture of the glass, the cement contains fluoride that is released into the surrounding tooth structure after placement. There is a strong release initially, which reduces over the first 2 months, but it has been shown to still be present after at least 5 years (Chapter 8, page 82). The fluoride content can be continually 'recharged' from topical applications. As a result, this material has a strong resistance to the development of recurrent caries and there will be little plaque formation on the surface.

Glass–ionomer is available in a number of forms, depending on powder : liquid ratio, particle size and the chemistry of the setting reaction. It is used extensively as a luting material for crowns and bridges as well as a lining and a dentine substitute under other restorative materials. Each of these versions is fast setting and develops an early resistance to water contamination. One of the most useful versions is the restorative cement which has an acceptable degree of translucency and colour matching and, because of its adhesive potential, there is no need to modify the cavity design to develop mechanical retention.

Both the Type II restorative cement and the Type III lining cement are available in a light-activated form (resin modified or dual cure) as well as the original chemically activated (autocure) system. Dual-cure has been made possible through the addition of further resins, including HEMA and photo-initiators, and the main advantage is resistance to water contamination immediately the cement is set. The original acid–base reaction, which allows the development of adhesion to the tooth, and is therefore the key to the

glass–ionomer system, is still present but is protected by the umbrella-like presence of the dual-cure resins.

Disadvantages

The main limitation is a relatively low fracture resistance, such that glass–ionomer cannot be used alone to withstand undue occlusal load. It is not suitable for rebuilding marginal ridges or incisal corners but, providing it is well supported by surrounding tooth structure, its physical properties and abrasion resistance are sufficient to withstand considerable load. Solubility is also low but, on occasion, translucency in the chemically activated (auto-cure) cements may not be sufficient for colour matching, and lamination with composite resin may be required for a satisfactory end-result.

COMPOSITE RESIN

Advantages

Summary

Composite resin

Advantages
- Excellent aesthetics
- Accepts good polish
- Variety available for different tasks
- Wear factor acceptable
- Relatively inexpensive

Disadvantages
- Placement techniques require high skill
- Difficult to restore full anatomy
- Difficult to bond to dentine
- Basic resin is hydrophilic, takes up water over time
- Longevity not great

Restorations with excellent aesthetics can be built with composite resin, using the modern light-activated varieties in particular. When the resin is placed incrementally, and properly light-activated at each stage, variation in both colour and translucency can be incorporated and anatomical form reproduced reasonably accurately. Much work has been carried out in recent years on the filler particles incorporated within the resin and there is considerable variation between products marketed by different manufacturers. Physical properties and translucency are affected by the filler content, and the ability of a material to take and retain a smooth polished surface also varies.

Properly placed its physical properties can be sufficient to withstand moderate occlusal load as far distally as the bicuspids and the wear factor of the more heavily filled types is sufficient for these restorations. Relative to ceramic restorations it is inexpensive but it has a notably shorter potential lifespan.

Disadvantages

Placement techniques require patience and a high degree of skill. One of the main problems at present is the overall shrinkage of the resin mass during the curing phase. The chemically cured composites shrink towards the centre of the restoration, thus tending to pull away from the walls of the cavity but towards the floor. When cured by light activation, shrinkage will occur towards the light, pulling the resin off both the floor and the walls (Chapter 9, page 98). Careful incremental placement will minimise the total shrinkage but it is still sufficient to place considerable stress on the bonding of the restoration to either the tooth or a cement base. These restorations are therefore subject to microleakage especially in relation to margins placed on dentine. In the presence of microleakage the pulp may become inflamed unless it is adequately sealed and protected with a glass–ionomer base.

The bis-GMA resin, which is the basis of most composite resins, is relatively hydrophilic and takes up water over time. This will lead to a degree of breakdown, particularly under occlusal load, so the wear factor can be significant particularly if the restoration is expected to maintain posterior support. On the other hand, some of the composite resin formulas containing large particles may cause wear on the enamel of opposing teeth.

Union between the filler particles and the resin matrix is developed through adding a silane coating to the filler particles. This is expected to lead to a chemical union throughout the restoration. However, this bond represents a potential weakness, because it may be incomplete or hydrolyse and break down, thus releasing the particles and increasing the wear factor.

Allergies to some of the ingredients have been reported by both operators and staff, as well as patients. Methyl methacrylate and HEMA have both been identified as allergens since resins were first used many years ago for the construction of dentures. Particles of barium or strontium glass may be released as a result of wear and the long-term effect of their ingestion is not yet known. Formaldehyde can also be a by-product of the setting reaction.

AMALGAM

Advantages

Over many years, particularly in small restorations, amalgam has been shown to have a very satisfactory history of longevity with a potential half-life of up to 25 years. It is relatively easy to handle through standardised methods and seems to be very tolerant of less than ideal placement techniques. Properly placed, it has physical properties which are sufficient to maintain occlusal stresses and it is a very economical material to work with and therefore cost effective. Although it does not have any caries resistant properties in itself, it will corrode in the oral environment, and the corrosion products will seal the margins against microleakage within the first 3 weeks after placement. It is therefore highly resistant to recurrent caries.

Summary

Amalgam

Advantages
- Relatively easy to handle
- Relatively tolerant of poor handling techniques
- Excellent longevity in small to moderate lesions
- Inexpensive

Disadvantages
- Poor aesthetics
- Difficult to restore full anatomy
- Wear factor too great for large restorations

Disadvantages

The main disadvantage of amalgam is that it is aesthetically undesirable. The material itself is dark grey in colour and as it corrodes it darkens and releases metallic ions into the surrounding dentine, leading to a blue discoloration in the remaining tooth structure. Corrosion is therefore both an advantage and a disadvantage. In modern formulations with a high copper content the corrosion potential has been reduced sufficiently to minimise the disadvantages although there is still enough corrosion product available to seal the margins against microleakage.

Reproduction of occlusal and proximal anatomy is difficult when placing all the direct plastic restorative materials and the problems increase as the cavity gets larger. Relatively sophisticated matrix techniques are available but reproduction of full proximal anatomy, particularly in relation to the marginal ridge and contact area, is problematical.

Occlusal anatomy can be restored for the smaller restoration but becomes a more onerous task as the cavity extends, particularly if a cusp needs to be protected. It is not possible to determine the success of the reconstruction of the anatomy until the restoration has been completed and the patient is able to close the mouth and check the occlusion. The wear factor of amalgam is slightly greater than that of enamel, and, therefore, if the restoration is extensive and the occlusal load is heavy, the occlusion may not remain stable over long periods.

Mercury safety issues are discussed in Appendix 1, page 255, and Chapter 10, page 113.

GOLD

Advantages

The physical properties of gold alloys are variable, with four types of alloys being available for the restoration of teeth using either direct or indirect techniques (Chapter 12, pages 156). Direct gold restorations are placed in the form of gold foil, which is pure gold leaf. This will cold weld to a uniform mass through malleting directly into a cavity. In addition there are three types of gold for tooth restoration

Summary

Gold

Advantages
- Wide range available
- Highly accurate fit
- Reinstates complete anatomy
- Wear factor similar to that of tooth structure

Disadvantages
- Multistage production
- High skill required at each stage
- Relatively high cost
- Aesthetics doubtful

using indirect techniques – types A, B and C – which range in hardness upwards from type A which is the softest. With this range available it is possible to select a relatively ideal material for restoration of any situation. It must be noted that the wear factor with gold is very similar to that of natural tooth structure.

Modern casting techniques allow for very high accuracy in fit and the inherent strength and ductility of gold means that it can be utilised in thin section to protect remaining tooth structure. It is a noble metal and will not corrode and, because of its highly polished surface texture, it is resistant to plaque formation and therefore shows a very high tissue tolerance.

One of the major advantages is that, when a restoration is produced by an indirect technique in the laboratory, it is possible to reinstate both the occlusal and proximal surfaces to the full anatomy of the original tooth. This is difficult indeed with any other material, except possibly ceramics.

Disadvantages

Placement of direct malleted gold foil is relatively time consuming and is indicated for small, one-surface restorations only. Gold inlays and crowns, constructed by indirect techniques, involve complex laboratory procedures as well as rather lengthy chairside operations. They are, therefore, relatively expensive in the first instance although their longevity will readily justify the initial outlay. In addition the multistage production routines allow the introduction of errors at any one of these stages and it is essential that skilled operators are available at each stage, both in the clinic and the laboratory. The error, or accumulation of errors, will often only be detected at the final insertion appointment and may require repetition of the entire procedure.

In the current era of aesthetic dentistry the acceptability of the appearance of gold restorations is becoming debatable. Not all patients are opposed to them but many request more aesthetic materials.

CERAMICS

Advantages

Summary

Ceramics

Advantages
- Perfect aesthetics available
- Reinstate complete anatomy
- Accurate fit

Disadvantages
- Multistage production
- High skill at each stage
- Relatively high cost
- Wear factor high on natural teeth

The art and science of dental ceramics has reached a very high level and it is the material of choice for aesthetic restorations (Chapters 12, page 158). With careful attention to detail ceramic crowns can defy detection by the naked eye. Because plaque will not readily accumulate on a fully glazed ceramic surface, tissue tolerance is very high and a skilled technician can reproduce the anatomy of both the occlusal and the proximal surfaces with great accuracy.

The physical properties of glazed ceramics are of a high order and their abrasion resistance is such that the opposing teeth is more likely to wear than the restorations. The cost of these restorations to the patient is high, but the initial outlay can be justified because of the longevity and superior aesthetics available.

Disadvantages

Because of the many stages involved in the production of ceramic restorations there is a high potential for the introduction of errors. All stages of production in both the clinic and the laboratory must be completed to the highest possible standard if success is to be assured.

The fracture resistance of ceramics is not high and restorations are prone to cracking and chipping, particularly if the occlusion is not properly developed. Repair and replacement is expensive and failure will generally require complete reconstruction. In addition, the wear factor of ceramics against both natural tooth structure and gold is rather high, particularly if the porcelain has lost its glaze. If the material is to be used it is better to oppose ceramics to ceramics rather than to oppose it to any other material.

FACTORS GOVERNING THE SELECTION OF A RESTORATIVE MATERIAL

Taking into account the advantages and disadvantages of the available restorative materials as listed above, the following rationale can be applied in any given situation with the materials discussed in order of preference.

Restoration and maintenance of physical properties of a tooth

- Gold is the material of choice inasmuch as it can be used in thin section to protect and reinforce remaining tooth structure. Also, constructed by indirect techniques, it is possible to re-establish the ideal contour and anatomy of a tooth and rebuild occlusion with a high degree of accuracy.
- Ceramic restorations also are built by indirect techniques and therefore it is possible to rebuild anatomy and occlusion with a high degree of accuracy. However, they are too brittle to be designed in thin section and therefore, generally, more of the remaining tooth structure must be removed to allow sufficient room for the restorative material.
- Both amalgam and composite resin are confined to intracoronal restorations and therefore it is generally not possible to restore strength to remaining tooth structure. Adhesion with resins is only as strong as the tensile strength of the component parts of the system and neither composite resin, resin bonding agents nor enamel are consistently strong in tension. Cavity modifications and an acid-etch union between enamel and resin can provide a degree of protection to weakened cusps, but not substantial reinforcement.
- The adhesion available with glass–ionomer cement will restore some of the lost physical properties but the cement itself has a relatively low tensile strength and cannot therefore be relied upon to offer a significant reinforcement to remaining tooth structure.

Restoration and maintenance of occlusion

- Gold is the material of choice because, depending on the alloy selected, the wear factor is almost identical to that of natural tooth enamel. Because the restoration is built through an indirect technique, occlusion can be refined to a high degree and will subsequently be maintained over many years, almost without change.
- Ceramic restorations are useful for restoring anatomy and occlusion because they must be built indirectly. However, the technique is more demanding and the wear factor is much greater than for gold. The porcelain surface will not flow and create the Beilby veneer which is seen with metals and therefore ceramic restorations abrade opposing surfaces, particularly as the porcelain loses its glaze. It is desirable to occlude porcelain to porcelain and not porcelain to natural tooth structure or any other restorative materials.
- Amalgam, composite resin and glass–ionomer cement are not suitable for the restoration and maintenance of the occlusion because the wear factor is too great with all three. In addition it is almost impossible to reliably recontour the occlusal surface in these materials directly in the mouth with restricted access and vision and,

generally, there is no opportunity to add to the restoration if it has been inadvertently carved out of occlusion during placement.

Restoration and maintenance of aesthetics

- Ceramic is the material of choice for restoration of the larger lesion because it is possible to simulate the original tooth in colour, translucency and character with a high degree of accuracy. However, in many cases, it is necessary to be relatively destructive of remaining tooth structure to make room for the porcelain. With the advent of reliable adhesion to sound enamel through resin bonding techniques it has become possible to produce ceramic veneers to restore the labial surfaces of anterior teeth with minimal removal of enamel. Care must be taken to avoid over-contouring because this may compromise gingival health.
- With careful attention to detail it is possible to restore aesthetics using composite resin. More conservative techniques can be utilised but the integrity of the margin depends entirely on the availability of sound, well-supported enamel which can be etched so the resin can be bonded to it.
- Glass–ionomer is a useful aesthetic restorative material with the main limitation being an inability to withstand heavy occlusal load. It is the material of choice for an erosion lesion or for any lesion where involvement of the occlusal surface is at a minimum. If the load is expected to be too great, the glass–ionomer can be laminated with composite resin; this combination has been shown to restore reasonable strength to the remaining tooth structure.

Choice of restorative material according to size of lesion

Natural tooth structure is the best defence against further caries. It can be remineralised and generally the patient can be re-educated in dietary and hygiene procedures (Chapter 3, page 20). Remineralised tooth structure is just as hard as the original tooth material and is more resistant to further caries attack. Therefore, even though the surface may be mildly disfigured and stained, the most conservative approach to cavity design should be adopted. The following recommendations are offered as a rational approach to the choice of cavity design and the subsequent selection of the restorative material.

Site 1 lesion – pits and fissures on smooth surface
- Newly erupted immature tooth with deep fissures
Use an unfilled resin or a glass–ionomer fissure seal. No instrumentation will be required.
- Mature tooth with small carious dentine involvement
Open into the caries very conservatively. Follow out remaining fissures only where stained or there is a possibility of caries. Restore with glass–ionomer cement.
- Moderate-size cavity with no undue occlusal load
Open conservatively and restore with glass–ionomer base

and composite resin laminated over in areas of heavy occlusal load.

- Large cavity in a molar with extensive occlusal involvement

Restore with amalgam over a glass–ionomer lining using a protective cavity design where required to overlay cusps and prevent further breakdown.

Site 2 lesion – contact area, posterior

- New lesion only just involving dentine

Restore using glass–ionomer as the principal restorative material. Laminate only if the occlusal surface is widely involved and the load is heavy.

- Larger lesion with marginal ridge involved

Use a conservative modified cavity design. If the occlusal fissure is not carious, restore the proximal box with composite resin over a glass–ionomer base and seal the fissure with resin. If the occlusal load is heavy, particularly in molars, restore with amalgam. When replacing a failed restoration in a position where the occlusal load is acceptable use glass–ionomer as a dentine substitute and laminate with composite resin.

- Extensive lesion leaving undermined and weakened cusp(s)

Use protective cavity design modified for restoration with amalgam or gold inlay to provide protection over those cusps requiring support. Gold is the most conservative material when used as an inlay because it can be placed in thin section to protect remaining cusps. However, the design must be such as to relieve stress on cusps that are already split and retentive elements must be in the gingival one-third of the crown.

- One or more cusps already lost

The cavity design is now complex and extensive. Additional retention must be provided using grooves and ditches or, occasionally, pins in the gingival one-third of the remaining tooth structure. Restore with amalgam as the primary restoration, with a gold or ceramic extracoronal restoration to follow.

Site 2 lesion – contact area, anterior

- Initial lesion

Glass–ionomer is the material of choice for the restoration of all such cavities. Wherever possible the lesion should be entered from the lingual thus minimising problems of aesthetics, for both the present and the future.

- Large lesions or replacement restorations

Glass–ionomer remains the material of choice for the primary lesion. However, once the incisal edge and the labial surface is involved and aesthetics is compromised the cement will need to be placed as a dentine substitute and laminated with composite resin.

Site 2 lesion – involving incisal corner

- Small initial lesion

The small lesion in this classification is likely to occur only as a result of trauma. If the enamel only is involved it may

be sufficient to bevel the enamel and restore with composite resin. If there is any dentine involvement it should be protected with a glass–ionomer first before lamination to provide pulp protection and adhesion to the dentine.

- Larger lesions or replacement restorations

Restore the entire lesion with a glass–ionomer cement. Immediately cut back the cement sufficiently to expose the entire enamel margin on the labial and sufficient of the lingual enamel to ensure a union strong enough to withstand the anticipated incisal load. If the enamel is weak along the gingival margin leave the cement covering that margin to a depth of about 2 mm. Bevel the enamel margins, etch and laminate with composite resin.

Site 3 lesion – cervical margin

- Erosion lesion

A Type II.1 restorative aesthetic glass–ionomer cement is the material of choice under most circumstances. No instrumentation is required and the lesion should be cleaned with pumice and water only, to remove the pellicle before being conditioned and restored. The aesthetic result should be checked after 1 week and if it is unsatisfactory the cement can be cut back lightly and laminated with composite resin. The resin-modified glass–ionomers are generally aesthetically satisfactory.

- Carious lesion or replacement restoration

The cavity should be instrumented only as far as is essential to remove active caries. Mechanical retention is unnecessary and demineralised enamel may remain unless badly undermined. Glass–ionomer is the material of choice and the cavity will need to be conditioned before restoration. If the aesthetic result is still unsatisfactory after 1 week, the cement can be cut back and laminated with composite resin.

Extracoronal restorations

- Porcelain or composite resin laminate veneers

Application of a laminate veneer can be regarded as a relatively conservative method of modifying the shape or aesthetics of anterior teeth. As at least half the thickness of the labial enamel must be removed to avoid over-contour, this restoration should not be regarded as reversible. Also it must be noted that, as it is almost impossible to determine the thickness of remaining enamel, the labial surface should not be cut back to an arbitrary depth for fear of inadvertently removing it all and leaving a bond to dentine only. This applies particularly to the gingival margin where it is most difficult to achieve a good bond to dentine.

Any existing restoration should be fully upgraded first using glass–ionomer cement and nonvital teeth should be bleached as close as possible to their correct colour. Composite resin may be the preferred material for minor modifications to one or two teeth only but indirectly built porcelain veneers are recommended for extensive modification of several teeth at a time.

- Three-quarter veneer

This is the most conservative of the extracoronal restorations and it is valuable for reinforcing posterior teeth in particular. Gold is the correct material to use because it can be cast with a high degree of accuracy and used in very thin section. Underlying restorations should be fully upgraded first using amalgam or glass–ionomer. Skilful cavity preparation will minimise the gold display and in many cases the aesthetic result is entirely acceptable.

- Full crown

A full coverage restoration is required where either the remaining tooth structure is so badly broken down that no other method will adequately restore the tooth or it is necessary to upgrade aesthetics or occlusion. If aesthetics is of no concern gold is the material of choice because remaining tooth structure can be conserved to a greater degree and also the occlusal wear factor is the same as for tooth structure. Construction of a porcelain crown will require removal of a greater amount of tooth structure to allow bulk in the crown for both fracture resistance and aesthetics.

Existing restorations should be fully upgraded first and, in view of the fact that retention of such restorations is gained in the gingival one-third of the remaining tooth, amalgam is the material of choice for such work. Glass–ionomer may be sufficient to make-good relatively small deficiencies, particularly on an anterior tooth but composite resin does not adhere to dentine so it is inadequate for this purpose.

FURTHER READING

Barnes DM, Holston AM, Strassler HE, Shires PJ. Evaluation of clinical performance of twelve posterior composite resins with a standardised placement technique. *J Esthet Dent* 1990; **2**:36–43.

Bryant RW. Posterior composite resin restorations – a review of clinical problems. *Aust Prosthodont J* 1987; **1**:41–50.

Davidson CL, Kemp-Scholte CM. Shortcomings of composite resins in Class V restorations. *J Esthet Dent* 1989; **1**:1–4.

Dawson AS, Makinson OF, An alternate philosophy and some new treatment modalities in operative dentistry, Part II. *Aust Dent J* 1992; **37**:205–10.

Dawson AS, Makinson OF. Dental treatment and dental health: Part I. A review of studies in support of a philosophy of minimum intervention dentistry. *Aust Dent J* 1992; **37**:126–32.

Hawthorne W, Smales R, Webster D. Long term survival of restorative materials in private dental practice [Abstract]. *J Dent Res* 1994; **73**:747.

Lambrechts P, Williams G, Van Herle G, Braem M. Aesthetic limits of light cured composite resins in anterior teeth.

Int Dent J 1990; **40**:149–58.

Mount GJ. Methods of restoration – a decision. *N Z Dent J* 1977; **73**:135–42.

Mount GJ. The problem – towards a resolution. *N Z Dent J* 1977; **73**:10–14.

Mount GJ. A review of newer restorative materials. Part I. *Dent Today* 1989; **5**:1–6

Mount GJ. A review of newer restorative materials. Part II. *Dent Today* 1990; **6**:1–8

Pink FE, Minden NJ, Simmonds S. Decisions of practitioners regarding placement of amalgam and composite resin restorations in general practice settings. *Oper Dent* 1994; **19**:127–32.

Sheth JJ, Fuller JL, Jensen ME. Cuspal deformation and fracture resistance of teeth with dentine adhesives and composites. *J Prosthet Dent* 1988; **60**:560–9.

Tyas MJ. Adhesive dental restorative materials and systems. *Ann Roy Aust Coll Dent Surg* 1989; **10**:101–7.

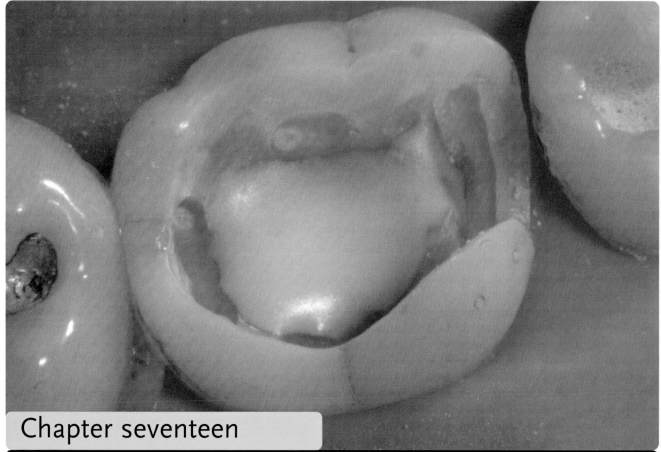

Chapter seventeen

Pulp protection during and after tooth restoration

W.R. Hume

In Chapter 5 the dynamics of disease within the pulp were outlined. This chapter is concerned with the measures that can be taken when restoring teeth to prevent pulpal damage, which may cause pain for the patient or lead to the death of the pulp.

The pulp can be damaged and may die as caries advances through dentine, probably because of the effects of bacteria or their metabolic by-products. Immediately after tooth restoration, the pulp can show damage, probably because of trauma directly related to the preparation and placement of a restoration. Also, the pulp may die months or years after restoration, probably because of the effects of bacterial microleakage.

AVOIDANCE OF PULP DAMAGE CAUSED BY CARIES

Most pulp death is caused either directly or indirectly by dental caries. Therefore, those strategies that prevent the ≠ initiation of carious lesions are likely to preserve pulp vitality at the same time as they conserve tooth tissue. Because the pulp will be involved almost immediately after caries penetrates through the enamel and reaches the dentine, early interceptive therapy to arrest and cure carious lesions will protect the pulp from damage. Dietary control, appropriate administration of fluoride (both systemic and topical), fissure sealing, maintenance of salivary flow and good oral hygiene are, therefore, all pulp-protective measures.

In the presence of active caries, placement of a restoration is designed to arrest, or at least slow down, the progress of the disease; it will therefore contribute to the protection of the pulp. As a general principle, a small restoration is less likely to damage pulp than a large one. The early diagnosis and accurate prognosis of active caries, followed by conservative restoration placement, when indicated, are therefore in the interest of the survival of the pulp, even when total control of the disease is not possible.

AVOIDANCE OF PULP DAMAGE DURING CAVITY PREPARATION

There is good evidence that cutting dentine damages or kills odontoblasts. The odontoblastic processes may be cut, and the sudden movement of fluid, even in the cell-free areas of the tubule, may damage the contents of the odontoblast or disrupt the cell membrane. Deep or extensive cutting of dentine is therefore more likely to cause pulpal damage and should be avoided wherever possible.

Generation of heat
The generation of heat during tooth cutting has considerable potential for damaging pulpal cells. The use of air–water spray coolant (Chapter 6, page 49) is essential when using high-speed rotary cutting instruments to clean, lubricate and cool both the tooth and the cutting instrument. The handpiece and the bur must also be in good condition and running concentrically, because vibration can also cause damage to the pulp.

Drying the dentine

Be aware

Drying and dehydration

There is a difference between drying and dehydration.
- Drying lightly is acceptable.
- Dehydration may damage the pulp.

Dentine is traversed by tubules that normally contain both plasma ultrafiltrate (dentinal fluid) and odontoblastic processes. Cut dentine is therefore naturally wet. However, it is necessary for the surface of dentine to be relatively dry for the successful placement of some restorative materials. It can be dried using either a jet of high-pressure air at ambient temperature, or warm air at a lower pressure from a triple syringe. Organic liquids such as acetone and ether can also be used take surface water into solution as they wash the dentine, then evaporate. Each method of drying brings with it the possibility of aspiration of odontoblastic cell bodies into dentinal tubules followed by cell rupture. Prolonged drying is more likely to cause damage than drying that is relatively brief and gentle; and a risk–benefit assessment may need to be made. The long-term benefit may be a more effective bonding of a resin restorative material to the dry dentine surface, whereas the short-term risk is pulpal damage through excessive dehydration.

Recovery
Odontoblast damage may therefore be inevitable during the preparation of a tooth before placement of a restoration, and it may be an acceptable risk, relative to the overall benefit to the patient. If the pulp is free of bacteria at the time of injury, there is a strong possibility that the inflammation, which will certainly follow cell damage, can fulfil its physiological function and the tissue will heal, although it may leave some degree of 'premature ageing'.

PROTECTIVE MEASURES DURING RESTORATION PLACEMENT

Bacterial microleakage

Be aware

Bacterial microleakage

This is the greatest risk to the pulp. All restorations must be resistant to microleakage.

There is strong evidence that bacteria can grow beneath restorative materials and that either bacterial by-products or bacteria themselves can move through dentine, inducing pulpal damage, inflammation and death. This concept is generally described as bacterial microleakage. A positive correlation has been demonstrated between the presence of bacteria immediately beneath restorations and pulpal inflammation. For example, the species *Prevotella intermedia* and *Prevotella melaninogenica* are known to be able to produce lipopolysaccaride, which may then diffuse through dentine, causing a chronic inflammatory response in the pulp, possibly leading to cell death.

Those restorative materials that are most often associated with pulpal problems following clinical placement are known to permit bacterial microleakage. Therefore, those materials that are most effective in protecting the pulp probably do so because they provide a seal that is proof against such bacterial invasion.

Placement of a lining

If it is necessary to place a restorative material that does not develop a union with dentine, a primary barrier should be laid down first using a varnish, a lining or a base (such as glass–ionomer) that adheres fully to the tooth structure. It may also be beneficial first to treat the cavity surface with an antibacterial agent to kill residual bacteria before commencing restoration, so long as the agent itself does no harm to the pulp.

Chemical toxicity

Notes

Toxicity

All chemicals are toxic depending upon concentration in relation to the relevant tissue. Dentine is an excellent buffer against chemical diffusion.

It must be understood that all chemical substances are toxic – it just depends upon the concentration of a substance in relation to a particular tissue. It must also be noted that dentine is an excellent buffer and will limit the diffusion rate of even the strongest acid to the extent that the pulp will suffer no ill effects, providing there is a reasonably substantial barrier of sound dentine between the diffusing chemical and pulp.

However, dentine is not a universal barrier, and some restorative materials release chemicals that can diffuse through and damage the pulp. Because of the presence of toxic chemicals from the resin, moderate to severe pulpal inflammation may occur within 2–3 days after placement of an unfilled bonding resin against deeply etched dentine. Low-viscosity resin luting cements, which are placed under considerable pressure during crown seating, can also bypass the protective barrier effect, particularly if the tubules have been opened by acid etching. There are a number of restorative materials that can be placed with relative safety on intact dentine, but are sufficiently toxic to cause moderate but reversible pulpal damage if placed directly on exposed pulp tissue because the concentration is then high on that tissue.

Recovery

Healthy pulp tissue is able to tolerate mild or moderate physical or chemical damage to the odontoblast layer so long as bacteria and their toxins are not present. Usually, in the absence of bacteria, the death of a limited number of cells will induce a transient, acute inflammation. New cells differentiate from the adjacent pulp to replace those that have died and the patient may only be aware of mild symptoms of pulpitis for a few days.

CHEMICAL DIFFUSION AND FLUID FLOW THROUGH DENTINE

The movement through dentine of bacterial toxins, bacteria themselves, or low-viscosity water-soluble chemicals under pressure, are all possible contributors to adverse pulpal responses. It is therefore worthwhile to review briefly what is known about the potential pathways of movement through dentine.

Permeability of dentine

Summary

Dentine permeability

This is affected by a number of factors
- diameter of tubules
- density of dentine
- length of tubules
- smear layer
- secondary dentine
- topical applications

Dentine behaves as an impermeable solid traversed by water-filled tubules. Fluids can diffuse through dentine only via the tubules and motile bacteria can grow and move within the tubule fluid. The term permeability is used to include all three types of potential movement: diffusion, fluid flow and bacterial passage through dentine.

The degree of dentine permeability is determined by:
- tubule diameter – the diameter decreases with age
- density – there are fewer tubules at the dentino-enamel junction
- length – proximity of cavity floor to the pulp
- presence or absence of a smear layer
- coagulated protein or calcific deposits; for example, secondary dentine
- restorative materials; for example, cements, resins or varnishes may modify permeability.

Modifying factors

Irrespective of other factors, the permeability of cut dentine is substantially increased by a factor of 4–5 times by removal of the smear layer, which occurs during cavity preparation. Smear layer can be removed rapidly with strong acid etchants, such as phosphoric acid, and a little more slowly with weaker acids, such as ethylenediamine-tetraacetic acid (EDTA) or polyalkenoic acids. Although complete smear layer removal may increase the potential bond strength of some adhesive restorative materials to

! Be aware

Removal of smear layer
- allows increased fluid flow
- allows increased chemical diffusion
- allows possible microleakage.

✴ Summary

Glass–ionomer
- Initial low pH
- Well buffered by dentine
- Seals dentine tubules
- Prevents microleakage

dentine, it also increases the potential for chemical diffusion from such materials through dentine to the pulp. It will also allow an outward fluid flow through dentine, and this may prevent the development of an effective seal for the restorative material, thus leading to later ingress of bacteria or their by-products. This means that the decision whether or not to remove smear layer involves an assessment of the risk–benefit ratio.

The relative area of dentine occupied by tubules increases as the cavity floor approaches the pulp. The number of tubules in coronal dentine is approximately:
- $20\,000$ per mm^2 at the dentino-enamel junction; that is, 1% of dentine area
- $45\,000$ per mm^2 close to the roof of the pulp; that is, 22% of dentine area.

! Summary

Cross-sectional area of dentine tubules
- 1% at dentino-enamel junction
- 22% near the pulp

Dentine permeability increases as remaining dentine thickness decreases towards the pulp because:
- tubules are tapered and become larger in diameter
- they converge and become more densely packed
- they become shorter.

Dentine is dense at the enamel–dentine junction, but becomes markedly more permeable over the pulp horns, where tubule density is highest and dentine is thinnest. It is also more permeable through the axial walls of prepared cavities than beneath the occlusal floor. The depth of the cavity, the location of the walls and floor relative to the pulp horns and the surface condition of dentine therefore control the potential for pulpal damage during preparation and restoration placement, and must influence decisions concerning the need for pulp protection.

RISKS TO THE PULP FROM PLASTIC RESTORATIVE MATERIALS

Glass–ionomer cement

Although glass–ionomer cement is inherently chemically toxic, the major toxin, unreacted acid, is well buffered by hydroxyapatite after placement into a cavity. Also, the ion-exchange union between the cement and the underlying

tooth structure leads to the development of an ion-enriched layer at the interface that effectively seals the tubules. Any subsequent failure of the union will be cohesive in the cement, rather than adhesive at the interface, leaving a fine layer of cement still attached to the tooth, sealing the tubules and preventing microleakage.

Composite resin

✴ Summary

Composite resin
- Releases chemical toxins
- Adheres well to enamel
- Short-term adhesion to dentine

Composite resins present two major problems for the pulp. They may release chemical toxins, particularly in the first few days after placement, and, because they do not reliably adhere to dentine, they may be subject to continuing microleakage. There is some variation between composites in toxin-release patterns, and the degree of damage caused by these toxins will depend on the variables discussed above that influence dentine permeability.

There is also likely to be some variation according to the cavity geometry. In an intracoronal box-form cavity that is directly filled with a single increment of composite resin, there is a strong likelihood that a gap will form at one or more cavity walls because of the setting contraction of the resin. This is particularly true with the light-activated composite resins and the problem needs to be controlled by careful incremental packing and curing. Also, the larger the cavity, the greater the problem.

It has been shown that triethylene glycol dimethacrylate (TEGDMA) (a low-molecular-weight diluent used in most composite resins) can be released in biologically significant quantities through dentine in the first days after placement. Also, most resin restorative materials, particularly those that are light activated, contain various quantities of hydroxyethyl methacrylate (HEMA), which is toxic in tissue culture. The dentine will modify the diffusion to the extent that the pulp response will be mitigated, but there should be a degree of caution exercised. The following points should be noted:

- dentine that has just been debrided of active caries is more permeable
- thickness of remaining dentine is very significant
- acid etching of dentine will reduce its buffering effect.

It is therefore desirable first to place a base capable of sealing the dentine tubules. Glass–ionomer is the most effective material because it develops an ion-exchange adhesion that is proof against microleakage. Use the strongest material available to ensure optimal physical properties, because it counters the setting shrinkage of a light-activated composite resin. The whole of the dentine should be covered so that the cement acts as a dentine substitute and thus provides protection against both chemical toxicity and microleakage. If the lesion is very deep and close to the pulp, carry out an indirect pulp cap routine first (Chapter 18). This will lead to remineralisation of affected dentine with subsequent retention of the maximum thickness between the pulp and the restoration. Removal of all affected dentine from the floor of an active carious lesion is strongly discouraged.

Dental amalgam

Summary

Amalgam

It has a very low toxicity to the pulp and can be sealed very readily by application of:
- copal varnish
- remineralising solution
- glass–ionomer
- resin bond.

Amalgam has a low potential for chemical toxicity, and seals the interface between restoration and tooth structure through corrosion, which commences shortly after placement. There is a moderate marginal gap in the first weeks after placement, but this decreases because of the formation of corrosion products and because of the calcification of surface pellicle and other organic materials. If amalgam is used alone as a restorative material without a primary layer of resin, varnish, liner or base, there may be pulpal inflammation in the days following placement caused by early microleakage. Thereafter, because an effective seal will be developed through corrosion, the pulpitis is likely to subside.

Copal varnish has been recognised for many years as providing an effective seal from microleakage in the short term and, as it washes out, the amalgam corrodes and develops its own organic seal. A low-viscosity resin or a thinly mixed glass–ionomer has now been suggested, and either will be effective over the longer term.

RISKS TO THE PULP WITH LUTED RESTORATIONS

When indirectly fabricated rigid restorations (such as crowns or inlays) are cemented into place, the luting agent may be a potential source of chemical toxicity and will generally be the factor that determines whether or not bacterial microleakage will occur. Zinc phosphate cement, polycarboxylate cement and glass–ionomer cement are the commonly used luting agents; none of these will release chemicals in sufficient concentrations to harm pulpal cells so long as the dentine is intact and the smear layer has not been removed. The liquid for each cement is a low-pH acid, but the hydroxyapatite of intact dentine is capable of acting as an effective buffering agent. Undue cleaning or etching of the dentine immediately before cementation, however, will open the tubules and, under the high hydraulic pressure that might arise during cementation, may allow some penetration of the liquid through the tubules, leading to pulpal irritation. Some of the resin cements, as well as some of the resin-modified glass–ionomer luting cements, contain materials with a potential for toxicity or allergy, such as HEMA, and these may find their way into the pulp if subjected to such pressure.

Clearly, pulpal problems in teeth that require restorations of this magnitude may well be caused by preoperative conditions such as large carious lesions, failing and leaking existing restorations or mechanical trauma during preparation procedures. If there is a pre-existing chronic inflammation, then the superimposition of further acute inflammation may well precipitate ultimate pulp death. However, sometimes pulps that appeared to be healthy immediately before the preparation phase become painful or die shortly thereafter. The cause is not always easy to determine.

Retention of smear layer

Be aware

Luting crowns and bridges

Either leave smear layer intact or seal smear layer into place with:
- mineralising solution
- two layers of varnish
- resin–dentine bond.

Retention of smear layer over the surface of a crown preparation is desirable because this occludes the tubules and prevents penetration of the cement liquid, despite relatively high hydraulic pressures that can be developed during cementation. If smear layer is removed the tubules will be opened, and a low-viscosity mix of cement may be forced through the tubules into the pulp space, thus by-passing the buffering effect. The result may then be postinsertion sensitivity. Rather than remove the smear layer, it is better to seal the tubules with a dentine-bonding agent, particularly one containing a polyalkenoic acid, or a mineralising fluid such as ITS solution (Causten & Johnson). This is best carried out immediately after preparation of the tooth and before taking the impression and making a temporary crown. The preparation will then be completely sealed from microleakage and will remain more comfortable and secure through the further stages, leading to the cementation appointment.

Unfilled resin cements

Unfilled resin cements can be used for luting crowns and inlays; they have a very low solubility and can be regarded as durable at the margin. However, they do not flow well, so the ultimate film thickness is usually greater than desirable. If the dentine is etched, there will be a micromechanical adhesion, but these cements do not unite chemically with dentine so they are not proof against future microleakage. Also, cleaning and acid treatment of dentine before crown cementation will open the tubules and increase the chance of resin components being forced down tubules under the hydraulic pressures involved with cementation, thus damaging the pulp.

Dissolution of luting cement

Each of the conventional luting cements appears to provide an adequate seal against bacterial microleakage for several years after placement, but the possibility of eventual dissolution of the cements poses a long-term risk to the pulp. Zinc oxide and eugenol cements tend to hydrolyse and convert to a zinc eugenolate; they should not be regarded as long-term cements. Glass–ionomer cement will last much better and has one additional advantage inasmuch as the ion-exchange layer will remain and will continue to seal the tubules, even after the loss of the cement.

 Notes

Dissolution of the luting cement

This is a serious long-term risk to the dental pulp.

The rate of dissolution may be related to plaque and dietary factors, because cement dissolution tends to be higher in an acidic environment. So long as the crown margins are well adapted and accurate, the dissolution will be slower, and it is possible that in some mouths the developing gap may be occluded by calcified debris, or colonised by relatively benign bacteria. However it is not unreasonable to expect pulp death to occur, in some cases many years after the placement of indirectly fabricated restorations on vital teeth. The best defence is to protect the dentine with an insoluble and impermeable intermediate layer as described above.

MATERIALS USED IN PULP PROTECTION

Varnishes and other surface treatments
Varnishes
A varnish is a material of very low viscosity, containing a relatively large proportion by volume of a volatile solvent, and its prime use is for application to dentine to decrease permeability. However, because of the high proportion of solvent, and subsequently the large volume reduction on drying, the ultimate film is relatively porous and therefore not very effective. It relies to a degree on the presence of an intact smear layer, with which it may combine, to reduce permeability. There are many versions on the market; they were originally used to decrease the early microleakage around amalgam restorations and then wash out to be replaced by corrosion products; this remains their best use.

Resin sealants
The light-activated, unfilled resins may be used as cavity primers or bonding agents with composite resins; they seal dentine more effectively after the smear layer has been removed. Most are relatively viscous and do not set through loss of solvent, but by either chemical action or light activation. Some systems are relatively complex and require several sequential applications to achieve the desired bond. Correctly applied, they reduce the potential for ingress of bacteria or their by-products. Whether the brief chemical risk they pose to odontoblasts is outweighed by their possible longer term benefits, by enhancing the seal against microleakage, is yet to be determined.

Remineralising solutions
Several chemical treatments using topical fluoride or oxalate salts are designed to reduce dentinal permeability and therefore the risk of ingress of bacteria and their products. Most of these will successfully reduce dentinal sensibility, but the long-term benefits of such treatments for pulp health have not yet been established.

Liners and bases
The main differences between a liner and a base is the thickness and strength. The term 'liner' is used for a thin wash. A base is a relatively thick material strong enough to provide resistance form and to become an intrinsic part of the ultimate restoration. A base can be regarded as a dentine substitute.

Calcium hydroxide

 Notes

Calcium hydroxide is applied only to the exposed pulp and then sealed with glass–ionomer.

Calcium hydroxide was introduced for direct pulp capping on the assumption that it would promote calcification in the wounded tissue against which it was placed; for example, an exposed pulp. It was expected that calcium hydroxide would provide calcium ions, thus aiding remineralisation, but this has since been discounted. In fact, because it is strongly alkaline at pH 12–13, there will be a degree of necrosis in adjacent soft tissue but, at the same time, bacteria fail to thrive in its presence. Therefore, it will counter bacterial microleakage and, as it is not unduly toxic, exposed and relatively healthy pulp tissue in the vicinity usually survives. Calcific scar tissue may be laid down beyond any area of necrosis and may successfully bridge the lesion if no bacteria remain.

However, over time, calcium hydroxide is likely to be washed out from under any restoration that does not have a complete marginal seal, so its effect may be transitory. Because of this, it is not recommended as a liner or base. Its use should be limited to protection of an actual pulp exposure only. A very small quantity of an autocure cement should be placed over the area of soft-tissue exposure, then a seal created over it with a glass–ionomer.

Zinc phosphate cement

! Be aware

Zinc phosphate has limited value as a lining cement.

This cement has been used for many decades as an 'insulating' base material beneath metallic restorations and also as a luting agent. Despite its acid nature, it is well tolerated by the pulp if placed on intact dentine, presumably because of buffering of the unreacted acid by hydroxy-apatite. There may be immediate and short-term pain if it is placed on the dentine of an unanaesthetised tooth, probably because of osmotic effects on dentinal tubule fluid. Because it has no therapeutic effect upon the pulp, there seem to be few indications for its use as a lining or base material.

Zinc oxide–eugenol

✴ Summary

Zinc oxide–eugenol
- Anti-inflammatory
- Antibacterial
- Mildly anaesthetic
- Good seal to cavity wall

Therefore, it should be used as a short-term temporary and/or indirect pulp cap.

Zinc oxide–eugenol is a useful part of pulp therapy in the management of deep, active carious lesions and has also been used as a lining and base material. Like glass–ionomer, it provides an effective antibacterial seal, probably because any gap between the cement and dentine will contain a high concentration of eugenol, which is strongly bactericidal. Any available eugenol may also inhibit bacterial metabolism within dentine, and if the material is placed on intact dentine it is unlikely to harm pulp cells. It is also possible for it to promote local anaesthetic and anti-inflammatory reactions in adjacent pulp tissue. Despite these therapeutic benefits, the cement slowly hydrolyses with time, leaving a residue of soft zinc hydroxide. Also, eugenol will inhibit the polymerisation of composite resin, so it must not be used anywhere before, or in relation to, resin restorations or resin luting cements. Nor should it be used in direct contact with exposed pulp tissue, as the release of eugenol by hydrolysis is markedly greater because of the wetness of the tissue. A concentration of eugenol sufficient to kill pulpal cells may develop rapidly in adjacent vital tissue and the level may be sustained for several days.

Indications for the use of zinc oxide–eugenol are limited to those situations where the dentine is intact and some form of indirect pulp therapy or caries therapy is required. For example, zinc oxide–eugenol is an effective temporary restoration in those situations where it is intended to remove infected surface caries and leave demineralised affected caries behind. Generally, within 3 weeks it will be safe to proceed with a permanent restoration. Because of the problem of long-term hydrolysis, the use of zinc oxide–eugenol should be limited to less than 6 months as a long-term temporary restoration.

Glass–ionomer cement

✴ Summary

Glass–ionomer

Excellent dentine substitute because:
- ion-exchange layer seals dentinal tubules
- it is mildly antibacterial
- it has adequate physical properties.

As noted above, glass–ionomer, when placed without pressure on intact dentine, poses no chemical risk to the pulp and, with the development of the ion-exchange layer, it creates an effective antibacterial seal. It shows a very low solubility, and therefore appears to be the material of choice for use as a base, or dentine substitute, beneath all plastic restorations.

Glass–ionomer also has considerable potential as a long-term temporary restoration in the treatment of active caries. Following removal of infected dentine a strong mix of glass–ionomer is placed in the cavity over the remaining affected dentine and allowed to set. In the presence of dentinal fluid from the affected dentine there is likely to be a reasonable release of fluoride as well as calcium and phosphate ions from the cement and these will be useful in the remineralising process. Glass–ionomer will adhere to remaining tooth structure through the ion-exchange mechanism and, in addition, it is apparently mildly antibacterial because of fluoride release.

It is the material which has been recommended for use in the ART technique (Chapter 18, page 213) and it has been shown to be very effective in stimulating remineralisation of affected dentine over a short period of time. So long as it is used with a high powder content, recent versions with high physical strength may be retained as a permanent restoration in the presence of high caries rates. If the occlusal load is expected to be high it can be laminated at a later time to ensure longevity.

FURTHER READING

Brannstrom M, Vojinovic O. Response of the dental pulp to invasion of bacteria around three filling materials. *J Dent Child* 1976; **43**:15–21.

Brannstrom M. *Dentin and pulp in restorative dentistry.* London: Wolfe Medical Publications Ltd; 1987.

Causten BE, Johnson NW. Improvement of polycarboxylate adhesion to dentine by the use of a new calcifying solution. *Br Dent J* 1982; **152**:9–11.

Cox CF, Keall CL, Keall HJ, Ostro E, Bergenholtz G. Biocompatibility of surface sealed dental materials against exposed pulps. *J Prosthet Dent* 1987; **57**:1–8.

Cox CF, Suzuki S. Re-evaluating pulp protection: calcium hydroxide liners vs. cohesive hybridization. *J Am Dent Assoc* 1994; **125**:823–31.

Fusayama T. A simple pain-free adhesive system by minimal reduction and total etching. *Ishiyaka Eur Am* 1993; 6 and 74.

Gerzina T, Hume WR. TEGDMA elution from resin composite through dentin *in vitro*. *J Dent Res* 1993; **71**:162–8.

Hamid A, Hume WR. Diffusion of monomer through carious dentin *in vitro*. *Endodontics and Dental Traumatology* 1996; **13**:1–5.

Hamid A, Hume WR. The effect of dentin thickness on diffusion of resin monomers *in vitro*. *J Oral Rehab* 1997; **24**:20–25.

Hume WR, Mount GJ. In vitro studies on the potential for pulpal cytotoxicity of glass–ionomer cements. *J Dent Res* 1988; **67**:915–18.

Hume WR, Gerzina TM. Release of monomers from bonding resin – composite resin combinations through dentin in vitro. *J Dent Res* 1994; **73**:224–6.

Hume WR, Gerzina TM. Bioavailability of components of resin-based materials which are applied to teeth. *Crit Rev of Oral Biol and Med* 1996; **7**:172–9.

Hume WR. Pulpal responses to restorative materials. *Dent Today* Spring 1989; **5**:1–7.

Johnson GH, Powell LV, Derouen TA. Evaluation and control of post-cementation pulpal sensitivity. *J Am Dent Assoc* 1993; **124**:39–46.

Mount GJ. Lessons from the early days. In: Hunt PR, ed. *Glass–ionomers: the next generation.* Philadelphia: 1994:92.

Pashley DH, Depew DD. Effects of the smear layer, copalite and oxylate on microleakage. *Oper Dent* 1986; **11**:95–102.

Pashley DH, Michelich V, Kehl T. Dentine permeability; effects of smear layer removal. *J Prosthet Dent* 1981; **46**:531.

Snuggs HM, Cox CF, Powell CS, White KC. Pulpal healing and dentinal bridge formation in an acid environment. *Quintessence Int* 1993; **24**:501–10.

Trope M, Orstavik D. Biologic responses of the pulp to restorations. In: Hunt PR, ed. *Glass–ionomers: the next generation.* Philadelphia: 1994;131–42.

Zander HA. The reaction of dental pulps to silicate cements. *J Am Dent Assoc* 1946; **33**:1233–44.

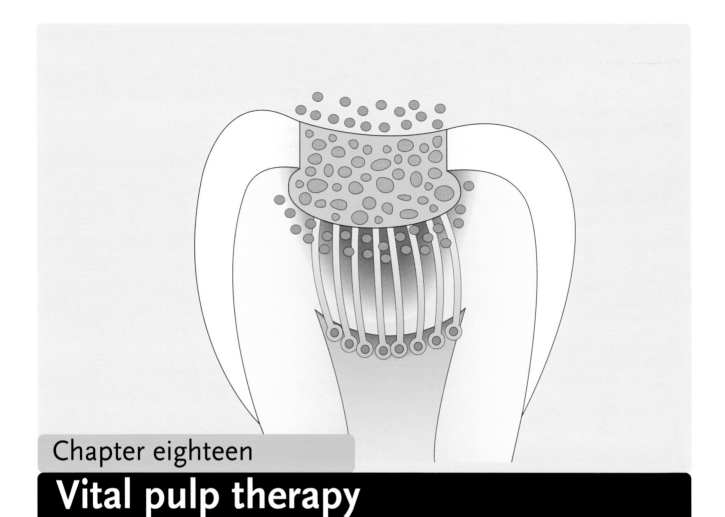

Chapter eighteen

Vital pulp therapy

W.R. Hume • G.J. Mount

In addition to procedures designed to keep the pulp alive by avoiding pulpal damage, there are several routine measures available that are designed to help heal a damaged pulp. Whether the damaged pulp will heal with the aid of a particular therapy will depend to a large extent upon the balance between the damaging factors and the host response.

It is impossible to predict accurately the outcome of a particular therapy when the principal pulpal irritant is microbial, because both the microbial mix and the host response vary greatly. These two factors can vary between individual patients, between teeth and, with time, in the same patient. Despite this, several therapies have been applied with sufficient likelihood of success to have made them accepted and reasonable parts of the practice of dentistry.

INDIRECT PULP THERAPY

Exposure of the pulp to the oral environment carries major risks to the survival of the tissue, so it is desirable to keep the pulp covered, so long as this can be done without compromising other treatment goals. It must be recognised that there are at least two clearly defined zones (**Fig. 18.1**) within a normal carious lesion.

'Infected layer'
The superficial surface of a carious lesion, adjacent to the oral cavity, is heavily infected by microorganisms and consists largely of denatured and unstructured enamel and dentine debris.

'Affected layer'
Beneath the infected layer a zone of demineralised dentine that retains the basic dentine structure but relatively free of bacteria except possibly for a few pioneer bacteria. Under magnification, the original dentinal tubules are apparent, supported mainly by the collagen matrix and this may, under normal circumstances, be remineralised. It is desirable, then, to regard it as 'pre-carious' and to retain the affected dentine.

The removal of the superficial infected dentine is a major component of the surgical treatment of an advancing carious lesion and this is relatively simple to accomplish. The affected zone is not always easy to define because it is relatively soft, generally colourless and its complete removal may result in exposure of the pulp. Caries-disclosing solutions are reasonably reliable inasmuch as they will define the infected layer and leave the affected dentine unstained. Exposure of the pulp tissue is highly undesirable because it will render it liable to bacterial contamination. Therefore, caries control in an extensive lesion should be carried out in two stages.

- Perform limited debridement to remove the infected dentine only and to clean the walls around the periphery of the lesion. Now, place a temporary restoration, using a material which is capable of providing a complete marginal seal. Leave in place for at least 3 weeks.

- Remove the temporary and complete the debridement before finalising cavity design and placing a definitive restoration.

The first stage allows time for the inflammation to subside and for the pulp to lay down reparative dentine in those areas close to exposure. If the pulp survives the inflammation and retains its vitality, there will be a degree of remineralisation in the affected demineralised zone. Secondary dentine formation will follow within the pulp chamber because the tissue fluid in the pulp is naturally supersaturated with calcium and phosphate ions (**Fig. 18.2**).

Temporary restoration
The main function of the temporary restoration is to provide a complete seal so that any remaining bacteria will be deprived of nutrition and will not be able to produce sufficient acid for demineralisation to continue. Further advantages will accrue if the temporary cement has an anti-septic or antibacterial effect on the remaining micro-organisms and if it helps stimulate remineralisation.

Longevity of the temporary
The temporary restoration should remain for a minimum of 3 weeks, but no longer than a maximum of 6 months, after which the lesion should be investigated again. By this time, pulpal inflammation will have subsided and there will have been some degree of secondary dentine formed within the pulp chamber. Under glass–ionomer there may be some discoloured, demineralised dentine remaining, but this can often be left on the floor of the cavity. In fact, no attempt should be made to clean the lesion down to a hard shiny dentine surface, because it is unnecessary and may result in a pulp exposure.

This two-stage sequence of debridement and covering for a period of time is known as 'indirect pulp therapy', because it is designed to avoid pulp exposure while allowing the tissue to heal. It has also been called 'indirect pulp capping' because it is intended that the potential pulp exposure will be 'capped' by secondary dentine before the area of the potential exposure is reached during the second stage of debridement.

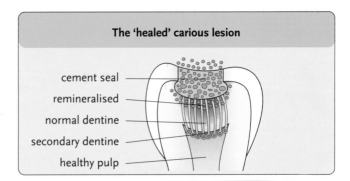

Fig. 18.1 Active caries. The two layers in a carious lesion. Infected layer: completely denatured and infected. Affected layer: demineralised but capable of being remineralised. There may be a few pioneer bacteria present.

Fig. 18.2 The 'healed' carious lesion. After a minimum of 3 weeks following sealing, the carious process will be arrested. Bacterial activity will cease, pulpal inflammation will resolve and secondary dentine will form in the pulp chamber. Any remaining denatured dentine can be safely removed without exposing the pulp.

Choice of temporary

The temporary restoration that was used for many years was a zinc oxide–eugenol paste.

- It provides an adequate seal, excluding most if not all dietary substrate from the remaining microorganisms in dentine.
- It releases eugenol into adjacent dentine, the rate of release being determined by the wetness of the tissue.
- Eugenol is probably effective in killing residual bacteria.
- Sufficient eugenol may diffuse through the dentine to the pulp space to inhibit inflammation and pain, as will be described in detail below.

The principal shortcomings of zinc oxide–eugenol in this role are its limited mechanical strength and its limited durability for the longer term because it becomes degraded through hydrolysis. Various resins have been included to increase both strength and durability, but expectations are still limited.

Glass–ionomer is now the material of choice, because it is more durable and has the added advantage of fluoride release.

- Glass–ionomer is relatively insoluble.
- It is sufficiently strong to withstand reasonable occlusal load.
- It is easily placed and relatively easy to remove.
- It releases fluoride which has the potential to kill bacteria in dentine.
- The release of fluoride and other ions promotes remineralisation of adjacent hard tissues.

The 'ART' technique

The term ART stands for 'Atraumatic Restorative Treatment'; this is a treatment method that has been developed for use in under-developed countries where full dental care is not always available. In some of these communities, Western-style dietary routines had been adopted before the development of preventive dental measures, with a resultant high caries rate. The only alternative dental treatment to date has been extraction of affected teeth leading, usually, to further dental problems.

The system takes into account the use of the indirect pulp therapy through placement of a fast-setting glass–ionomer for the stabilisation of rampant caries. It can be carried out simply, in the first instance, using hand instruments to gain access through the enamel and spoon excavators to remove the superficial infected dentine. Care must be exercised to clean the walls of the cavity only, leaving a substantial layer of affected dentine over the pulp chamber. The cavity is then conditioned with polyacrylic acid for 10 seconds, washed with wet cotton pellets and dried. A high-physical-property, auto-cure glass–ionomer is then placed in the cavity and allowed to set. A gloved finger can be used to apply pressure for positive placement as well as to keep the cement isolated during the setting phase (**Figs 18.3–18.6**).

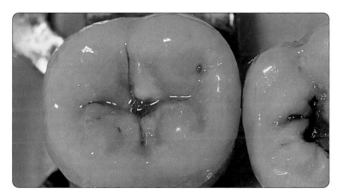

Fig. 18.3 Atraumatic restorative treatment. A lower molar tooth with an extensive cavity that may result in a pulp exposure if all affected dentine is removed.

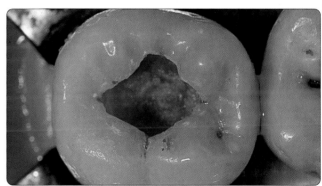

Fig. 18.4 Cavity opened. The infected dentine has been spooned out using hand instruments.

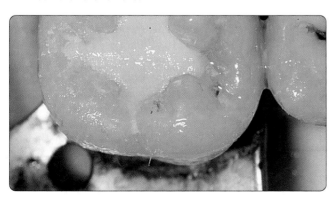

Fig. 18.5 Cavity sealed. The cavity has been sealed with a strong glass–ionomer only.

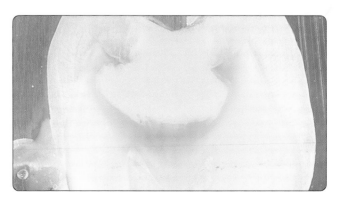

Fig. 18.6 Cross-section. A cross-section of the finished restoration showing the close adaptation of the cement.

This routine has been used in several countries to stabilise cavities regardless of the position on the tooth crown. Site 1 lesions are the easiest to treat but it is reasonably successful for Site 2 and Site 3 lesions so long as they are not too extensive. In restoring a Site 2 lesion, it is usually not possible to restore a normal contact area or to build up a marginal ridge, which means that these restorations must be regarded as having a limited life potential.

However, so long as the lesion is not too extensive, Site 1 and Site 3 restorations can be expected to show acceptable longevity. Logically, if normal dental services become available, such restorations should be carefully assessed and replaced as required. Results over recent years suggest acceptably high short-term success with the potential for saving many teeth. The only difference between this technique and that recommended for use in general practice is that the cement can be replaced with a longer term restoration at a predictable time in general practice. This may not always be possible in situations where the ART technique is used.

TREATMENT OF PULPITIS UNDER INTACT DENTINE

A transient acute pulpitis may occur because of a long-term insult, such as an advancing carious lesion or microleakage under a restoration, and some form of interceptive therapy would be appropriate. A similar pulpitis may occur after a traumatic injury, or may be caused by exposure of extensive areas of healthy dentine during crown preparation. However, in the absence of an acute bacterial infection, no treatment is required because it should normally resolve in 1–2 days.

The most effective therapy in these cases is to remove the insult. If the pulp is still alive and not infected, the potential for resolution of the inflammation and its symptoms is excellent. Two types of material can be applied to dentine to help overcome or suppress pulpal inflammation.

Suppression of pulpal inflammation
- Eugenol is antibacterial, and has a direct effect upon pulpal inflammation and pain. It inhibits the synthesis of prostaglandins as well as reducing nerve action potentials. A brief application of eugenol to dentine, or the sustained release of eugenol into dentine from a zinc oxide–eugenol base or temporary filling, results in concentrations of eugenol in the outer layers of the pulp tissue sufficient for these effects to develop.
- Corticosteroids are widely used in medicine for the temporary suppression of inflammation. The same effect occurs in inflamed pulp tissue. However, a lining or base containing a corticosteroid will not have any long-term effect because all the steroid will be released within the first 3 days.

TREATMENT OF THE EXPOSED PULP

Pulp tissue may be exposed to the oral environment as a result of direct mechanical trauma fracturing both enamel and dentine or, alternatively, exposure may occur during cavity preparation. Various materials may be placed directly on the exposed pulp, but whether the pulp will then survive depends upon the following factors.
- The age of the patient – because of a relatively high vascularity, the younger the patient the more likely it is that the tooth will survive.
- The state of the pulp, including its cellularity and vascularity – previous injury or insult may have led to the development of fibrous repair tissue, thereby reducing vascularity and the ability of the tissue to recover.
- The nature and number of contaminating microorganisms – the presence of any microorganism is undesirable and attempts at sterilisation with antibacterial agents may cause further tissue damage. However, in the presence of high vascularity, the pulp tissue may survive minor infection with relatively benign bacteria.
- The material applied – if the pulp tissue is healthy and the area of exposed tissue relatively small, and if contaminating bacteria are either absent or benign, calcific healing will occur adjacent to many materials. Effectiveness of the seal over the long term with prevention of further ingress of bacteria should therefore be the principal consideration. Glass–ionomer cement will create such a seal under most circumstances and the pulp may heal in direct contact with it. However, the response may be better if the soft tissue only is covered with an autocure calcium hydroxide cement first, and then sealed with the glass–ionomer.

PULPOTOMY

In young individuals, the preferred treatment for a small area of uninfected pulp, such as a pulp horn, that is exposed by tooth fracture, is a 'Cvek pulpotomy' – named after the dentist who first described the technique. The problem is most likely to occur in permanent upper anterior teeth of teenagers and young adults during sport, rough play or fighting and it is likely that, at this age, the pulp tissue will be free of fibrous degenerative tissue and the blood supply will be rich.

Cvek pulpotomy
A Cvek pulpotomy should be carried out as soon as possible after the injury is sustained to minimise the penetration of bacterial contamination. Isolate the tooth with rubber dam and clean gently with air–water spray. Under local anaesthesia, a small amount of pulpal tissue and adjacent dentine is then surgically removed with a high-speed bur to a depth of approximately 1 mm. This will remove the surface layer of pulp, which is the area most likely to be contaminated with bacteria. The wound is washed, bleeding controlled and calcium hydroxide applied directly to the pulp tissue. The remainder of the tooth defect is then restored, using conventional techniques. Use a material, or combination of materials, which will develop an effective antibacterial seal

while restoring function and aesthetics. The high success rate in young patients is probably the result of a combination of factors, including the low level of bacterial contamination and good response to trauma in that age group.

Deciduous pulpotomy

If larger areas of pulp tissue are removed the response is generally not so effective. A total pulpotomy, in which the entire coronal pulp is removed, is used as an alternative to full root canal therapy in deciduous teeth, and is acceptable because failure is often slow enough to allow natural exfoliation after space retention for several years. In permanent teeth, however, the predictability of the success of pulpotomy is so uncertain as to contraindicate the procedure, except as a temporary or economic expedient. Root canal therapy is therefore indicated.

FURTHER READING

Brannstrom M. *Dentine and pulp in restorative dentistry.* London: Wolfe Medical Publications; 1982.

Cvek M. A clinical report on partial pulpotomy and capping with calcium hydroxide in permanent incisors with complicated crown fracture. *J Endodontol* 1978; **4**:232–7.

Massler M. Preventive endodontics: vital pulp therapy. *Dent Clin North Am* 1967; **12.2**:663–73.

Mertz-Fairhurst EJ. Cariostatic and ultra-conservative sealed restorations: six year results. *Quintessence Int* 1992; **23**:827–38.

Pashley DH. The effects of acid etching on the pulpo-dentine complex. *Oper Dent* 1992; **17**:229–42.

Stanley HR. The effect of bonding and conditioning agents on the pulp. *J Esthet Dent* 1993; **5**:208–13.

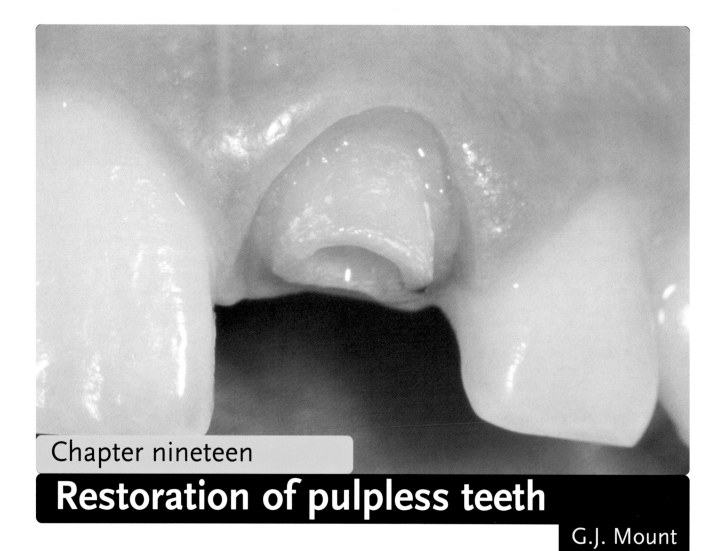

Chapter nineteen

Restoration of pulpless teeth

G.J. Mount

Loss of vitality reduces the physical properties and translucency of remaining tooth structure. Depending to some degree upon the cause of pulp death and the history of the endodontic treatment, there will usually be a colour shift towards grey or brown. There will inevitably be a reduction in the fracture resistance of remaining tooth structure and the strength of the remaining crown of the tooth will be reduced by the need to open into the crown to carry out root canal therapy.

Restoration of nonvital teeth will need to take all these factors into account.

PHYSICAL PRINCIPLES

Anterior teeth

In general, the direction of the load on upper anterior teeth is upwards and outwards, moving the crown of the tooth in a labial direction out of the arch, adjacent teeth giving no support. In most cases, the central dentine core of the crown will have been weakened by preparation of the access cavity for root canal therapy, and possibly by caries as well. This means the main stress will be accepted by the remaining dentine at the labial gingival margin. Unless there is considerable bulk of dentine in that area, simple restoration of the coronal form may be insufficient to reinforce the tooth. Even the use of adhesive restorative materials such as glass–ionomer is of no help, because these materials are weak in tension and that will be the greatest stress applied.

It is generally necessary, therefore, to reinforce the crown by placing a post into the root canal, so moving the potential point of fracture from the gingival margin of the crown some distance up the root towards the root apex.

The load applied to lower anterior teeth is usually in the opposite downwards and inwards direction; this will tend to close the arch, and the crown will gain some support from adjacent teeth. Reinforcement through placement of a post is therefore not as important. However, the crown is relatively small and preparation of the access cavity will leave little of the original dentine, so placement of a post may still be desirable.

Posterior teeth

The usual cause of loss of vitality of a posterior tooth is extensive caries or microleakage beneath a large restoration. Therefore, much of the central dentine core of the tooth is missing and the remaining buccal and lingual enamel is undermined and weakened. In essence, the length of the cusps will now be extended through the entire length of the crown to the gingival margin or beyond. Simple restoration of the crown of the tooth is rarely adequate to impart sufficient strength to withstand laterally directed occlusal load. The tensile strength of glass–ionomer is not great enough to reinforce the crown, and the use of composite resin in an attempt to unite the remaining cusps is dependent upon the strength of the remaining enamel. This enamel is generally rather weak and ill-supported by dentine. It is also subject to microcracks around the margins and its soundness should, therefore, not be relied upon. It is desirable, therefore, to rebuild a posterior tooth with amalgam to support the posts before placing a crown to tie the remaining tooth together.

Retentive elements

The use of pins or the development of retentive grooves and ditches in the cavity design will be of some value in aiding retention of a coronal restoration but they are rarely adequate on their own and each may also further weaken the remaining tooth structure. Self-threading pins tend to produce microcracks, even in vital dentine, and these will propagate even further into nonvital tooth structure. Ditches and grooves will help, but often there is so little dentine remaining it is not possible to place them.

Point of rotation

If placement of an extracoronal restoration is planned for upgrading aesthetics or for reinforcement, more coronal tooth structure will be lost while cutting the preparation. With an intracoronal restoration, the point of rotation of the restoration out of the crown, as a result of a buccal or lingual component of forces, is at the most buccal-gingival or lingual-gingival point angle of that restoration (Chapter 13, page 168). Placement of pins or ditches and grooves does not alter this point of rotation to a significant degree; as the amount of dentine is reduced in these critical areas, the more significant will be the weakening factor. Pins have very little intrinsic strength and bend readily around the axis of rotation. Self-threaded pins have some resistance to being withdrawn from the side opposite the point of rotation but, in the presence of microcracks, further caries is likely to develop and they will eventually be released (**Figs 19.1** and **19.2**).

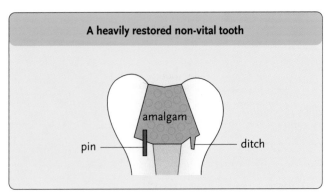

Fig. 19.1 A heavily restored non-vital tooth. If a tooth is heavily restored and non-vital, the strength of the remaining tooth structure is severely compromised.

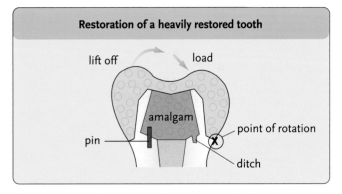

Fig. 19.2 Restoration of a heavily restored tooth. Following restoration for a crown, neither ditches nor pins will offer any substantial advantage to counter potential rotational forces.

Lateral forces

An opposing tooth in contact with the central fossa can exert a buccal or lingual component of force sufficient to split a cusp at the gingival margin. It must be noted that an intracoronal inlay type of restoration is entirely dependent upon the strength of the weakest of the remaining cusps, even though the cusps may be veneered with a protective-style design. Placement of an extracoronal restoration minimises splitting stresses on buccal or lingual cusps and extends the life of the tooth.

Value of posts

Placement of posts in one or more root canals is desirable to move the potential point of fracture from the gingival margin of the crown as far as possible up the root of the tooth towards the apex of the root. Placement of a post alone, however, does not relieve the cusps from occlusal load. If either the buccal or lingual cusps are weakened or already split, a post should be placed followed by an extracoronal restoration to keep the point of rotation well up the length of the root (**Figs 19.3–19.5**).

However, there are inherent risks in the placement of a post as given below.

- A post is essentially an intraradicular restoration and therefore relies on the strength and integrity of the remaining root structure to retain it in place.
- The larger the diameter of the post, the weaker the remaining root.
- The thinner the post, the more likely it is to bend.
- The longer the post, the greater the risk of lateral perforation.
- The shorter the post, the less the retention.
- Great care is required in the preparation of the post hole to ensure that it follows the root canal, does not deviate laterally and does not disturb the root canal filling.

PRINCIPLES OF RESTORATION

In light of the above points, it is essential to retain as much tooth structure as possible, particularly in the gingival one-third of the crown. The access cavity to a root canal should be very conservative and the canal should be reamed open no further than is essential for adequate obturation. Obturation should be carried out in such a way that subsequent development of a post hole is relatively simple and straightforward so minimising the risk of lateral deviation and perforation of the root. Optimal physical properties will be retained only if the post passes straight up the middle of the root.

Anterior teeth
Preservation of remaining tooth structure
On occasion, with a tooth that has become nonvital with no loss of coronal tooth structure, it may be possible to bleach it and restore only the access cavity with glass–ionomer. If, however, the dentine is weakened to any degree in the

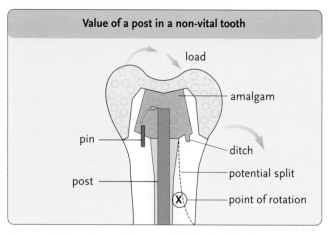

Fig. 19.3 Value of a post in a non-vital tooth. This diagram emphasises the value of a post to assist in placing the point of rotation down the root of the tooth, so making the most of remaining tooth structure. The restoration is essentially intraradicular, with support coming from the root only. The point of rotation is now one-quarter of the distance up the root from the apical end of the post; the potential fracture line is shown. Load on the pins or grooves is now minimal.

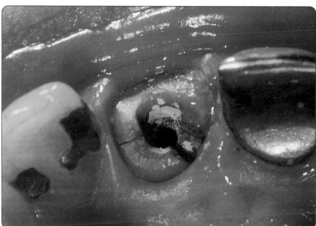

Fig. 19.4 Split root. The crown has been lost twice in a period of 12 months and the split is now clearly visible.

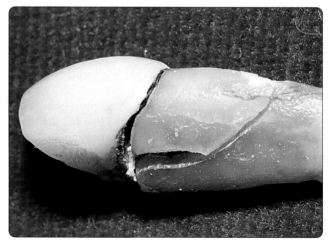

Fig. 19.5 Split root. The tooth has been extracted and the classic anatomy of a split becomes apparent.

gingival one-third of the crown, it may be wise to place a threaded parallel-sided post first to accept some of the incisal load before sealing the access cavity.

If the crown is broken down any further, a full crown becomes the restoration of choice and it is essential to maintain as much as possible of the gingival one-third of the crown, because this will be an important element in retention. Remove any remaining caries or old nonadhesive restorations and replace with glass–ionomer cement. Remove the incisal two-thirds of the crown and prepare the remainder according to the type of crown to be placed. The labial gingival margin will almost invariably be prepared as a flat shoulder all the way from the midline at the mesial to the midline at the distal at a level approximately 0.25 mm below the gingival crest. Preparation of the lingual margin will vary depending upon whether the crown is to be porcelain bonded to metal or all-ceramic. Whichever type of crown is to be placed, it is essential to preserve as much of the cingulum as possible so that the crown can form a cuff around the dentine and offer some resistance to the labial stresses to which it will be subjected.

Having completed preparation of the gingival margin, remove any remaining coronal dentine that is too thin or weak to be of significant help in retention.

Preparation of the post hole

Ideally the coronal one-half of the post hole will have been left open at the time of obturation. If not, care must be taken to avoid deviation from the canal while opening it to accept a post. Assuming the canal has been sealed with gutta percha, guidance can be obtained by softening the root filling with a heated instrument. A reamer can then be inserted to remove the softened material and the direction of the canal identified. The use of magnification and a fibre-optic light is helpful in following progress. The length of the post should be at least the length of the proposed crown as measured from the labial gingival margin to the incisal edge, with a minimum of 10 mm. Having opened the canal to the required depth, it can be reamed to the appropriate size to accept a post.

It has been suggested that there is a need to include an antirotation device at the entry to the canal to reduce tensile stresses on the cement. Generally, an anterior root canal is ovoid in section and will still be ovoid after endodontic treatment is completed. It is sufficient, therefore, to develop a cuff at the entry to the post hole that follows the anatomy of the canal to a depth of about 2.0 mm. This will both reinforce the post at that point and act as an antirotation device. It is unwise to weaken the top of the root by the placement of pins or grooves in this area because this is the section of the root that requires the greatest strength if the crown is to survive.

Selection of the post

There is a great variety of materials from which a post can be made, as well as a number of preformed post systems available. It is possible to take an impression of the post hole and cast a post in a hard gold alloy to fit accurately through its full length. Alternatively, preformed posts, both tapered and parallel sided, are available onto which a core can be either built direct or cast. A root and the canal within is usually tapered from the crown to the apex, so that a newly reamed canal is also tapered. Because it is possible to exert considerable splitting stresses on the remaining root when cementing a tapered post, the preferred design is a parallel-sided post with a groove along one side to act as a release channel for excess cement. Additional advantages in retention can be gained by incorporating horizontal grooves or threads up the sides of the post to give mechanical attachment to the cement.

There are two anatomical problems in the preparation of such a parallel-sided post hole which, when mechanically reamed, will necessarily be round in cross-section.

1. The root is tapered towards the apex, so the further a parallel-sided post hole is reamed up the canal, the closer the post will come to the external surface. Certainly, the larger the diameter of the hole, the greater the risk and the weaker the tooth.
2. The root of a tooth is not necessarily round in cross-section through its full length. In fact, many roots demonstrate a reverse curve on the mesial surface, distal surface, or both, particularly those with two canals such as lower anteriors and the mesial roots of lower molars. These anatomical variations do not show clearly in radiographs and their presence must be assumed.

There is an inherent risk in preparing any post hole and the risk–benefit ratio must be taken into account. As the cement is always the weakest link in the chain, the post must be a reasonably accurate fit, particularly at both the apical and the coronal end. The post must be of a sufficient diameter to resist bending stresses at the coronal end of the post where it joins the core. It can be reinforced to a degree at that point by casting a cuff around the post or building an amalgam core. As the resistance to bending is directly proportional to the diameter of the post, it must be as thick as possible. However, the remaining tooth structure is already weakened by loss of vitality and the reaming of the post hole. The remaining root suffers all the problems of a crown with an intracoronal restoration, and it is not surprising that a split in the root is an occasional problem. The point of rotation of a post crown is approximately one-quarter of the way from the apical end of the post; the split will commonly occur from that point upwards to the mesio-distal midline of the coronal end of the root (see **Fig. 19.5**).

Construction of the core by indirect method

The core for an anterior tooth should closely resemble the design of a preparation for a similar crown for a vital tooth. It should be of sufficient length to allow for optimal retention while allowing room for incisal coverage with the restorative material. The sides should be no more than 10° from parallel. It should engage the remaining dentine around the cingulum to provide a ferrule effect to counter labial stresses. The main support will generally be provided by the root itself, but there are situations, such as the presence of a long fracture up the lingual surface of the root, where the core should incorporate the lingual surface of the root – the crown margin will then be on the core. It is important that the core is evenly positioned so that there will be an equal thickness of crown all around it.

The core can be constructed indirectly on a master model and cast in a Type III gold (Chapter 12, page 157) or it can be built direct in the tooth using plastic restorative material. The advantages of the indirect technique are that the correct positioning and dimensions are readily achieved and the gold can be heat treated to obtain optimal physical properties. As it is, essentially, an intraradicular restoration it should be cast by a technique that will ensure a small percentage reduction in size in contrast to the usual technique for a full crown, which incorporates an element of expansion. The limitation is that if the post does not seat fully into the root canal the final crown will not seat completely. Some operators prefer to cast and cement the post first before taking the master impression for the crown to avoid this problem.

Construction of the core by direct method

An alternative technique is to build the core in a plastic restorative material direct in the mouth. A stainless-steel post can be cemented into a correctly designed post hole and any deficiency in the crown made good with amalgam, composite resin or glass–ionomer. Amalgam has the best physical properties, particularly in tensile strength and it can be condensed into the top of the root canal to give additional support to the post. Composite resin is limited by its lack of adhesion to the dentine and its relative flexibility. Glass–ionomer lacks tensile strength, but it does adhere to dentine and has a fluoride release that can be valuable. With any of these materials, remaining tooth structure should be retained as far as possible to act as a

guide for correct placement and contouring of the core and to compensate for their limited physical properties. In fact, if the entire crown of the tooth is already missing as far as the gingival margin, none of these materials is very satisfactory and a cast core is the method of choice.

Design of crown

There remains a limited choice for the final crown restoration of a nonvital anterior crown. If very little tooth is lost, bleaching alone may be sufficient, with the access cavity restored using glass–ionomer. It will adhere to the dentine with no microleakage or colour change and offer a minor degree of reinforcement to the crown.

If there is still a considerable amount of sound tooth structure remaining that has bleached satisfactorily, it may be sufficient to place a post and restore with glass–ionomer laminated with composite resin. Also, with this type of foundation, it may be possible to place a resin or porcelain laminate veneer. However, it must be noted that the further the tooth needs to be prepared to make room for the restoration, the less natural tooth structure will remain and therefore the weaker the crown will be. Composite resin laminate veneers must rely upon sound etched enamel to provide attachment.

A gold three-quarter crown can be designed to preserve labial enamel but, in a nonvital tooth, the enamel is usually aesthetically poor and is best removed. This means that full crowns are usually the restoration of choice; the design and construction of these is dealt with in Chapter 13, page 172 (**Figs 19.6** and **19.7**).

Posterior teeth
Preservation of remaining tooth structure
It is desirable when dealing with a posterior tooth to follow procedures that will preserve tooth structure before root canal therapy is commenced. In the absence of an acute emergency, so long as the patient is not distressed or in

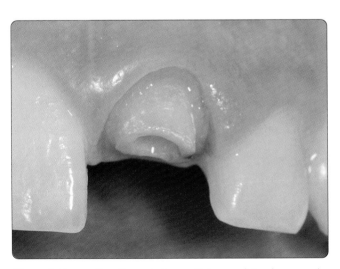

Fig. 19.6 Preparation for post. A nonvital upper lateral prepared for a post. Note retention of maximum amount of dentine.

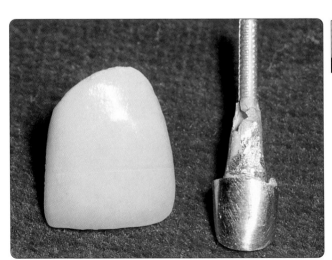

Fig. 19.7 Post and core for crown. Note that the post is at least as long as the crown, has parallel sides and fits accurately at the top and the apex.

pain, it may be best if the tooth is fully restored initially with one of the plastic restorative materials and then access gained through the restoration. Amalgam is the material of choice because it will seal its own margins and will withstand occlusal stress. Also, it will become a satisfactory foundation for the ultimate crown. Glass–ionomer can be used for smaller defects where it will not be subjected to undue load.

Following rubber-dam isolation, all old restorative material should be removed and active caries cleaned up. Access to the pulp chamber is not essential at this point and should be avoided if possible. If the pulp chamber is exposed, it should not be entered but sealed with a suitable sedative type base. All the cavo-surface walls should be completely cleaned so that the new restoration will be soundly based with no microleakage.

Construction of the core

If there is sufficient natural tooth structure remaining, it is desirable to build the core before endodontic therapy, as discussed above. Complex matrix techniques may be required. Every attempt should be made to develop good proximal contacts to avoid food impaction and maintain patient comfort, but the core does not need to provide a full occlusal contact with the opposing tooth. The patient may be more comfortable with the tooth free of the occlusion until the endodontics is completed.

On the other hand if there is little or no coronal tooth structure remaining it may be necessary to carry out the endodontic therapy before building the core. Isolation of the root may well pose a problem but is not impossible to achieve. The construction of the post and core will follow the stages set out for an anterior tooth. The core can be made of amalgam, but the matrix technique will be more difficult to carry out. A copper band matrix, supported with green stick compound, is probably the simplest to use. A cast-gold core is an alternative and, with care and good technical support, allowance can be made for post holes that are not parallel by using a sectional post (**Figs 19.8–19.11**).

Preparation of the post hole

The same principles apply as those set out for an anterior tooth. The anatomy of the roots varies, and this variation is not always easy to detect with radiographs. Remove the gutta-percha with a hot instrument and watch carefully for deviation using magnification and a fibre-optic light. Continue the post hole as far up the root canal as possible extending at least as far as the height of the crown. The diameter of the post hole will be dictated by the diameter of the root at the apical extension of the post hole. In multirooted teeth, place a post hole in each root and vary the size according to the diameter of the root.

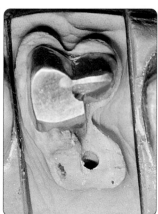

Fig. 19.8 Split post and core. The molar has divergent roots so a two-part cast core has been made for it. The buccal section has been placed on the model. Note the mechanical interlock between the sections.

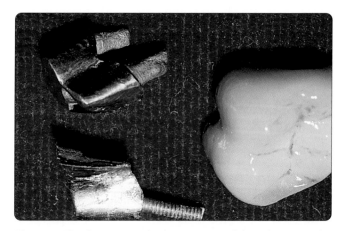

Fig. 19.9 The three parts. The two sections of the split post with the crown.

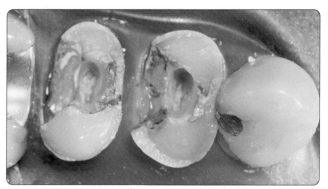

Fig. 19.10 Core build-up. Two nonvital bicuspids prepared for core build-up. Preformed posts will be cemented into the root canals and a cermet cement core will be placed.

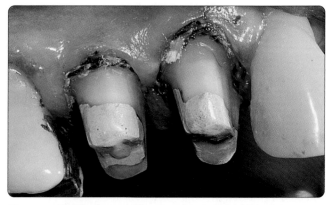

Fig. 19.11 Finished cores. The completed cores. Note the amount of sound dentine retained at the gingival margin.

Selection of the post

Preformed parallel-sided posts are preferred because they apply less stress during cementation. They are relatively straightforward to use, particularly from the prematched kits available, which include reamers with posts of a slightly smaller diameter. They are made in either stainless steel or titanium to resist corrosion and they are generally threaded and vented for ease and efficiency of cementation.

Design of crown

Because of the relatively large amount of destruction that has usually occurred with nonvital tooth intracoronal restorations, such procedures are now rarely indicated. As noted, intracoronal restorations are only as strong as the weakest element in the remaining tooth. A limited amount of reinforcement or protection can be derived from an intracoronal amalgam or gold inlay but, if either buccal or lingual cusps are undermined or fragile, an extracoronal restoration is indicated. Simply covering cusps with an inlay will not alter the position of the point of rotation of the restoration out of the tooth from the buccal-gingival or lingual-gingival point angle and weakened or split cusps will fail (see Chapter 13, page 168).

Providing the remaining buccal cusp can be returned to a satisfactory colour a three-quarter gold crown is the most conservative restoration. Having placed a post and built an amalgam core around it, a minimal preparation can be undertaken. The buccal cusp of an upper posterior tooth needs to be lightly covered because it is usually poorly supported at this stage. Also, the gold should be wrapped around the distal as far as aesthetics will allow, for additional support. As the buccal cusps of lower molars are working cusps and under heavy occlusal load they will need more generous protection still.

In most cases, the remaining tooth is so weak and the aesthetics so poor that a full crown is the restoration of choice. Gold is the more conservative material to the extent that it can be placed in very thin section and therefore does not require undue preparation of the tooth. Preparation for a ceramic crown, on the other hand, requires the removal of considerably more tooth structure particularly on the buccal side, to the extent that often there is no enamel left. This situation reinforces the recommendation that a post should always be placed in a nonvital tooth because, following crown preparation, there may be insufficient natural tooth left to support a crown by itself.

FURTHER READING

Andreasen JP, Andreasen FM. *Essentials of traumatic injuries to the teeth.* London, Denmark: Laursen A/S; 1989.

Chan RW, Bryant RW. Post core foundations for endodontically treated posterior teeth. *J Prosthet Dent* 1982; **48**:401–6.

De Sort KD. The prosthodontic use of endodontically treated teeth – theory and biomechanics of post preparation. *J Prosthet Dent* 1983; **49**:203–6.

Gutman JL. The dentine-root complex; anatomic and biologic considerations in restoring endodontically treated teeth. *J Prosthet Dent* 1992; **67**:458–67.

Shillingburg AT, Kessler JC. *Restoration of the endodontically treated tooth.* Chicago: Quintessence; 1982.

Sorensen JA, Martinoff JT. Clinically significant factors in dowel design. *J Prosthet Dent* 1984; **52**:28–35.

Turner CH. The retention of dental posts. *J Dent* 1982; **10**:154–65.

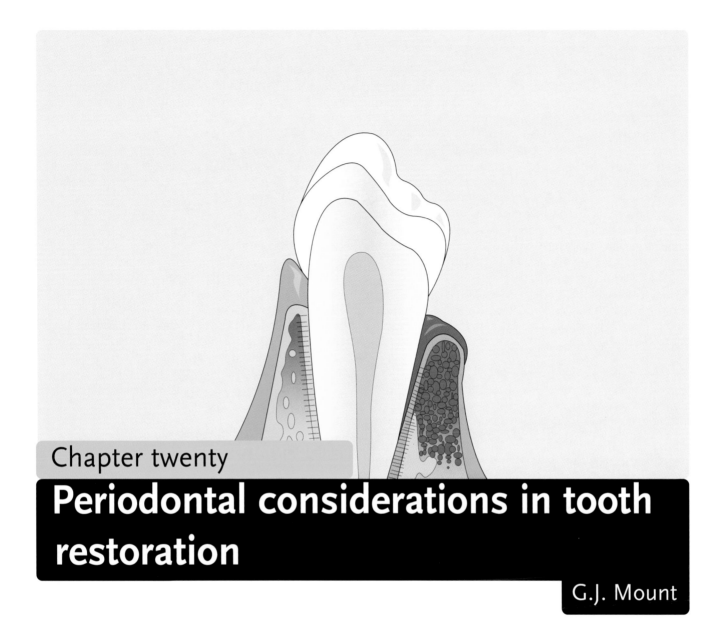

Chapter twenty

Periodontal considerations in tooth restoration

G.J. Mount

The significant factors that require consideration are those situations which can compromise the health of the gingival tissues as the result of operative procedures undertaken for the restoration of a diseased or broken tooth. It is necessary to be able to recognise variations from normal before commencement of treatment as well as to be aware of the changes that may take place following restorative procedures. Consideration must also be given to actions that may cause irreversible damage during treatment.

NORMAL GINGIVAL TISSUE

Normal healthy gingival tissue is usually described as firm, coral pink with a stippled surface and a smooth knife-edge margin around the circumference of each tooth. There is expected to be a zone of gingival tissue attached firmly to the underlying alveolar bone on the buccal and lingual aspects of each tooth, varying in width from 1 mm to 5 mm, and a crevice about 2 mm deep around each tooth that can be traced with a fine probe. At the base of the crevice lies the epithelial attachment representing a firm biological attachment of the gingival tissue to the root surface. The epithelial attachment normally begins immediately at the cemento-enamel junction of each tooth and is about 2 mm wide towards the apex (**Figs 20.1** and **20.2**).

Any divergence from the above description is regarded as a disease state that requires diagnosis and treatment. However, as with all pathology, there is a wide variation of acceptable levels as well as a wide variation in treatment method.

Epithelial attachment

It is accepted that, at the time of eruption of a tooth, the epithelial attachment is located at the cemento-enamel junction, but initially the pocket around the tooth above the junction will be very deep. By the time the tooth is fully erupted, however, it should be only 2 mm in depth. The pocket can remain at that depth for life, but the site of the epithelial attachment may migrate down the length of the root for a variety of reasons, not all of which are properly understood. It is not essential that this happens, and patients of advanced age may show no change at all. It is also accepted that the zone of attached gingival tissue at the buccal and lingual aspects of each tooth can be reduced to 1 mm without any indication of pathology and, in a few patients, it can be absent entirely without any untoward result.

Abnormal situations

Reasons for apparent aberrations are not clearly understood; it is suggested that the only indication of pathology or alteration from normal that is significant and requires treatment is the presence of inflammation. Occasionally situations arise wherein migration of the epithelial attachment or loss of attached gingiva is accompanied by severe loss of supporting bone, to the extent that the life of a tooth is compromised and surgical intervention is warranted. However, this occurs in association with a generalised periodontal condition, which is beyond the scope of this book.

PROBLEMS THAT COMPROMISE PERIODONTAL TISSUE

Gingivitis

Gingivitis can be identified as a change in the colour, texture and contour of the gingival tissue around part or all of the circumference of a tooth. The earliest signs are a subtle change in colour and a tendency to bleed from within the gingival crevice following gentle probing. These changes can progress to hypertrophy of the tissue with a major change in colour to a dull red and a tendency to be easily damaged by tooth brushing or even eating. The gingival crevice may increase through hypertrophy in an occlusal direction to a depth of 3–4 mm, but the position of the epithelial attachment may remain at the cemento-enamel junction, particularly in the early stages of gingivitis (**Fig. 20.3**).

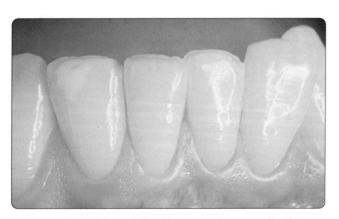

Fig. 20.1 Gingival tissue in health. A typical picture of healthy gingival tissue in a patient aged 35.

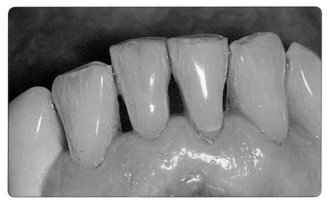

Fig. 20.2 Gingival tissue in health. This patient is aged 92; note the similarity of the tissue to Figure 20.1, despite the advanced age.

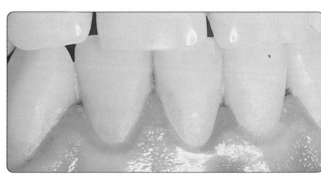

Fig. 20.3 Chronic gingivitis. Note the presence of plaque around the gingival areas of the teeth and the presence of a low-grade chronic gingivitis that shows as slightly swollen, glazed, red gingival margins.

The role of plaque

The cause of gingivitis is bacterial activity. Bacteria attach to the surface of a tooth or restoration and become organised to the extent that they form a soft mass referred to as bacterial plaque. If the plaque is allowed to remain in the vicinity of the gingival tissue, this will inevitably result in an inflammatory reaction in response to the presence of toxins from the bacteria. The pathogenic potential of plaque can vary from one individual to another and from one area of the mouth to another. It is accepted that the inflammation is an immunological defence mechanism and investigations are still being undertaken to determine if the body responds to a greater degree to one bacterial group or another (**Figs 20.4** and **20.5**).

Treatment

Treatment of gingivitis consists simply in the removal of plaque or calculus, or of both. Achievement of this aim is not always easy because, over time, the plaque matures and takes up additional calcium and phosphate ions and turns into calculus, a hard accretion on the surface of the tooth which is difficult to remove. However, if plaque is to be removed effectively on a daily basis, the teeth must be maintained in a cleansible condition. Any situation that compromises the ability of the patient to remove plaque must be avoided or eliminated. This includes maintenance of the correct contour of the crowns and the roots of the teeth, the avoidance of prosthetic replacements that are not cleanable and the elimination of areas of crowding of teeth that compromise the effectiveness of cleaning techniques.

Periodontitis

Periodontitis is the usual sequel to untreated gingivitis. It is essentially an extension of the inflammatory process into the connective tissue and the bone surrounding the teeth leading to the progressive destruction of those tissues. It has been suggested that periodontal disease progresses in bursts of activity, ranging in length from a few days to a few months (**Fig. 20.6**).

Migration of epithelial attachment

The first stage involves the loss of the epithelial attachment at the cemento-enamel junction. The crevice surrounding the tooth becomes deeper and the patient's ability to remove plaque from the depths of the crevice on a daily basis is reduced. There is normally only a distance of about 2 mm from the base of the epithelial attachment to the crest of the alveolar bone surrounding the root, so the bone itself is rapidly involved in the inflammatory process. It cannot withstand the presence of bacterial activity and resorbs rapidly, developing a pocket around the root within the alveolar bone. By this time, the marginal gingival tissue may have resumed a relatively normal appearance with very little obvious inflammation, although the destructive process may continue into the deeper structures.

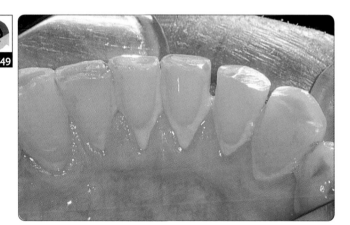

Fig. 20.4 Calculus accumulation. Typical accumulation of calculus on the lingual of the lower anteriors with resultant inflammation in the gingival tissues.

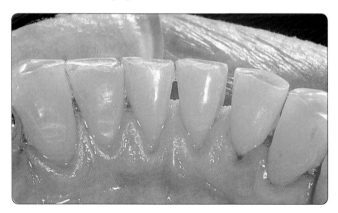

Fig. 20.5 Recovery of gingival tissue. One week after removal of calculus, the gingival tissue has recovered.

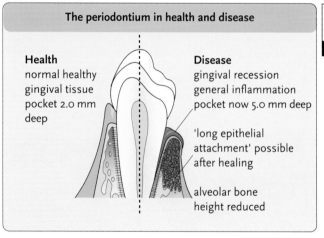

The periodontium in health and disease

Health
normal healthy gingival tissue pocket 2.0 mm deep

Disease
gingival recession general inflammation pocket now 5.0 mm deep

'long epithelial attachment' possible after healing

alveolar bone height reduced

Fig. 20.6 The periodontium in health and disease. The periodontal attachment as it should be in health, with a pocket of only 2.0 mm depth and the alveolar bone crest about 2.0 mm below the pocket floor. After inflammation, the pocket will deepen and alveolar bone will migrate away from the inflammation. Even after restoration of health, the epithelial attachment will remain extended and the alveolar bone will not return to its full height.

Ultimately, the loss of bone may progress to the point where the root has lost mechanical support and the tooth becomes mobile and has to be extracted (**Figs 20.7** and **20.8**).

Treatment

Treatment of periodontal disease is essentially the same as treatment of gingivitis in that removal of the cause, the plaque and calculus, is of primary importance. However, resolution of the damage arising from the disease is often very complex. It has proved impossible to date to redevelop a normal epithelial attachment and very difficult to regain bone height to support the roots of teeth. Therefore, it is accepted that periodontal disease can be terminal for remaining teeth unless vigorous treatment procedures are undertaken before bone loss has advanced to the stage where mechanical support for the teeth has been lost.

Removal of the plaque and calculus will allow rapid resolution of the inflammatory response. After the soft tissue has regained health, at least superficially, steps can be undertaken to ensure that the root surface is entirely free of calculus and that the width of attached gingiva has been reinstated to a reasonable extent.

'Long epithelial attachment'

The epithelial attachment will not regenerate in its original form without surgical intervention, because the epithelial cells propagate down the inside of a wound very rapidly and prevent the development of a normal tissue attachment on the cementum of the root surface. The result, often, is a so-called long epithelial attachment which, although not entirely physiological, can remain healthy and free from further inflammation in the presence of careful plaque-control routines. Ideally, the bone should be regenerated and the epithelial attachment restored to its original dimensions, but surgical techniques are required to achieve this latter end.

EFFECT OF RESTORATIVE DENTISTRY ON GINGIVAL TISSUE

In view of the potential for the ultimate loss of the dentition through periodontal disease, it is important to consider all the implications of restorative dentistry on the periodontal tissues. There are three different aspects to this problem.

Prior assessment and treatment

It is important that the condition of the periodontal tissues is assessed before restoration of the teeth and that all necessary measures are undertaken to restore normal health (**Figs 20.9** and **20.10**).

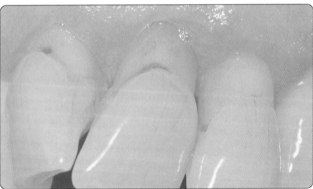

Fig. 20.7 Apparently healthy periodontium disguises an infra-boney pocket, mesial to tooth #22. After treatment, the tissue appears healthy but a pocket is still present within the alveolar bone.

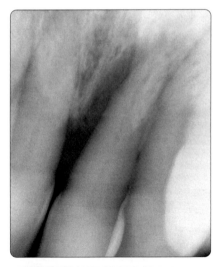

Fig. 20.8 Radiograph showing deep pocket on mesial aspect of tooth #22.

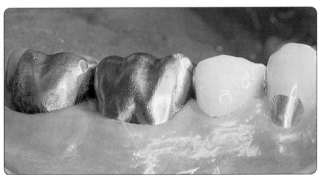

Fig. 20.9 Response to restorations. Gingival tissue around quality amalgam, gold, porcelain and gold foil 10 years after placement.

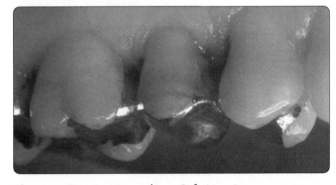

Fig. 20.10 Response to amalgam. Soft tissue in response to amalgam restorations 8 years after placement.

Minimal trauma during treatment

At the time of carrying out restorative procedures, care must be taken to minimise trauma to the gingival tissues. If the tissue is healthy to begin with, it can be expected to heal rapidly and uneventfully. However, it is possible to traumatise the tissues to such a degree during restorative procedures that normal healing cannot take place and some degree of permanent alteration to gingival contour will result.

Restore original contour for plaque control

It is imperative to maintain the teeth in such a condition and contour that plaque control can be achieved readily on a daily basis. The natural contour of the coronal anatomy of a tooth is usually such that hygiene procedures are relatively effective. However, over-contour in any dimension will pose problems in plaque removal. Lack of contour is less of a problem so long as it does not lead to food impaction between teeth or under prosthetic appliances. It is generally accepted that it is impossible to achieve a perfectly smooth union between a restorative material and the tooth being restored so, wherever possible, it is desirable to maintain the restoration margin outside the gingival crevice. A further reason for keeping margins supragingival is that some of the common restorative materials, such as composite resin, have a tendency to encourage plaque formation.

Treatment procedures

Improvement of gingival tissue

Restoration of the gingival tissues to a normal healthy state before commencing restorative procedures is essential, particularly if the cervical margin of a restoration must be placed subgingivally. In many cases, it is adequate to carry out a thorough prophylaxis with removal of plaque and calculus and the topical application of a fluoride gel. The fluoride remineralises the enamel and dentine and also decreases the wettability of the surface of the tooth, therefore reducing future plaque formation. There is rarely any justification for the surgical removal of hypertrophied tissue at this point, because elimination of the inflammation will lead to resolution of the soft tissue with the result that surgery may no longer be required.

Improvement of existing plastic restorations

Existing restorations that are over-contoured should be recontoured as far as possible at this time even if they are to be removed subsequently. In particular, old corroded amalgam restorations and over-contoured composite resins should be contoured and polished to the extent that the patient can use dental floss or inter-proximal brushes to improve the quality of the gingival tissues. Recontouring can be achieved with very fine tapered diamond stones at intermediate high speed under air–water spray followed by reciprocating diamond blades in a special handpiece to produce a reasonable polish on the surface. Local anaesthesia is not required, even though there is often a copious flow of blood resulting from the gingival inflammation. Removal of the entire restoration at this point is not recommended because it is very difficult to replace it with a final restoration in the presence of gingival inflammation. Temporary intra-coronal restorations are not very successful because of the problems of achieving and maintaining proper inter-proximal contour and as most of the temporary restorative materials are relatively fragile (**Figs 20.11** and **20.12**).

Improvement of existing rigid restorations

Recontouring of ceramic crowns and gold restorations is more difficult but should, nevertheless, be attempted. Diamond burs are indicated on porcelain crowns, but multi-bladed tungsten carbide burs remove gold more efficiently. There is a tendency to gouge into the restoration and it is difficult to achieve a perfect result. Therefore, if the original

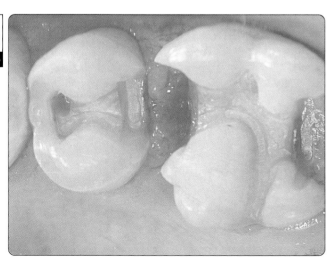

Fig. 20.11 Gingival response to amalgam overhang. A minor overhang on old amalgam in the mesial proximal box of the first molar. Gingival response is apparent upon its removal.

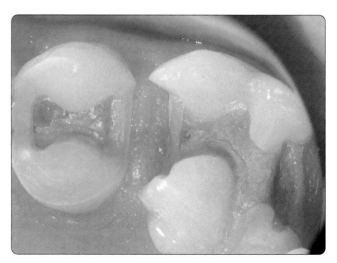

Fig. 20.12 Soft-tissue recovery. After 2 weeks with a correctly contoured temporary restoration, the gingival tissue shown in figure 20.11 recovered.

restoration is to be retained; recontouring must be done with great care. If it is intended to eventually remake the crown, the construction of a high-quality temporary crown may be justified while treatment of the periodontal condition continues. However, the gingival tissue will respond rapidly to the initial recontouring and within 1 week it may be possible to determine the final contour of the gingival margin and therefore construct a better temporary crown (**Figs 20.13** and **20.14**).

Maintenance of occlusion

There are two factors in relation to the occlusion that are significant to the periodontal tissues and these must be taken into account when restoring posterior teeth.

Functionally opening contact

Impaction of food debris between two teeth can have a devastating effect on the interproximal periodontal tissues. The cause may, on occasion, be poor contour in relation to the marginal ridge, but more commonly the problem arises because of deflective inclines on the occlusal surface of adjacent or opposing teeth. For example, when the patient

closes towards the centric relation position during mastication of a food bolus, a distally facing incline on a lower molar may engage a mesially facing incline on the opposing molar. The result may be that the upper molar moves distally and opens the contact between it and the adjacent tooth, allowing ingress of fibrous food debris. On opening the mouth and relieving the load, the tooth will move mesially again and entrap the food debris. This situation occurs most commonly with the terminal tooth on the arch but it is possible for it to arise elsewhere in the arch.

Therefore, in the presence of chronic food impaction, it is necessary to examine the relationship of the opposing teeth to determine the presence or absence of such contacts, particularly as the teeth approach each other in the centric relation position. Occasionally there may be a dominant cusp occluding directly into the contact area of two opposing teeth – a situation that has been described in the past as a 'plunger cusp'. However, mostly the problem arises from cuspal inclines not directly related to the contact area at all. Modification of the appropriate cusp inclines will overcome the problem (**Figs 20.15** and **20.16**).

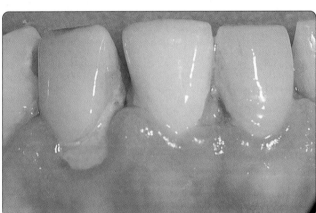

Fig. 20.13 Overhangs on crowns. Crowns on teeth #42 and #43 have gross overhangs and rough margins. Note gingival response.

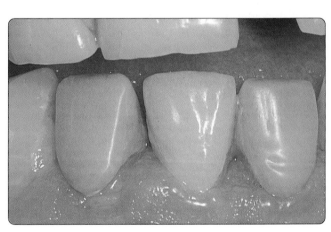

Fig. 20.14 Soft-tissue recovery. One week after recontouring, gingival tissue has recovered sufficiently to consider redesigning the crowns.

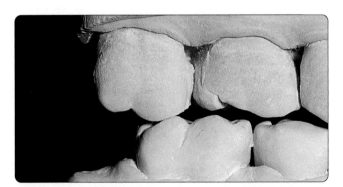

Fig. 20.15 Functionally opening contact. As the patient closes in retruded contact position the initial contact is on the cusp inclines.

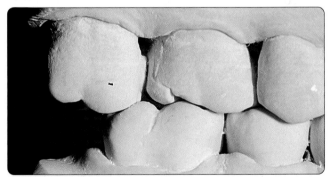

Fig. 20.16 The contact opens. To achieve centric occlusion, the molar is moved distally, thus opening the contact and allowing food impaction.

Notes

Functionally opening contact

This term is more accurately descriptive of a food-impaction problem than the previously used term, 'plunger cusp'.

Maintenance of posterior support

As discussed in Chapter 21, page 239, a lack of posterior support can lead to undue load on remaining teeth and, if there is already periodontal disease present, such disease may be severely exacerbated. Maintenance or regeneration of the minimum eight units, in conjunction with treatment of the periodontium, will stabilise the situation.

Placement of the gingival margin relative to the gingival tissue

A number of factors need to be taken into account before deciding upon the final placement of the gingival margin for any restoration. Because of the potential for accumulation of plaque along the interface between restoration and tooth structure, it is desirable to keep the margin out of the gingival crevice. However, the following factors affect the decision.

Strength of remaining tooth structure

After caries debridement there may be weakened, undermined dentine or enamel along the gingival margin. Because this will not be subjected to occlusal load it need not be totally removed, but fine acute angles of dentine should be flattened off and rough fragile enamel should be lightly planed with a gingival margin trimmer. With care it may then be possible to avoid entering the gingival crevice.

Retention of the restoration

The strength of retention of a restoration is dependent upon the area of the vertical walls of the preparation. This is less significant when placing a plastic restorative material in an intracoronal cavity, because grooves and ditches can supplement retention. However, it is very important for both inlays and extracoronal restorations. The situation may often arise where it is necessary to enter the gingival crevice to develop sufficient length to ensure retention. Very occasionally, gingival surgery with recontouring of the alveolar bone may be indicated, but this is undesirable because of the difficulty of redeveloping a normal epithelial attachment.

Aesthetics

Particularly when designing extracoronal restorations on the upper arch, it will be necessary to compromise the position of the gingival margin to develop satisfactory aesthetics. So long as the gingival tissue is healthy in the first place, the gingival margin of the preparation can be placed up to 0.5 mm into the gingival crevice without provoking an adverse tissue response. Care must be taken, particularly with tissue retraction techniques for impression taking, to minimise tissue damage at the time of operation; skilled technical work is required to develop a smooth union between the restoration and the tooth, with the ideal emergence profile, to minimise plaque retention.

Summary

Placement of gingival margin

The following factors control placement of the gingival margin:
- strength of remaining tooth structure
- retention of restoration
- aesthetic appeal

Procedures during restorative work

It is desirable to return the gingival tissue to full health before embarking on restorative procedures so that the position of the gingival contour will be predictable. After any damage to the gingivae, there will be inflammation in the periodontal tissue, even if it was perfectly healthy to begin with. The heat, redness and swelling that will arise may alter the gingival contour, and subsequent resolution of the inflammation will modify the shape again, making it impossible to predict the ultimate contours (**Figs 20.17** and **20.18**).

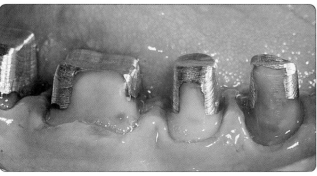

Fig. 20.17 Healthy gingivae. The gingival tissue was in excellent condition before preparations.

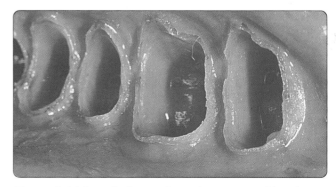

Fig. 20.18 High-quality impressions. These are possible only in the presence of healthy tissue.

The following methods can be utilised to maintain gingival health.

Rubber dam and wedges

The most effective method of preventing the damage is proper protection. The routine placement of rubber dam is strongly recommended even though dam, by itself, does not guarantee protection. The dam will displace the soft tissue to some degree but it is still possible to tear the dam or have an instrument pass through it. When preparing a gingival margin, a further precaution is to place a wooden wedge between the teeth, thus displacing and protecting the dam as well. A wedge will serve multiple purposes inasmuch as it will also move teeth mesially and distally sufficiently to enhance access and improve the strength of the contact between teeth after restoration.

Retraction cord

An alternative method of protecting gingival tissue is to displace the gingival crest laterally by packing a short length of an astringent gingival retraction cord into the gingival crevice. When placed with care, the tissue will be displaced out of the way of rotary cutting instruments such as diamond stones.

Localised removal of excess gingival tissue

Low-grade chronic gingival inflammation, sustained over a long period, may resolve into relatively healthy but over-contoured fibrous tissue. If this tissue is allowed to remain, it may compromise the anatomy of a restoration; also, it is easily damaged during operative procedures and will haemorrhage freely. There are several methods of removing such tissue or, at least, of controlling the haemorrhage.

A brief application of trichloroacetic acid arrests the bleeding very effectively and resolves some of the tissue overgrowth (**Figs 20.19** and **20.20**). Electrosurgery or laser therapy can be used to remove larger areas of excess tissue (Chapter 14, page 177).

Additional scaling during restorative procedures

Despite following the recommended procedure of thorough scaling and cleaning at the time of recontouring old restorations, before embarking on final restoration calculus is often found on the interproximal surfaces immediately below the gingival margins of old restorations. A hand instrument or an ultrasonic scaler should always be passed over the root face below the gingival margin before proceeding with the new restoration. Also, the opportunity should always be accepted for polishing the proximal surface of an adjacent restoration that has become accessible during restorative procedures.

Placement of matrices

Assuming the gingival tissue is in good health, very little damage will be sustained through the placement of a matrix. However, care must be taken to ensure a firm fit with good support for the band using wooden wedges as well as green-stick compound as required. Trim the matrix to contour and polish roughened edges. Achieve a degree of separation between the teeth with a wooden wedge so that the ultimate contact with adjacent teeth will be firm and positive.

Correct approximal anatomy

Because of the overriding need to control plaque development and retention in the oral cavity, there must be considerable emphasis placed on maintaining the correct anatomy of each tooth. As indicated previously, over-contour of any part of the tooth anatomy enhances plaque retention, particularly in the vicinity of the gingival margin.

The term 'emergence profile' refers to the contours of the tooth at the gingival margin as it appears out of the gingival crevice. If this profile is over-built in any way, plaque removal will be more difficult. An overhanging margin on a restoration of any material is probably the most dangerous alteration to the emergence profile inasmuch as it is almost impossible to clean under it. Even

203, 208

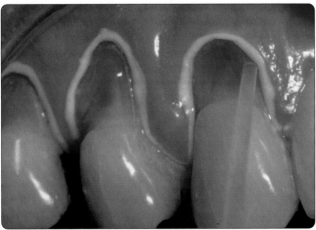

Fig. 20.19 Trichloroacetic acid treatment. There was minor gingival haemorrhage along the margin, so a drop of trichloroacetic acid was applied and washed off after 30 seconds, leaving an eschar.

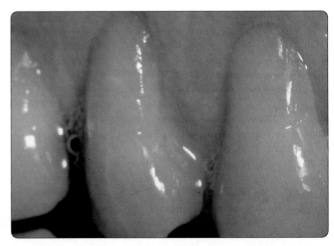

Fig. 20.20 One week after the trichloroacetic acid treatment described in Figure 20.19, the tissue was completely healed without showing any inflammatory response.

a smoothly curved and polished over-contour in a plaque-resistant material such as porcelain is undesirable because of the increased problems of plaque removal.

Contact area

The contour of the proximal surface of the crown of a tooth, particularly in the contact area, is also important and is difficult to redevelop when using the direct plastic restorative materials. It is desirable that the surface is smooth and polished, but it is also essential that there is a positive area of contact with the adjacent tooth. The following factors are important (**Figs 20.21** and **20.22**).

- The contact area (CA) in a posterior tooth should be approximately 1–2 mm below the greatest height of the marginal ridge.
- The CA should be no more than 1–2 mm in height occluso-gingivally and extend bucco-lingually approximately 25% of the width of the adjacent teeth.

- In the upper arch, the CA is generally placed slightly to the buccal side of the mesio-distal midline.
- In the lower arch, the CA is in the midline.
- In the young patient, the CA is narrower bucco-lingually.
- As the patient ages, the CA will broaden.
- The interproximal space should be open as wide as possible commensurate with the presence of a sound CA and a smooth vertical emergence profile to allow optimal plaque removal.

Correct occlusal anatomy

The occlusal anatomy is equally important, particularly in the area of the marginal ridge (**Fig. 20.23**).

- The marginal ridge should rise above the contact area and be smoothly rounded to allow ease of access of dental floss.
- Usually, there are shallow grooves running out to the buccal and lingual of the marginal ridge to guide the food bolus away from the contact area and off the height of the cuspal inclines.
- In youth, the cuspal inclines tend to be steep but, as the patient ages, the occlusal anatomy assumes a flatter profile.
- Deep intercuspation between opposing arches is undesirable because of the lateral stress that can be imposed on cusp inclines, particularly nonworking cusps.
- It is important to adjust both opposing occlusal surfaces as required during restorative procedures to minimise the intercuspation because deep intercuspation may lead to the development of both balancing-side and working-side interference during lateral excursions.

Modification to gingival architecture
Surgical modification

The ultimate aesthetic result of restorative dentistry is important to both the patient and the operator, particularly in relation to the anterior teeth. A lack of balance and symmetry in the gingival margins may be significant.

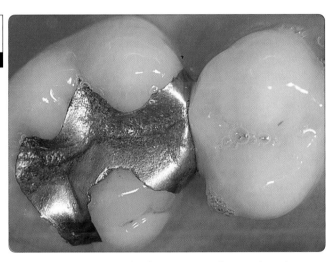

Fig. 20.21 Poor interproximal contour. Poorly carved amalgam with a grossly over-extended contact area.

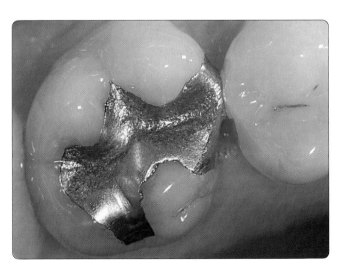

Fig. 20.22 Proper contour. Interproximal amalgam has been recontoured without replacing the restoration.

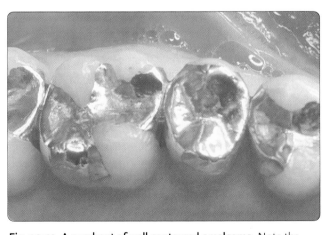

Fig. 20.23 A quadrant of well-contoured amalgams. Note the position and dimension of the contact areas, the well formed cuspal inclines and the pronounced marginal ridges, which will deflect the food bolus from the contact areas.

Surgical techniques have been developed which include recontouring both the bone and the soft tissue. These must be carried out before designing the gingival margins of the ultimate restorations, and temporary restorations of very high quality should be constructed to ensure maintenance of gingival health during the healing process.

Orthodontic modification

There are occasions where orthodontic movement of a tooth or teeth is desirable before restoration. However, the gingival tissue is likely to remain in the same position relative to the cervical margin of the crown of the tooth following movement and surgical intervention may be required for adjustment of irregularities.

Orthodontic eruption of the remainder of a root after trauma or extensive subgingival caries is always accompanied by migration of the gingival margin. The gingival tissue will need to be repositioned and often some degree of alveolar bone recontouring will be involved. The restoration of the crown is further complicated in this technique as the dimensions of the root face are notably smaller than those of the desirable aesthetic configuration of the crown and a compromise is usually necessary, particularly in relation to the emergence profile.

In view of the difficulty of re-establishing a normal epithelial attachment, it is suggested that the advantages of such surgery must be weighed carefully against the likely modification to gingival anatomy, and surgery should be undertaken only when essential. The techniques come into the realm of periodontal surgery and will not be discussed further in this treatise.

FURTHER READING

Behrend DB. Crown margins and gingival health. *Ann R Australas Coll Dent Surg* 1984; **8**:138–45

Block PL. Restorative margins and periodontal health; a new look at an old perspective. *J Prosthet Dent* 1987; 57:683–9.

Brunsvold MA, Lane JJ. The prevalence of overhanging dental restorations and their relationship to periodontal disease. *J Clin Periodontol* 1990; **17**:67–72.

Burch JG. Periodontal considerations in operative dentistry. *J Periodontol* 1975; **34**:156–63.

Eismann HF, Radke RA, Noble WH. Physiologic design criteria for fixed dental restorations. *Dent Clin North Am* 1971; **15**:543–68.

Grasso JE, Nalbandian J, Sandford C, Balit H. Effect of restoration quality on periodontal health. *J Prosthet Dent* 1985; **53**:14–19.

Jameson LM, Malone WFP. Crown contours and the gingival response. *J Prosthet Dent* 1982; **47**:620–4.

Leon AR. Amalgam restorations and periodontal disease. *Br Dent J* 1976; **140**:377–82

Leon AR. The periodontium and restorative procedures; a critical review. *J Oral Rehab* 1977; **4**:105–17.

Mount GJ. Crowns and the gingival tissue. *Aust Dent J* 1970; 4:253–8.

Newcomb GM. The relationship between the location of sub-gingival crown margins and gingival inflammation. *J Periodontol* 1974; **45**:151–4.

Ramfjord SP. Periodontal aspects of restorative dentistry. *J Oral Rehabil* 1974; **1**:107–26.

Van Dijken JWV, Sjostrom S, Wing K. Development of gingivitis around different types of composite resin. *J Clin Periodontol* 1987; **14**:257–60.

Youdelis RA, Weaver JD, Sapkos S. Facial and lingual contours of artificial complete crown restorations and their effects on the periodontium. *J Prosthet Dent* 1973; **29**:61–6.

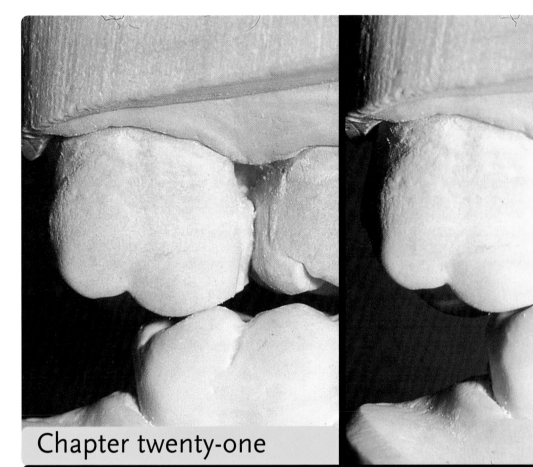

Chapter twenty-one

Occlusion as it relates to restoration of individual teeth

G.J. Mount

When the anatomy of the occlusal surface of a posterior tooth or of the incisal or lingual surface of an anterior tooth is to be modified in any way as a result of restoration of that tooth, or of an opponent, such modification must be carried out with an understanding of the potential for change in the occlusal relationship between the arches.

Any change must maintain the overall pattern of occlusal harmony.

BASIC PRINCIPLES OF OCCLUSION

Posselt (1962) stated that 'a knowledge of occlusion and the articulation of opposing dental arches is of great practical value: hardly a day passes in dental practice without the dentist having to articulate teeth, coincidentally coordinating the jaw muscles and joint components.' Strictly speaking, occlusion is a static term describing the relationship of opposing teeth in contact. However, it has evolved into common terminology to mean also the movement of opposing teeth during the function of mastication.

The basic parameters of articulation have been set out clearly in Hanau's 'Quint', of which the following are the guiding components.

- 1 – angle of the condyle paths
- 2 – angle of incisal guidance
- 3 – occlusal plane
- 4 – occlusal curve
- 5 – angle of the cuspal inclines.

Several factors can be varied or modified during reconstruction of the teeth, but the path of the condyles will remain constant, although they can change slowly over time. The inclination of the incisal path can vary as a result of restoration, abrasion or attrition, or of a combination of these factors. The curvature of the occlusal plane is difficult to change through the simple restoration of individual teeth, but random loss of posterior teeth with subsequent over-eruption of unopposed teeth or depression of overloaded teeth may lead to change. The inclination of the cuspal inclines can be changed very readily and the curvature of the occlusal plane can also change as a result of repeated alteration to the occlusal surfaces of posterior teeth.

THE INTERCUSPAL RELATIONSHIP OF NORMAL TEETH IN THE ADULT

Although there is an infinite variation possible in the relationship of opposing teeth, it is accepted that certain descriptive positions can be referred to as 'normal'. The terms 'centric occlusion' and 'intercuspal position' are interchangeable and refer to the position at which the teeth are in normal contact with each other, with the cusps at maximal intercuspation and, more importantly, when the musculature of the temporomandibular joints is unstressed. Normally, all teeth will be in contact with others, although in some situations, not necessarily regarded as malocclusive, the anterior teeth may be apart, such as in the 'Angle Class II, division 1' situation. If a tooth becomes unopposed because of the loss of an opponent, it may over-erupt or drift, particularly if it is periodontally involved, and thereby modify the centric occlusion position. Also, if the occlusal anatomy of a tooth is altered by deepening the central fossa or lengthening the cusps or increasing the angle of the cuspal inclines, the tooth may drift or tilt to improve its intercuspal relationship with its opponent and further modify centric occlusion. Such modifications may

lead to alteration in the tooth to tooth relationship during excursive movements. All mandibular movements are discussed as commencing from the centric occlusion position and consist of one or a combination of the following (**Fig. 21.1**).

The envelope of movement
Centric relation position
The 'centric relation position' or 'retruded contact position' is regarded as the most retruded position that the mandible can achieve with the condyles in their most upward and forward position within the fossae. In this position, the teeth should be in contact among the posteriors and this contact should be even on both sides and the mandible should be able to move forwards and upwards to the intercuspal position without deviation to either side. Interference to this position or movement may lead to parafunction with muscle stress and excessive attrition on individual teeth or groups of teeth. The areas of attrition will not always be clearly related to the interference or initial contact.

Lateral excursions
From the centric occlusion position the mandible should be able to make lateral movements for several millimetres in all directions without undue stress or interference from the teeth. For the first millimetre or so in an excursive movement, the teeth may remain in contact. Thereafter guidance should be derived from the anterior teeth only, particularly the canines, with no contact between the posteriors at all.

When moving into a lateral excursion the lower canine should move smoothly down the lingual incline of the upper canine and the posterior teeth should become

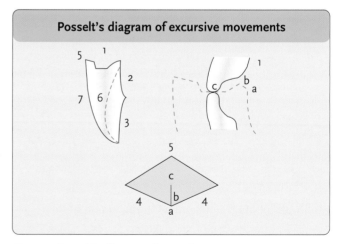

Fig. 21.1 Posselt's diagram of excursive movements.
1 Movement of lower incisors: a, terminal hinge; b, intercuspal position; c, edge-to-edge position. 2 Opening from hinge. 3 Further posterior opening. 4 Lateral excursions. 5 Extreme protrusion. 6 Habitual closing arc. 7 Extreme opening arc.

totally discluded on both sides. Under these circumstances very little stress can be exerted on the teeth or the musculature.

On the other hand, if contact is maintained, during movement, on the opposite nonworking or balancing side, considerable muscular pressure can be applied because of the relative triangulation between the teeth and the joint.

Protrusive movement
Similarly, during a protrusive movement the posteriors should be discluded, thus minimising the amount of muscular pressure that can be developed. The lower anterior teeth should move smoothly down the lingual surface of the upper anteriors with an even contact on both sides of the midline and the posterior teeth should immediately disclude.

The significance of correct guidance
The factors outlined above in 'Hanau's Quint' will normally be in balance when the occlusion first develops. As tooth wear occurs throughout life, this balance should be maintained. However, the introduction of iatrogenic modifications to the relationship will be likely to introduce undesirable stresses and pressures that may lead to excess wear and muscle stress. In the presence of anterior guidance, the musculature cannot exert undue pressure on either the teeth or the joint. There can be no fulcrum around which the mandible can rotate distally, and the lever arm is so long as to be inefficient in the application of pressure on to the joint.

Proprioception appears to be designed around cuspid guidance of the mandible as it approaches the maxilla, so cuspid guidance is regarded as normal. However, in the presence of interference in the envelope of movement, or the development of triangulation between both sides of the mandible and the joint, there is likely to be a subconscious attempt to remove the source of the interference by parafunctional actions such as clenching and grinding and this may lead to the development of bizarre wear patterns.

Factors which may modify anterior or lateral guidance
Changes to cuspal inclines
Three factors commonly lead to alteration of the angle of cusp inclines, with the potential for complicating the occlusal relationship between the arches. Any change that makes the cuspal inclines steeper will result in deeper intercuspation with opposing teeth sufficient to lead to interference in lateral excursions through the development of balancing-side contacts (**Fig. 21.2**).
* When placing a restoration in amalgam or composite resin there is a temptation to deepen cuspal inclines in an attempt to 'improve' the aesthetics of the occlusal surface of a posterior tooth.
* Both amalgam and composite resin wear away more rapidly than natural tooth structure.
* Routine re-polishing of the occlusal surfaces of amalgam or composite resin will bring about further change to occlusal anatomy with deeper intercuspation.

Changes to anteriors
Modifications to the incisal edges of anterior teeth can alter anterior guidance and should be undertaken with care.
* Adjustment of the incisal edge of a lower anterior tooth to allow greater thickness in a crown on an upper anterior tooth can alter the curvature of the occlusal plane or change the inclination of the incisal path, and may lead to protrusive interference.
* Aesthetic modifications to the incisal edges of either upper or lower anterior teeth may have a similar effect and should be carried out with care and attention to possible sequelae.

Uncontrolled changes are undesirable because the sequelae of undue change may be complex and can include such things as wear facets in unusual places, split cusps, split roots, lost restorations, broken prostheses, migration of periodontally involved teeth and temporomandibular joint pain–dysfunction syndrome. Every restoration should be placed with care to reinstate normal occlusion and avoid undue change. Any sign of unusual wear or failure of tooth structure or restoration without obvious cause, should be carefully explored to detect changes to occlusion.

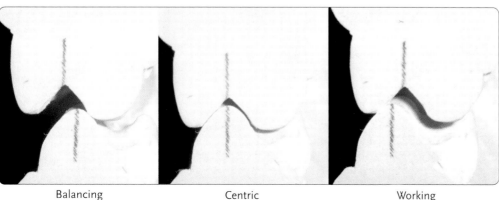

Balancing   Centric   Working

Fig. 21.2 Posterior contacts in lateral excursions. With deep intercuspation, there may be contacts in posteriors in both lateral excursions. This may lead to clenching and parafunction with undue wear on anteriors as well as posteriors and possibly split cusps. Note contacts with both buccal and lingual cusps on working side excursion.

FACTORS LEADING TO OCCLUSAL CHANGE

Where there is a relatively intact dentition, a number of factors come into play which may lead to excessive wear and subsequent changes to occlusion.

Orthodontic movement

Orthodontic movement that does not reinstate a correct cuspid rise and anterior guidance may lead to bruxing and excessive wear. Correction of orthodontic anomalies should be directed not only to aesthetics, but also to function because, whether the patient is conscious of the problem or not, they may subconsciously attempt to arrange their own correction by parafunction.

Wear on occlusal surfaces and incisal edges

A restorative material occupying a reasonably large area of the occlusal surface, should have a wear factor that closely resembles that of the opposing and adjacent tooth structure. As a restoration wears away, deeper intercuspation may develop with the opponent, with the potential for a locked occlusion, for balancing-side contacts in lateral excursions

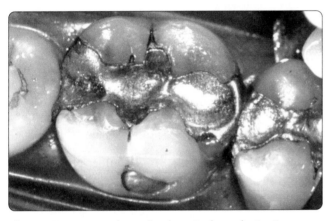

Fig. 21.3 Wear on amalgam. Amalgam in the molar is 28 years old and has worn deeply in the distal fossa.

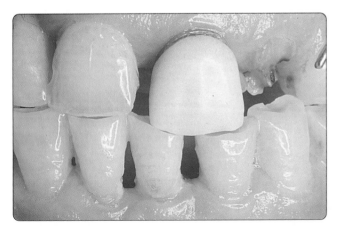

Fig. 21.4 Wear from porcelain. Porcelain crown approximately 30 years old; it has worn the lower anteriors to the extent that the occlusion is affected.

and, possibly, for split cusps. Excessive wear cannot be diagnosed simply by examination of the relationship of opposing teeth to see that they are still in contact, because continual eruption will generally maintain a contact. Serial measurement of study models of both arches taken at intervals is essential to be able to determine the speed and extent of wear and to decide whether this is taking place within the restoration or on the opposing tooth or restoration.

Of the current restorative materials, gold has a wear factor closest to that of enamel and some of the ceramics are the most abrasive. Amalgam wears a little faster than enamel and some of the composite resins have posed problems in the past (**Figs 21.3** and **21.4**).

Failure to replace a posterior tooth

When a posterior tooth is lost and not replaced, there is the potential for drifting or migration of opposing or adjacent teeth. Any movement will take place within the first year after loss of normal contact and will occur more readily and to a greater extent in the presence of active periodontal disease. Movement will then slow down and, in an otherwise healthy mouth, will cease. However, any alteration to the occlusal relationship between the arches may lead to alterations to contacts during lateral or protrusive excursions or to changes in the direction of the slide between centric relation and centric occlusion.

Loss of a lower first molar, for example, may lead to over-eruption of the opposing upper molar. The centric occlusion position may remain apparently comfortable, but the initial contact in the centric relation position may then be the distal marginal ridge of the lower second bicuspid against the mesial marginal ridge of the over-erupted upper molar. The mandible, in fact, may be thrust forwards, upwards and to one side to achieve a centric occlusion position and, in so doing, load the lingual aspect of the upper anterior teeth, leading to undue wear on the lingual surfaces or even tooth migration in the presence of periodontal disease (**Fig. 21.5**).

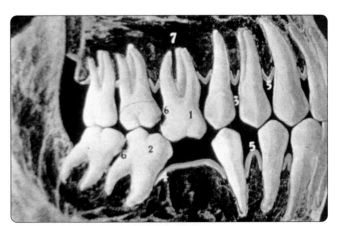

Fig. 21.5 Collapse of the arch. The classic sequelae likely to arise from the loss of a lower first molar. A similar pattern of tilting, drifting and over-eruption can be expected from loss of any single tooth that is not replaced. Functionally opening contacts and deflective inclines are inevitable complications to follow.

Also, if the upper molar erupts sufficiently far, it may act as a guidance in protrusive movements, making the mandible swing laterally as well as forwards, thus producing unusual wear patterns on the incisal edge of the contralateral central incisor tooth or even encouraging tooth migration, particularly in the presence of periodontal disease. There are many combinations of the above pattern and it is essential that the occlusion be examined with great care to establish the cause in any situation showing wear patterns outside of a relatively normal range (**Figs 21.6** and **21.7**).

Loss of posterior support

As more teeth are lost, the problems become further compounded. It is apparent that it is not necessary to retain 32 teeth and in fact the average patient has no more than 28 teeth in full function. Many get by comfortably and safely with fewer still. However, below a certain number it may not be possible to maintain a normal vertical dimension and

function without remaining teeth over-erupting or being depressed into the alveolus under excessive load (**Fig. 21.8**).

Minimum posterior support

A formula for defining the minimum amount of posterior support required to prevent loss of vertical dimension can be stated in the following terms. If molars are allotted two units and bicuspids and third molars are allotted one unit each, then a total of eight units in function is sufficient to maintain posterior support to the extent that, in a normal healthy mouth, the occlusion will not collapse. This assumes that the teeth oppose each other in a relatively normal relationship and that their periodontal status is acceptable. Although it is desirable to be able to record units on both sides of the mouth, it is not essential for stability. If less than eight units are present it is likely that, particularly in the presence of periodontal disease, the upper anterior teeth will migrate labially, the lower

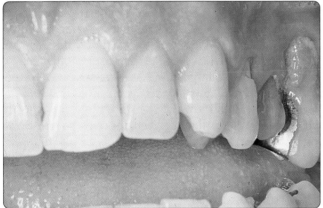

Fig. 21.6 Thieleman's diagonal law. The first molar is over-erupted giving guidance in protrusive. The contralateral central incisor has over-erupted as a result.

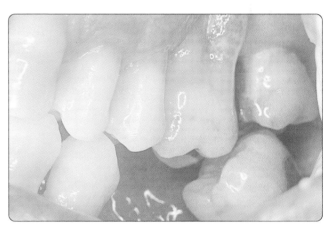

Fig. 21.7 Over-erupted molar. A similar patient to that discussed in figure 21.6 showing the extend of the over-eruption with tilting of the lower second molar.

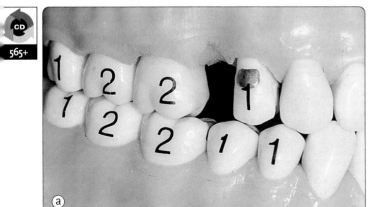

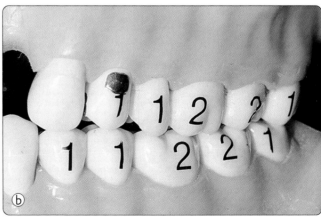

Fig. 21.8 Counting posterior units. The two sides of this model (**a**) and (**b**) show the units allocated to each posterior tooth.

A minimum of eight units is required to avoid loss of vertical dimension or intrusion of posterior teeth because of overload.

anteriors will tilt to the lingual and remaining posteriors will either drift under load or be depressed into the alveolus, leading to loss of vertical dimension.

Distal rotation of the mandible

An additional problem arising from loss of posterior teeth is the potential for a distal rotation of the mandible placing extra load on the condyle and the temporomandibular joint. It has been suggested that the fulcrum for this distal rotation lies about the second bicuspids in the average occlusion. In other words, as long as the second bicuspids are present in both arches, the mandible will not rotate. If all eight bicuspids are present and in normal occlusion the parameters of both theories are fulfilled (**Figs 21.9** and **21.10**).

INTERPRETATION OF WEAR FACETS

Careful examination of the occlusal surfaces and incisal edges of remaining teeth often reveals much useful information, and helps to lead to a diagnosis and treatment plan. Direct intra-oral examination with a good light source is essential and this should be supplemented with mounted study models. There is a further discussion on recognition and diagnosis of wear facets and their cause in Chapter 4, page 34.

Patient habits

Discussion of the problem with the patient may reveal further information. Both dietary and cleaning habits are significant, particularly in relation to erosion, and it is essential that the patient understands the chemistry of demineralisation. Stress and tension are factors in parafunction and,

although there may be little that a dentist can do to relieve this, simply discussing the situation may help the patient. In fact, it is important that the patient understand the whole cycle, because this will help to rationalise problems ranging from obvious wear patterns to split teeth and loss of cusps. Occasionally, it will be discovered that the patient can place the mandible in a bizarre position to produce a wear pattern that seems impossible to reproduce on an articulator.

Deflective inclines

Excessive wear on the lingual surfaces of upper anterior teeth or the incisal edges of lower anteriors may be the result of a deflective incline between the centric relation position and centric occlusion. This should be readily detectable, both in the mouth and on the articulator, and the cause defined. The problem frequently arises through under-contouring the mesial marginal ridge of an upper first bicuspid, allowing the opposing canine to erupt into the void. The situation will be exacerbated if there has been a collapse of the lower anterior segment because of loss of teeth or in the presence of a Class II, division 2 malocclusion. The wear pattern on the teeth seems to be dictated to a degree by which teeth lose the enamel first, the uppers or the lowers, and the wear may be excessive before being detected. In an extreme case, the anteriors may fit together so intimately that there appears to be no room in which to place a protective restoration. Elimination of deflective inclines in the posterior teeth between centric relation and centric occlusion may allow the mandible to move distally sufficient to make room for restoration and, at the same time, eliminate the cause (**Figs 21.11** and **21.12**).

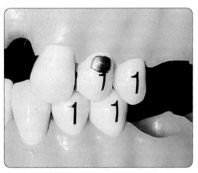
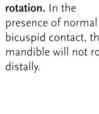

Fig. 21.9 Point of rotation. In the presence of normal bicuspid contact, the mandible will not rotate distally.

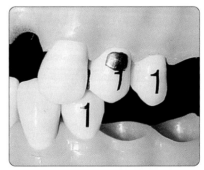

Fig. 21.10 Distal rotation. With the mandible medially displaced there is a greater chance of rotation placing pressure on the temporomandibular joint.

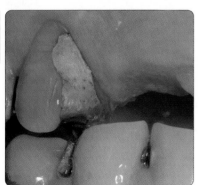

Fig. 21.11 Deflective incline. In retruded contact, the distal incline of the lower canine contacts an over-carved amalgam in the mesial of the upper first bicuspid.

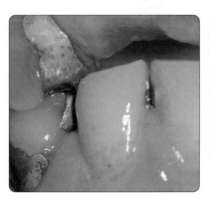

Fig. 21.12 Forward and upward slide. To achieve centric occlusion, the mandible is thrust forwards and upwards, putting stress on the lingual of the remaining upper anteriors.

Balancing-side interference

Excessive wear on canine teeth is usually the result of the development of a balancing-side interference. This interference occurs mostly on second and third molars and the further distal the contact, the greater the load and the leverage that can be applied. Deep intercuspation between upper and lower molars, particularly second or third molars, is usually caused by loss of canine guidance and cuspid rise. Conversely, it may arise from deep over-carving of the occlusal anatomy of a molar restoration, thus allowing over-eruption of the opposing tooth with the development of balancing-side interference, as well as a working-side interference, leading to parafunction and excessive wear on the canine.

Random loss of teeth

Uneven and bizarre wear patterns can usually be traced to serious irregularities in the occlusion caused by random loss of teeth, over-eruption, tilting and reduction of posterior support to below the prescribed eight units. Occasionally, there may be excessive wear from an isolated porcelain crown that has over-erupted because of abrasion and loss of tooth structure from the opponent and it may now cause an interference in the envelope of movement of the mandible.

Chemical erosion

Generalised wear patterns may arise because of chemical erosion, with abrasion and attrition as a secondary cause. The real cause may be difficult to detect because information from the patient is essential for a correct diagnosis and this is not always forthcoming. However, careful observation may lead to a diagnosis. For example, loss of enamel on the lingual surfaces of the upper posteriors as well as those of the upper and lower anteriors is often caused by highly acidic gastric reflux (**Figs 21.13** and **21.14**).

Loss of enamel on the labial surfaces of the upper anterior teeth as well as the lingual of the upper posteriors may arise from frequent ingestion of low-pH drinks such as citrus juices, cola drinks or wine.

DAMAGE ARISING FROM EXCESSIVE WEAR

Modification to aesthetics

Probably the most obvious effect of excessive wear is alteration to the aesthetics of the upper anterior teeth. These are the ones that the patient sees, and the ones to which they are likely to draw attention (**Figs 21.15** and **21.16**).

Wear on the incisal edges of anteriors, both upper and lower, will generally arise from parafunction and the cause must be identified first before treatment planning for

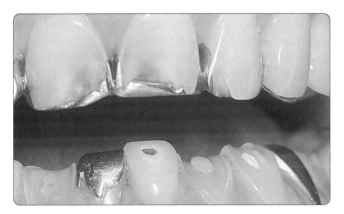

Fig. 21.13 Excessive wear. A combination of chemical erosion, toothbrush abrasion and, probably, attrition.

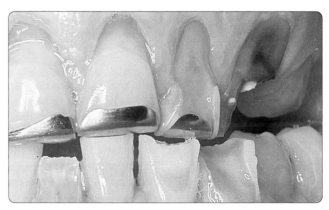

Fig. 21.14 Chemical erosion. Probably exacerbated by toothbrush abrasion.

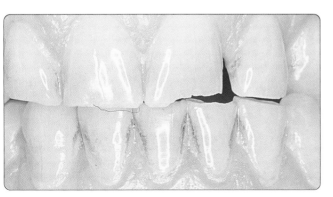

Fig. 21.15 Uneven wear. The left central incisor is probably worn because of a deflective incline in the right molars which leads to guidance in a protrusive lateral movement.

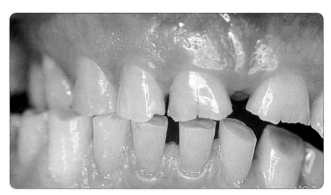

Fig. 21.16 Severe generalised wear. Generalised wear on incisal edges of all anteriors, possibly resulting from parafunction.

restoration. Restoration of the incisal edge without identifying the cause will inevitably lead to failure.

Split cusps

Split cusps are a common cause of pain and on many occasions alterations to the occlusion are a contributing factor. The initial symptoms are intermittent pain on pressure, and the patient has difficulty in determining the actual origin. Pain will become more frequent and eventually the tooth will become sensitive to change of temperature. Finally, the entire cusp will fail, leaving a surface that is temperature sensitive for a 1–2 days and then is comfortable except that it will probably be sharp and rough to the tongue.

Occasionally, the split will progress through the pulp chamber and this will lead to extreme pain and possibly loss of the tooth. Identification of the involved cusp is often difficult and may only be confirmed by removal of the old restoration. There are a variety of devices available for applying discrete pressure to individual cusps, and one of these may be useful, but it may require lateral stress applied in a particular direction to reveal the problem (**Figs 21.17** and **21.18**).

Functionally opening contact

A functionally opening contact is a common problem arising from altered occlusal patterns. These occur in relation to heavily restored teeth, most often the terminal tooth in the arch, where there has been a large restoration placed with a direct plastic restorative material. Recontouring the occlusal surface is difficult in these circumstances and is largely completed on the basis of guesswork. Arising from the atypical occlusal anatomy and the subsequent drifting and tilting of opposing teeth, there may be deflective inclines that have developed between the arches. As the patient then closes, the initial contact may be between a mesially facing incline of, say, an upper molar with a distal facing incline of the opposing lower molar. The upper molar will move slightly distally, opening the contact sufficiently to engage a

piece of fibrous food debris. As the patient opens, the upper molar will move mesially again, entrapping the food debris. This situation has, in the past, been called a 'plunger cusp' but this is a misnomer because simply reducing the height of an opposing cusp will not necessarily eliminate the problem. It is essential to observe the entire occlusion and identify deflective inclines in relation to the offending area and modify them to be successful in dealing with the situation (**Figs 20.15** and **20.16,** page 230).

RESTORATION OF OCCLUSAL HARMONY

Examination and monitoring of the intermaxillary relationship is an essential prerequisite for successful treatment. For a new patient, identify the initial contacts in the centric relation position and then observe the presence or absence of a slide to one side or the other as the patient moves into the centric occlusion position. Determine the cause of the slide. Now observe the lateral excursions and assess the presence or absence of a balancing-side contact. This is more difficult to determine, and examination of study models may be necessary. Reassess these movements periodically because the relationship is never static, even in the presence of an apparently stable unrestored dentition.

Working-side and balancing-side interference

Look carefully at each tooth, drying them off and varying the angle of the light to seek wear facets on surfaces that should not be worn. Working-side interference can be just as damaging as balancing-side contacts and must be identified. They may be reproduced on study models, but identification in the mouth will often yield more information than the model.

Careful observation of nonworking cusps on molars, in particular, is very important. They are not subject to the heavy load of working cusps and may be left unworn and therefore relatively high. They then become working-side interferences, with the potential for undue guidance in

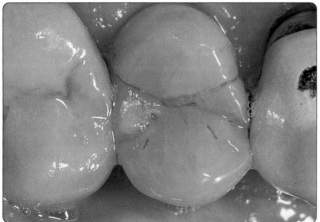

Fig. 21.17 Virgin tooth with split. A virgin unrestored bicuspid has split under load without involving the pulp.

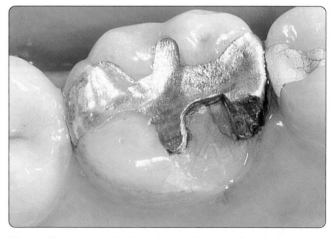

Fig. 21.18 Lost cusp. A relatively heavily restored molar has lost the mesiolingual cusp.

excursions, and they are very prone to develop a split at the base (**Figs 21.19** and **21.20**). In a situation such as the one seen in **Figure 21.19**, the distolingual cusp should be reduced and the cusp incline modified to reduce the stress and eliminate the possibility of interference in lateral excursions and the development of a split.

Adjustment directly in the mouth can be carried out before commencing restorative treatment but, on many occasions, the required adjustments can be achieved simply by altering cuspal inclines at the time of placing a restoration. If there is any doubt concerning the possible result of adjustment and alteration to cuspal inclines, carry out the modifications on study models first, including removal of inclines or the addition of anatomy to the occlusal surfaces, using a trial wax-up technique.

Restore anterior guidance

Restoration of anterior guidance and rebuilding cuspid rise is an essential part of reinstating occlusal harmony. The cuspid rise will probably eliminate balancing-side contacts, but, in some circumstances, restoration of the occlusal anatomy in a lower molar with, at the same time, reduction in the height of the palatal cusp of the opposing molar, may achieve almost as much freedom for the excursive movement. In the situation where there is excessive wear of the lingual of upper anterior teeth, removal of the deflective inclines in the posterior teeth often allows sufficient distal movement of the mandible to leave adequate room for restoration and protection of the upper anteriors without modification to the lower anterior teeth.

Orthodontic correction

Orthodontic correction may be an essential prerequisite for successful reinstatement of occlusal harmony. This may become more difficult as the patient ages but, conversely, it may be very important in some situations to include a degree of orthodontic correction. Prevention of relapse is then the main problem and fixed bridgework may be required.

Restore posterior support

Restoration of posterior support is essential for the badly broken down dentition when there has been random loss of posterior teeth. However, it is only necessary to rebuild the support until there are eight units present and stable, as described above. Fixed bridgework is usually necessary, because removable partial dentures are not very efficient as load bearers and the patient may not wear them conscientiously. A free-end saddle on a removable partial denture is not an effective load bearer at all, and a tooth-borne saddle must be very well seated and supported if it is to make any contribution to posterior support.

Restore vertical dimension

A judgement as to whether vertical dimension has been lost may be difficult to make and is often controversial. If there are less than eight units of posterior support remaining, there is almost certain to be some loss, but in the presence of an acceptable number of normal posterior units, it is difficult to make a decision. Restoration can be carried out simply; it is normally only a matter of determining the amount of space required to accommodate the new restorations, rather than to go to any length to determine what the patient will tolerate. So long as correct occlusal balance is maintained, with freedom of movement and proper guidance, the patient will accommodate very readily an increase of up to 1 cm or more without being aware of the change.

It is important to use fixed prostheses rather than removable partial dentures. Any tooth that is left out of occlusion in the process of restoration of the vertical dimension will erupt over a period of time and achieve a new occlusal contact. This may be done deliberately with success. For example, a lone molar tooth that has been under heavy load may be left out of a rehabilitation; within 1 year it will be in function. It is necessary under these circumstances to review the occlusion periodically to ensure that the new pattern is stable and acceptable.

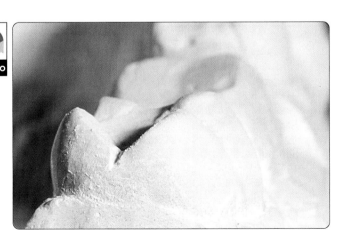

Fig. 21.19 Deep intercuspation. A large amalgam has been overcarved, allowing deep intercuspation and leaving the lingual cusp standing high.

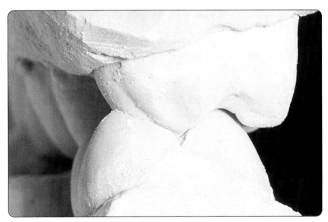

Fig. 21.20 Working-side interference. When the teeth are articulated, the working-side interference becomes apparent. The lingual cusp is at risk of fracture.

Use of a removable splint

The use of an occlusal splint to determine whether the patient will tolerate restoration of vertical dimension is not valid and may even deter the patient from receiving further treatment. It may be of value as part of an overall treatment plan for a patient with a grossly broken-down dentition, particularly if there are signs of a temporo-mandibular joint pain–dysfunction syndrome, but insistence on a trial period before rebuilding an occlusion cannot be justified. For a patient already wearing a partial denture it may be worthwhile modifying it at the proposed vertical dimension, but it must be noted that any tooth not fully engaged within the splint may move to the extent that, with the splint out, the occlusion will be unstable. Essentially, if a removable appliance is to be utilised at any stage, all teeth must be fully engaged when the splint is in the mouth and the occlusion must still be completely stable when the splint is out.

Restoration over time

Finally, it should be noted that development of a stable harmonious occlusion may well be a long-term project. Longevity is the key to success, so restorative techniques and materials should be chosen because their future is predictable. Use restorative materials with known wear factors and, where possible, oppose each material with a similar material. Recognise the long-term effect of alterations to the occlusion that may arise from using materials which wear faster than natural tooth structure. Be prepared to modify the occlusal surface of the opposing tooth when an old restoration needs to be replaced. Do not necessarily contour a new restoration to accommodate an existing opponent without contemplating the advantages of recontouring the opponent. Restore vertical dimension with care and ensure that all teeth are stable at all times. Observe patients frequently and reassess the occlusion, looking constantly for change. Carefully examine the occlusion after any breakdown to determine if the failure involves an occlusal component.

FURTHER READING

Hanau RL. *Full denture prosthesis. Intraoral technique for Hanau articulator model.* H Buffalo, 1930.

Kayser AF. Shortened dental arches and oral function. *J Oral Rehabil* 1981; **8**:457–62.

Kerveskari P, Alanin P. Association between tooth loss and TMJ dysfunction. *J Oral Rehabil* 1985; **2**:189–94.

Khera SC, Carpenter CW, Staley RM. Anatomy of the cusps of posterior teeth and their fracture potential. *J Prosth Dent* 1990; **64**:139–47.

Love WO, Adams RL. Tooth movement into edentulous spaces. *J Prosthet Dent* 1971; **25**:271–7.

Posselt U. *Physiology of occlusion and rehabilitation.* Oxford: Blackwell Scientific Publications; 1962.

Randow K, Glantz P-O, Zoger B. Technical failures and some related clinical complications in extensive fixed prosthodontics. *Acta Odontol Scand* 1986; **44**:241–5.

Rivera-Morales WC, Mohl ND. Relationship of occlusal vertical dimension to the health of the masticatory system. *J Prosthet Dent* 1991; **65**:547–53.

Wise MD. *Failure in the restored dentition: management and treatment.* London: Quintessence Publishing Company Ltd; 1995.

Witter DJ, Cramwinckel AB, van Rossum GMJM, Kayser AF. Shortened dental arches and masticatory ability. *J Dent* 1990; **18**:185–9.

Zarb GA, McKay HF. The partially edentulous patient: 1. The biological price of prosthodontic intervention. *Aust Dent J* 1980; **25**:63–8.

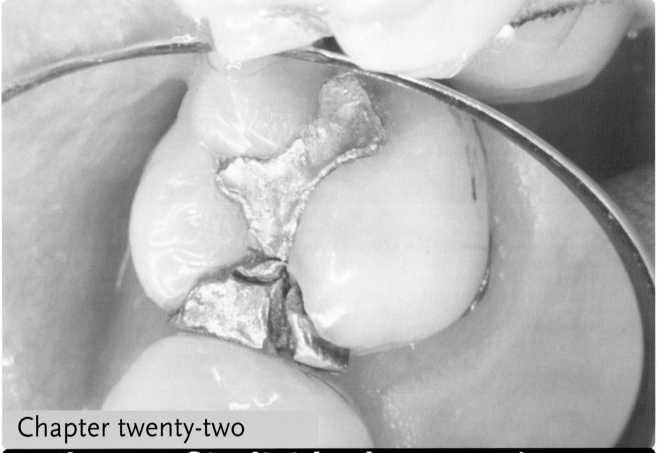

Chapter twenty-two

Failures of individual restorations, and their management

G.J. Mount

There are many reasons for failure of a restoration and there is always a temptation to replace a failed restoration entirely rather than repair it. However, each time a restoration is replaced there is, inevitably, further loss of tooth structure, and that structure which remains will be weakened. It is desirable, therefore, that all factors be taken into account before a decision is made to remove all remaining restorative material; in many cases, repair of the existing restoration may be adequate. Interpretation of failure should never be made on external appearance alone because this may be very deceptive.

First, it is essential that the cause of failure be assessed and, if possible, fully determined. This may pose problems, because the physical properties of the remaining restorative material cannot be assessed without its removal. Second, it is impossible in many cases to be certain that there is no recurrent caries under the restoration, or to make a valid assessment of the condition of the pulp. Some restorative materials can be repaired more readily than others but adequate access to the area of breakdown may be difficult.

FAILURE OF TOOTH STRUCTURE

Failure of the enamel margin

Wedge-shaped defects along the margins of a restoration caused by failure of the enamel generally arise because of incorrect cavity design. The margin may have been placed too far up the medially facing cuspal incline and, as a result, may be subjected to heavy occlusal load. Proper protection of the remaining enamel may now be required and this can usually be achieved only by replacement of the entire restoration (Chapter 11, page 142). There are occasions where the bulk of the restoration is sound and it is acceptable to rebuild one section only; however, if remaining enamel is not fully protected, it will fail again.

If the restoration is gold, it may be repaired with gold foil, although a small defect, which is not under undue occlusal load, can be sealed with glass–ionomer. Similarly, a minor defect from flaking of the enamel along an amalgam margin may be repairable so long as the load is not heavy. On the other hand, loss of enamel around a composite resin margin can rarely be repaired because of loss of adhesion; a complete redesign is generally required. Both amalgam and composite resin require bulk in themselves if they are to support the occlusion, and compromise is undesirable.

Failure of dentine margin

It is generally the gingival margin of a restoration that is embedded in dentine; detection of a fault and its repair poses problems. Often the cause is an operator fault, such as failure to adapt or condense the restorative material adequately at the margin. Probably the greatest problem is caused by leaving an overhanging margin on a restoration, because it will retain plaque and lead to recurrent caries. Root surface caries is a problem for the ageing patient following gingival recession, and the best restoration can fail as a result (**Figs 22.1** and **22.2**).

The decision on whether to repair the margin or replace the entire restoration depends on two factors. Access to the lesion is not always easy without undesirable destruction of remaining tooth or, alternatively, the main bulk of the restoration may be of low quality. Under these circumstances, the entire restoration should be redesigned. If the restoration is satisfactory, however, and access is simple, the margin may be repaired with a conservative restoration using glass–ionomer in one form or another (Chapter 8).

Bulk loss of tooth structure

Loss of an entire cusp is distressing for the patient. This situation often arises because the dentist has failed to take into account the weakened nature of the remaining tooth structure in an extensively restored tooth and failed to provide some form of protective restoration. It is necessary to continually monitor changes to the occlusal wear patterns, because loss of occlusal anatomy may result in a nonworking cusp, eventually standing high and becoming subject to lateral stress (Chapter 21, page 243).

The design of any restoration that involves preparation of a cavity into the dentine on the occlusal surface of a posterior tooth at least doubles the length of the cusps. Further preparation of a proximal box doubles the length again, leaving the tooth susceptible to splitting (**Figs 22.3** and **22.4**).

Repair of a lost cusp usually requires replacement and redesign of the entire restoration. Occasionally, a protective-type restoration is already in place, with the occlusion being sustained by the restorative material. Under these circumstances, it may be sufficient to repair the defect by adding to the existing material or placing a composite resin facing. However, there is now reduced support for the remaining restoration and it will need to be soundly based to accept the extra load. Also, it may be desirable at this point to explore the remaining tooth structure, because of the possibility of a split elsewhere requiring further protection. If the restoration is to be converted to an extracoronal design it is

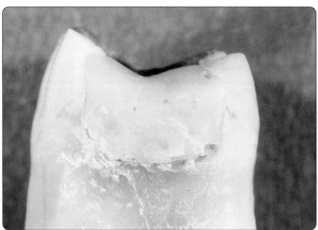

Fig. 22.1 Failed composite resin. The gingival margin in dentine has failed through poor placement and lack of adhesion.

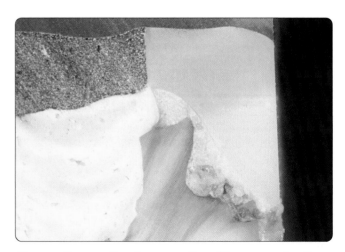

Fig. 22.2 Cross-section. A cross-section of the same restoration showing the poor adaptation and lack of adhesion of the composite resin that led to failure.

essential that the remaining primary restoration is very soundly based and firmly attached to underlying tooth structure with retentive grooves and ditches.

Split root

This usually occurs in the remaining root structure of a non-vital tooth that has been restored with a post crown. The post is essentially an intra-radicular restoration that relies on the integrity of the root to sustain it. It will naturally be subjected to considerable lateral stresses, particularly in an anterior tooth, and there is a need to reinforce the root against these forces if at all possible. Minimal enlargement of the root canal during endodontic treatment and preparation for a post is highly desirable and the best method of prevention. It is sometimes possible to place a cuff around the top of the root as part of the post and core design, but the most difficult area in which to prepare for this cuff is around the lingual–gingival margin. Considering the direction of the stresses, this is the area that requires the most reinforcement. A split in a root will allow the development of tensile forces on the cement that will eventually destroy the cement and lead to the loss of the crown (Chapter 19, page 219).

Diagnosis of a split root is very difficult and, almost invariably, terminal to the life of the tooth. When a post crown becomes uncemented, the remaining root must be carefully explored for signs of a split. The use of magnification and fibre-optic lighting to illuminate the tooth from various angles may be sufficient. A caries-detecting dye may help, or simply applying leverage may show percolation of gingival fluid on the root face. If the diagnosis is not conclusive, re-cement the crown, adjust the occlusion and warn the patient of a possible further failure at a later date. If the re-cementation lasts less than 12 months, the cause is almost certainly a split root.

After the diagnosis has been confirmed, it must be acknowledged that long-term repair is impossible, and an alternative restoration should be planned.

Loss of vitality

Assessment and treatment following the death of the pulp is dealt with in Chapter 19. Modification of the treatment plan will need to be made following loss of vitality, whatever the cause. There is likely to be a shift in the translucency or colour of the remaining crown and some further weakening following the enlargement of the root canal during root canal therapy. Any pre-existing restoration will need to be reviewed and, possibly, redesigned.

FAILURE OF RESTORATIVE MATERIAL

Failure of the margin of the material

Most of the restorative materials, other than gold, have a poor edge strength and therefore may not withstand undue occlusal load. It is important in designing a cavity to try to place the margin away from an area subject to direct occlusal load. Where the margin must be under load, the edge of the restorative material should have a cavo–surface margin close to 90°. There must be a compromise between strength in the material and strength in the enamel and the other properties of each material will have a bearing on final cavity design and therefore the potential life span of the restoration.

Amalgam

Amalgam has a relatively poor edge strength, and ditching along the margins is not uncommon. However, because the cavo–surface margin will seal as a result of corrosion in the amalgam, there will rarely be recurrent caries. Despite the average amalgam restoration looking less than ideal within a reasonably short period of time after placement, repair of the margins is not normally indicated. Ditching of the margin of a low-copper amalgam should be regarded as normal (**Figs 22.5** and **22.6**).

Repolishing the occlusal surface to improve the margins will result in alteration to occlusal anatomy and contact

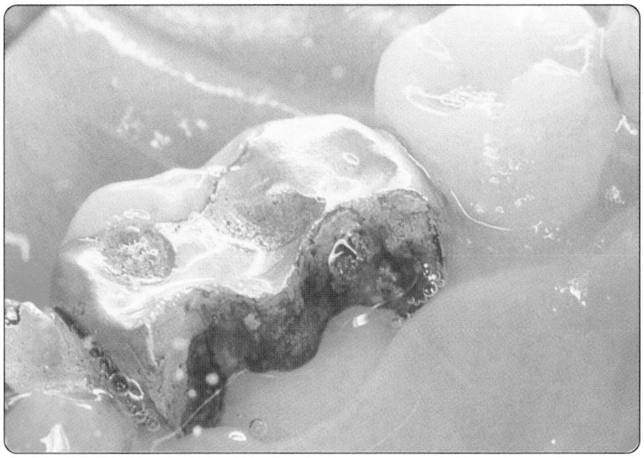

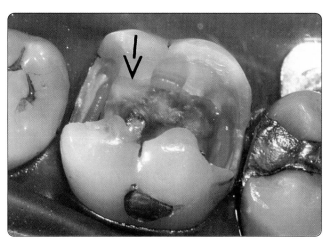

Fig. 22.3 Failed cusps. Both lingual cusps have failed in the presence of a large amalgam that offered no protection.

Fig. 22.4 Split leading to failure. A split is clearly visible at the base of the lingual cusps and failure is imminent if the cusps are not protected.

with the opposing tooth; it is strictly contraindicated (Chapter 21, page 237). There are differences between high-copper amalgams and other alloys in their resistance to marginal ditching and corrosion; these factors have been discussed in Chapter 10, page 114.

Composite resin

Composite resin has no resistance at all to recurrent caries so, therefore, failure at the margin requires immediate attention. If the margin is left open on the occlusal surface, plaque will be forced in to the gap under the high hydraulic pressure generated by mastication, and recurrent caries will develop rapidly. In view of the difficulty in obtaining long-term adhesion between composite resin and dentine, failure at the gingival margin is not uncommon. Repair is not normally appropriate and replacement of the entire restoration is usually indicated. The use of a glass–ionomer base is strongly recommended to avoid further breakdown (**Figs 22.7** and **22.8**).

Glass–ionomer materials

Because glass–ionomer should not be placed under heavy occlusal load, it is usually not subject to marginal or bulk failure. If such problems should occur, complete replacement is probably the best solution. However, the cause of failure must be determined first and an alternate material placed if the cause is not clear.

Gold

Occasionally, gold will fail along a margin as a result of further wear on the occlusal surface, particularly if opposed by a ceramic restoration with a high wear factor, and caries may progress very rapidly. Assuming the original cause can be eliminated, repair of the margin with gold foil may be adequate. If the occlusal load is not great, glass–ionomer cement can be utilised in a very conservative repair.

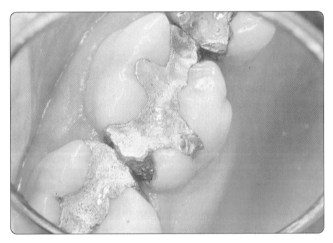

Fig. 22.5 Failed margin. A wedged-shaped marginal failure resulting from poor cavity design.

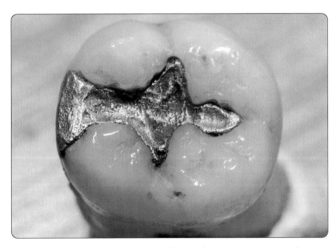

Fig. 22.6 Ditched margins. An old amalgam in an extracted tooth. Further polishing to eliminate marginal ditching alters the occlusal relationship with the opposing tooth

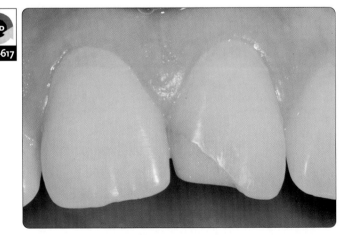

Fig. 22.7 Failure of composite resin. There has been overall loss of bulk and marginal leakage of a composite resin over 10 years.

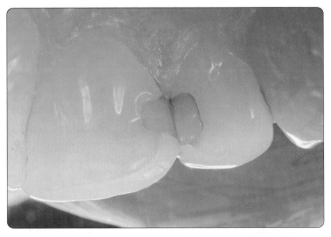

Fig. 22.8 Change of colour. Two small resin restorations have changed colour and leaked at the margin over 7 years.

Loss of luting cement

All indirectly fabricated restorations carry the risk of dissolution of the luting agent over time. The use of a low-solubility luting cement, combined with high-quality laboratory techniques to ensure an accurate fit in the first place, are the best methods of control. Repair is difficult because the margin is usually close to, or under, the gingival tissue. If caries is becoming active along the margin, repair can be attempted by opening conservatively and placing glass–ionomer. The alternative is replacement of the restoration.

Fracture or collapse of a restorative material

Fracture through the main bulk of a restoration is potentially dangerous, particularly if a segment is retained within the cavity after becoming mobile. Rapid caries will develop as a result of plaque being admitted under the mobile segment, because it will be forced into the dentinal tubules by occlusal pressure. It is preferable that the entire restoration be lost, but the directly placed plastic restorative materials are often retained because of the retentive design of the original cavity.

Amalgam

Bulk failure of an amalgam restoration is not uncommon and there are several possible causes (**Figs 22.9** and **22.10**). It is necessary for each section of a complex amalgam restoration to be individually retentive and the material must be properly condensed. The causes of failure are listed below.

- Inadequate retention in a section of the original cavity design.
- Failure at the isthmus of a Site 2, Size 2 (#2.2) restoration may occur because the proximal box is not locked into the dentine with retentive grooves and ditches. Apparent lack of bulk in the material at the isthmus and the design of the axio-pulpal line angle are of no significance.
- Placement of an inappropriate lining material. The use

of a lining material that hydrolyses and disintegrates may leave the amalgam without physical support.
- Multiple layers of lining materials, or one lining material in excessive bulk, will reduce the volume and therefore the physical properties of the final restoration.

Failure to condense the material adequately during placement, or contamination at that time abases the physical properties. Although amalgam is a very compliant material, attainment of full physical potential is rarely achieved. The only cure for this type of failure is complete replacement of the entire restoration.

Composite resin

Composite resin may fail in a similar fashion, although it is rather flexible and failure will normally occur at the margins rather than in bulk. If the resin has been placed over a glass–ionomer base as a dentine substitute, the risk of further caries immediately following failure is reduced over the short term because of the presence of the cement. However, replacement of the entire restoration is necessary. The cause of failure must be determined and a decision made as to the replacement material to be used.

Porcelain

Generally, gold does not break, but ceramic crowns, inlays and veneers are relatively brittle and therefore subject to bulk failure. A careful analysis of the reason for failure is essential if the replacement is to succeed. There are several possible causes.

- Occlusion – it is essential to maintain a properly balanced occlusion in the presence of porcelain restorations because irregularities may lead to parafunction on the restoration and bulk failure.
- Design – porcelain requires both adequate bulk and stable support. The marginal ridge of a molar crown should have a gold shoulder below it. The lingual aspect of an anterior crown should have adequate thickness of porcelain if it is to withstand occlusal load.

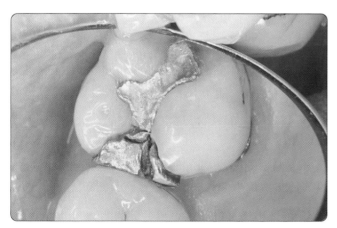

Fig. 22.9 Collapse of amalgam. The amalgam in the proximal box has collapsed.

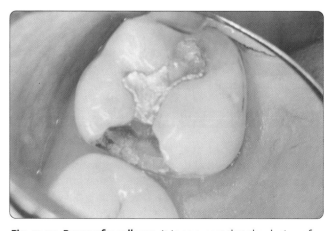

Fig. 22.10 Reason for collapse. It is apparent that the design of the box is nonsupportive and recurrent caries has left the amalgam completely unsupported.

Repair of porcelain is difficult and complete replacement is generally required. There are a number of proprietary products available for the repair of chipped or broken porcelain, but it is very difficult to match the colour properties of ceramic with any other material; adhesion between the two within the oral environment remains tenuous. Also, the wear factor is always greater with composite resin, so the lifespan of repairs with materials other than porcelain remains limited.

Total loss of a restoration

Rigid restorations

This is usually the result of loss of cementation of a rigid extracoronal restoration. The fault generally lies in incorrect cavity design, although poor handling of materials or bulk failure of tooth structure are contributory factors.

Extracoronal restorations should be retained by a fully retentive design, and the luting cement is utilised, essentially, to prevent microleakage between the restoration and the tooth. The physical properties of the cementing medium may be insufficient to withstand undue tensile stresses, although compressive properties are adequate to accept occlusal load. The main reason for cementation failure is improper mixing of the cement or contamination during placement of the restoration. Alternatively, the retentive features of the design may be inadequate. To avoid repeated failure, a careful assessment of the cause is required before re-cementation.

Direct plastic restorations

Amalgam and composite resin will rarely disappear entirely from a conventional cavity, but composite resin or glass–ionomer may be lost from erosion lesions without leaving a trace. The cause will generally be failure to develop the full adhesion potential of either material by leaving surface contamination on the cavity at the time of placement. Alternatively, abraction stresses may be involved, and the occlusion should be examined to assist in diagnosis. Develop a fresh surface on the dentine before attempting to replace the restoration, in case the existing surface is sufficiently demineralised to be unsuitable for chemical adhesion. Similarly, following loss of a composite resin there will be tags of resin remaining in the surface layer of enamel or dentine and it will be necessary to freshen the surface by removing up to $50\,\mu m$ of tooth structure to re-establish adhesion.

CHANGE OF RESTORATIVE MATERIAL

After the failure of any restoration, it is desirable to reassess the situation and decide if the current material is the material of choice under the circumstances. Each replacement means that there will be further loss of natural tooth structure and, clearly, this is a finite resource. None of the currently available restorative materials can be regarded as totally permanent in the true sense and therefore the longevity of each restoration is important.

Selection of the material for restoration of the initial lesion and then for each replacement should take into account such factors as:
- caries rate
- occlusal load
- ability to protect remaining tooth structure
- aesthetics
- size of the cavity; that is, the amount and strength of remaining tooth structure
- economic considerations.

No one factor should dominate this decision, apart from the patients long-term wellbeing and stability. The following factors should be considered.

Glass–ionomer

Indications

- Simple and inexpensive to use.
- Chemical union with tooth structure that is proof against microleakage.
- Continuing fluoride exchange throughout the life of the restoration.
- Adequate for aesthetics and it can be veneered with composite resin if necessary to enhance physical properties.
- Ideal for use in the presence of a high caries rate because of the chemical adhesion and continuing fluoride release.

Contraindications

- Unable to withstand heavy occlusal load and may require protection and support from remaining tooth structure or another restorative material placed over it.

Composite resin

Indications

- Satisfactory for the restoration of small lesions and areas under moderate occlusal load.
- Has excellent aesthetics, at least in the short term.
- Generally, physical properties are sufficient to accept moderate occlusal load, but the wear factor is less than ideal and it should be used on occlusal surfaces of molars with discretion.
- Can develop an excellent seal with etched enamel so long as the enamel is sound and well supported.
- Long-term union with dentine is doubtful. To develop sound dentine adhesion it should be used in conjunction with a glass–ionomer base.

Contraindications

- The proper placement of composite resin in the oral cavity is complex and demanding. It is therefore more expensive to place and has a relatively short clinical lifespan.
- Composite resin has limited ability to restore extensive cavities because of problems associated with achieving both proper interproximal contour and occlusal anatomy.
- It has a relatively large setting shrinkage, so the larger

the cavity the greater the total shrinkage, thus putting considerable stress on the margins and the union with remaining tooth structure.

- It has no built-in resistance to bacterial invasion and should, therefore, be used with caution in the presence of a high caries rate.
- It is based on methyl methacrylate, which is a known allergen, and contains materials such as HEMA, which can also cause an allergic reaction. The full degree of toxicity is not yet understood.

Amalgam
Indications
- Relatively simple, inexpensive to use and reasonably tolerant of careless placement technique.
- Physical properties are generally adequate to withstand occlusal load.
- Efficient and cost effective for the restoration of average to medium-sized cavities because carving and contouring direct in the oral cavity is straightforward in the presence of guidance from remaining tooth anatomy.
- Can be used to a degree to protect remaining tooth structure.
- Excellent in the presence of a high caries rate because it corrodes and seals its own margins and is economical to repair.

Contraindications
- Contains mercury, a known health hazard to dental staff.
- Poor aesthetics; tends to produce a blue–grey colour change in any tooth.
- Of limited use in the restoration of extensive cavities because of the difficulty of restoring correct occlusal anatomy directly in the mouth.

Gold
Indications
- When well constructed, gold restorations show the greatest longevity and this will often justify their use.
- Physical properties are ideal for the restoration of the occlusion.

- Indirect methods of construction are generally utilised and this allows for the ideal reconstruction of all aspects of anatomy, both occlusal and proximal.
- Can be used in very thin section for protection of remaining tooth structure.

Contraindications
- Gold restorations are complex to construct, with the potential for error at any one of a number of stages, and are therefore relatively expensive.
- Gold cannot be recommended in the presence of a high caries rate.
- Aesthetics is a matter of opinion and some patients regard this as unsatisfactory.
- Gold itself has no built-in resistance to bacterial invasion. However, a glass–ionomer luting cement will release fluoride and may provide some protection.

Porcelain
Indications
- Longevity may well justify its use.
- Excellent aesthetics available, at least over the medium term.
- Physical properties and indirect methods of construction are adequate for reconstruction of the occlusion.

Contraindications
- Ceramic restorations are complex to construct, with the potential for error at any one of a number of stages, and are therefore expensive.
- Porcelain may cause undue wear on natural tooth structure, and on other restorative materials as well, so care must be exercised in using it on an occlusal surface.
- Porcelain itself has no built in resistance to bacterial microleakage. However, a glass–ionomer luting cement will release fluoride and may provide a degree of protection.
- Cannot be recommended in the presence of a high caries rate or a heavy occlusion. It is important the occlusal problems be overcome first.

FURTHER READING

Anonymous. Recommendations on dental mercury hygiene. Revision of FDI Technical Report No. 7. *Int Dent J* 1988; **38**:191–2.

Bell GJ, Smith MC, dePont JJ. Cuspal failure of MOD restored teeth. *Aust Dent J* 1982; **27**:283–7.

Bergman M. Side effects of amalgam and its alternatives: local, systemic and environmental. *Int Dent J* 1990; **40**:4–10.

Council on Dental Materials, Instruments and Equipment. Council on Dental Therapeutics. Safety of dental amalgam – an update. *J Am Dent Assoc* 1989; **119**:204–5.

Department of Health and Human Services. *Dental amalgam: a scientific review and recommended public health service strategy for research, education and regulation.* Washington, DC: Department of Health and Human Services, Public Health Service; 1993.

Dodes JE. Amalgam toxicity: a review of the literature. *Oper Dent* 1988; **13**:32–6.

Eley B. *Dental amalgam; a review of safety* [Occasional paper, issue 3]. London: British Dental Association; 1993.

Jorgensen KD, Matona R, Shimakobe H. Deformation of cavities and resin restorations in loaded teeth. *Scand J Dent* 1976; **84**:46–50.

Mjor IA. Repair versus replacement of failed restorations. *Int Dent J* 1993; **43**:466–72.

Mount GJ. Failures in crown and bridgework. *Dent Outlook* 1985; **11**:53–8.

Mount GJ. Repair of porcelain fractures. *Dent Outlook* 1985; **11**:84–86.

Snapp KR, Boyer DB, Peterson LC, Svare CW. The contribution of dental amalgam to mercury in blood. *J Dent Res* 1989; **68**:780–5.

Appendix one
Hazards to the operator and staff
F.E. Martin

Modern dental practice is conducted in an atmosphere in which there is a constant element of risk to both operator and staff. It is not intended to over-emphasise the hazards but they cannot be ignored. High-speed handpieces move at speeds that lead to the generation of aerosols, which can readily distribute bacterial and viral infections.

Many instruments must be regarded as 'sharps' in current terminology and therefore have the potential for transfer of life-threatening diseases. The health of dentists and their staff has been the subject of many surveys and considerable investigation and, to date, the record has been excellent. But the risk remains and will, in fact, increase. At the same time the wellbeing of patients is just as important so it is imperative that dentists are seen to be taking all possible care to avoid transfer of infection to, or imposition of injury on those who avail themselves of dental health services. The dental surgery must not be seen to be a place for transfer of disease but rather as a place for its elimination and prevention.

AEROSOLS

> # Be aware
>
> **Aerosols are a hazard**
>
> Always wear a mask

Cutting teeth and removal of old restorations may create aerosols of particulate matter consisting of bacteria, viruses and fungi, fragments of dentine and enamel, or particles of dental materials. About 95% of aerosol particles have a diameter less that $5.0\,\mu m$ and these are capable of remaining suspended in air for over 24 hours. The major hazards from aerosols include spread of infection and damage to the respiratory system. The smaller the particles, the greater the potential for deep penetration.

- Particles of $0.5–5.0\,\mu m$ are regarded as fully respirable and capable of being deposited in the alveoli and bronchioles of the lungs.
- Particles of $5–10\,\mu m$ lodge in the nasopharynx, pharynx and trachea.
- Particles of $10–50\,\mu m$ trapped in the nose and upper airways.

The greatest risk is from particles lodged in the terminal alveoli. Microorganisms have the potential to cause infection and phagocytic cells may take several weeks to clear the alveoli because of the lack of ciliary transport. Elevated blood mercury levels can result from exposure to amalgam particles with subsequent mercury absorption.

Preventive measures to minimise aerosol risk

- Ventilation and good airflow.
- Delay the treatment of patients with respiratory infections, if possible, until they are fit again.
- Preoperative mouth rinse can significantly reduce the bacterial flora in the patient's mouth, thereby reducing the concentration of bacteria in the aerosol.
- Face mask and glasses protect both the dentist and assistant from inhalation and eye contamination. The face mask should fit well enough to provide an adequate seal and be effective at filtering small particles and bacteria. Commercially available masks vary in efficiency and many makes will filter to $5.0\,\mu m$ only and should be changed every hour.
- Use rubber dam and high-velocity aspiration.
- Rubber cups, finishing burs and rubber points carry a lower risk of aerosol production than polishing brushes.

Other pathways of bacterial transmission

Infection can also be spread by direct contact with fluids or tissues. As patients with transmissible infections cannot always be identified it is important to regard all tissues and body fluids as potentially infectious. Personal protection with glasses, gloves and mask is essential. Take care to prevent injury from local anaesthetic needles and other sharps during clinical use.

CHEMICAL HAZARDS

The main chemicals of concern are mercury, resin monomers and latex.

Mercury

> # Be aware
>
> **Mercury poses the greatest controversy**

Elemental mercury is a potential health hazard because mercury vapour can be taken up via the lungs or absorbed via the skin. Mercury vapour and uncharged mercury in the blood are lipid soluble and the latter can cross the blood–brain barrier (Chapter 10, page 113). After several minutes in solution, the mercury changes to the anionic form and cannot recross the same barrier. There is therefore potential for accumulation of mercury in the brain of those who inhale mercury vapour for prolonged periods. The recommended threshold limit for the maximum amount of ambient mercury vapour to which dental personnel should be exposed over a 40-hour week is 0.05 mg/m^3 air.

Although mercury is not uniquely toxic, at high tissue concentrations it is a nonspecific enzyme inhibitor and interferes with cellular function. Chronic exposure to levels in excess of the recommended threshold may produce central nervous system symptoms that include (with increasing concentrations) insomnia, physical weakness, irritability, loss of memory, nervous excitability, headaches, depression, speech disorders, impaired vision and muscular tremors.

Note on risk to patients

Available evidence suggests that, for patients, the placement and presence of amalgam restorations does not constitute a health hazard except in the rare case of hypersensitivity. Investigations of mercury vapour from amalgam and mercury concentrations in blood, urine and other biological specimens suggest that minute quantities of mercury are released from amalgams during mastication. However, these quantities are small compared with mercury from other sources, such as the diet. The amount of mercury in blood attributable to amalgam restorations has been quoted as $1.13\,\mu g/l$, which is well within the normal limits for the population, and from which no adverse health effects have been demonstrated. Physical evidence of toxicity begins to appear in the most sensitive adults at blood concentrations of $30\,\mu g/l$ and over.

A survey of over 4000 US dentists disclosed a mean urine mercury level of $15.3\,\mu g/l$, which was higher than the level reported for the general population of 1–3 μg/l. However, it was noted that the group exhibited no higher levels of morbidity or mortality than the general population. On the other hand, studies evaluating neurobehavioural performance in dentists found impaired reactions to cognitive, attention and perception tests with increasing mercury urine levels.

Release of mercury from amalgam restorations

The average daily dose of mercury from dental amalgam for patients with more than 12 restored occlusal surfaces has been estimated at up to 3 μg. This represents 10–15% of the normal daily intake of up to 20 μg of mercury from all sources for a person who is not occupationally exposed to mercury.

Mercury release has been quantified for a number of procedures:

trituration	1–2 μg
placement of amalgam restoration	6–8 μg
dry polishing	44 μg
wet polishing	2–4 μg
amalgam removal under water spray and high velocity suction	15–20 μg

The release of mercury is:

- greater for low-copper amalgams, because of corrosion-related loss of tin and increased porosity
- greater from unpolished surfaces
- increased by tooth brushing, which removes a passivating surface oxide film – although this re-forms rapidly.

Some of the released mercury enters the saliva and is either evaporated from the saliva and respired into the lungs or released into the environment. Alternatively, it may be ionised and bound in complexes and carried to the gastrointestinal tract.

In deep unlined cavities, detectable levels of mercury may be found in the dental pulp, reaching a maximum level in 7 days after placement of a restoration. It may irritate the pulp for a short period.

Mercury toxicity

 Be aware

Mercury toxicity

Because the release of very small quantities of mercury from amalgam has been demonstrated, there have been anecdotal reports of cases of mercury toxicity resulting from dental amalgams. The evidence has been subjected to scrutiny from multidisciplinary panels of experts, who report that 'although it is not possible to completely rule out adverse effects in a minority of susceptible patients, it is concluded that there is insufficient evidence to justify the claims that mercury from dental amalgam restorations has an adverse effect on the health of the vast majority of patients' (Eley and Cox, 1988).

Dental mercury hygiene

Recommendations from the World Dental Federation include the following.

1. All personnel involved in the handling of mercury should be alerted, especially during training, to the potential hazard of mercury vapour and the need to observe good mercury hygiene practices.
2. The workplace should be well ventilated, with fresh air exchange and outside exhaust. Air filters such as those in air conditioning systems may act as mercury reservoirs and should be replaced periodically.
3. The surgery atmosphere should be checked periodically for mercury vapour.
4. Do not lay carpet in dental surgeries. Continuous seamless sheet flooring carried up the walls for at least 10 cm is recommended.
5. Mercury should be stored in unbreakable, tightly sealed containers away from any source of heat.
6. Mercury and amalgamation equipment should be used only in areas that have an impervious surface with a lip along the leading edge so that spilled mercury or excess amalgam is confined and recovery facilitated.
7. Use single-use capsules rather than reusable ones or any other method of dispensing the alloy and mercury.
8. Reusable capsules should be kept closed between uses. Single-use capsules should be reassembled after use and immersed in used radiographic fixer solution. Alternatively store them in a screw-top container pending proper daily disposal.
9. Avoid the need to remove excess mercury before or during packing by selecting an appropriate alloy:mercury ratio.
10. Use only capsules that remain sealed during amalgamation.
11. Use an amalgamator with a completely enclosed activator arm.
12. Mercury dispensers should be handled with care and checked periodically for leakage.
13. The orifice of the mercury dispenser should be examined after use for residual mercury.
14. Mercury and unset amalgam should not be touched with the bare hands.
15. All amalgam scrap and free mercury should be salvaged and stored in a tightly closed container under used radiographic fixer solution.
16. Spilled mercury should be cleaned up immediately and placed in the scrap jar.
17. Do not heat mercury or amalgam or any equipment used with amalgam. Instruments contaminated with amalgam should be cleaned before heat sterilisation.
18. Do not use ultrasonic amalgam condensers.
19. Remove old amalgams and polish new ones under copious air–water spray with high-volume evacuation. The exhaust for the system should be outside the surgery.
20. Wear a mask which is fine enough to prevent the inhalation of amalgam dust.
21. Disposable materials contaminated with mercury or amalgam should be placed in a polyethylene bag, sealed and disposed of every day.
22. Waste systems that amalgam scrap may enter, (for example, cuspidors, sinks and suction systems) should have plastic traps from which the scrap can be recovered and stored as described in recommendation No. 15.
23. Skin accidentally contaminated by mercury should be washed thoroughly with soap and water.
24. Do not eat, drink or smoke in the surgery.
25. If a mercury hygiene problem is suspected, personnel should undergo urinalysis to detect mercury levels.

Sensitivity to amalgam restorations

Allergic response to the mercury associated with dental amalgam is rare but may be manifested in two ways. An immediate sensitivity may follow amalgam restoration with, skin lesions being more common than oral lesions. An urticarial rash may appear on the face and limbs and this may be followed by dermatitis. Once the amalgam has set and the level of free mercury is greatly reduced, the skin lesions resolve.

Alternatively, there may be a long-term response in the form of oral lichen planus or lichenoid reactions with erosive areas on the tongue or buccal mucosa adjacent to an amalgam restoration. Frequently these amalgam restorations are poorly contoured and corroded.

Any one of three factors may be related to persistence of the mucosal lesions.
- Allergy to mercury.
- Cytotoxicity related to the corrosion products.
- Trauma from the rough restoration.

Patients with lesions related spatially to amalgam restorations should be patch-tested for sensitivity to the constituents of dental amalgam by a dermatologist experienced in this field. If allergy is proved, the restorations should be replaced using another material. If there is no apparent allergy new amalgams should be placed to eliminate corrosion products and to improve the contour.

Replacement of an old amalgam with composite resin in a patient who has demonstrated an allergy should be undertaken with care. The patient should be kept under close observation because of the possibility of an allergy to the new restorative material.

Amalgam tattoo

The so-called amalgam tattoo, in which components of amalgam are trapped in the oral tissues, appears clinically as a macular or slightly elevated blue, black or grey pigmentation, generally in close proximity to an existing amalgam. Possible causes are as follows.
- Scraps of amalgam may fall into open surgical or extraction wounds.
- Excess amalgam may be left in the tissues following sealing the apex of a root canal with a retrograde amalgam.
- Pieces of amalgam may be forced into the mucosa.

Usually there is no local tissue response, although chronic inflammation and dystrophic calcification at the site have been reported.

Resin monomers

Notes

Allergy to composite resin monomers is becoming more common

Many resin-based restorative materials contain one or more methacrylate monomers. In concentrations encountered during restoration of a single tooth these methacrylates do not pose toxic risks to either dental staff or their patients. However, a cumulative effect may be seen after continuous or concentrated use.

The main risk is the possibility of developing an allergic response, seen as a contact dermatitis, principally in dental staff, but recently reported in a few patients. Some methacrylates can penetrate surgical gloves and have also been shown to traverse dentine tubules into the pulp chamber. Therefore all resin-containing materials should be handled using a 'no-touch' technique and patients should be observed for the possible development of a dermatitis.

Latex

Notes

Allergies to latex can be a hidden hazard.

Reports of hypersensitivity to latex products have increased in oral health care workers since the introduction of universal precautions in the early 1980s. Two types of allergic reactions may occur after prolonged exposure. Delayed hypersensitivity (type IV) is characterized by itching, redness fissures, and sores of the affected region. This reaction is attributed to the accelerators and anti-oxidants used in the rubber manufacturing process.

Immediate hypersensitivity (Type 1) reactions vary from urticaria and erythema to bronchospasm, hypotension and anaphylaxis. In this instance, natural rubber latex proteins are the causative agents, which can precipitate a response by direct contact or be adsorbed on the cornstarch powder used in gloves and dams, which facilitates air dispersion.

Treatment involves complete avoidance of the allergens which may be present in a range of products including gloves, rubber dam, bite blocks, orthodontic elastics, prophylaxis cups and anaesthetic carpules. Those staff and patients at risk must be identified by an adequate medical history including questions pertaining to latex exposure, medication and food allergies, atopia, and the frequency of childhood surgical procedures. Patch testing by an allergist or endocrinologist will assist in the diagnosis. Where necessary, all rubber products should be replaced by alternatives, such as vinyl gloves, silicone dam and bite blocks.

Chemical risk to eyes

A wide range of chemicals used in dentistry can damage eyes, as can particles turned into projectiles by dental cutting instruments. Protective measures include:
- education of personnel on the serious nature of eye injuries
- the operator, assistant and patient wearing protective glasses at all times.

PHYSICAL HAZARDS

Activator lights

Notes

Activator lights can be a hazard

High-intensity light is commonly used for initiating poly-merisation of composite resin materials, fissure sealants, bonding agents and glass–ionomer cements. Direct exposure to light with wavelengths in the band 400–500 nm can cause retinal damage by thermal injury that disrupts the photoreceptor cells. It can also induce photo-chemical processes resulting in the formation of reactive free radicals which, in the retina, can produce peroxides that denature the photoreceptors, damaging the retina and predisposing to cataracts. Factors that affect the degree of retinal damage include:

- the length of exposure to the light
- brightness of the light
- pigmentation of the fundus
- blood pressure
- genetic factors.

Protective cowls, glasses and shields are available for use with light-curing units to reduce incident light intensity.

Lasers

Be aware

Lasers require staff discipline and training

Dental lasers also have the potential to damage eyes irreversibly. Even the skin can be damaged by laser-generated light of certain wavelengths, and therefore great care must be taken to prevent the laser being reflected in unintended directions. Note that metal and metal-plated instruments can reflect the beam.

To ensure safe use of laser equipment:

- the operator must be adequately trained
- there must be a master control switch that will only function when a key is inserted and operated
- the laser must give an audible or visible warning when being operated
- foot switches used to operate the laser must be protected to prevent accidental operation
- all patients and staff must wear protective glasses suit-able for the particular wavelength of the laser being used
- the operator should verbally warn staff in the immediate area that the laser is about to be fired.

Management of 'sharps'

Summary

'Sharps' pose a hazard to
- Operators
- Staff
- Refuse collectors

Disposal of needles and other 'sharps' presents a problem because of the possibility of skin puncture of those handling the waste including those outside the dental practice. Several techniques for safe disposal have been suggested.

- 'Sharps' can be collected in metal cans or plastic containers. These receptacles help prevent injury during disposal but rely on the integrity of the container for safety.
- 'Sharps' can be autoclaved or chemically treated to reduce their infectivity but this does not reduce their potential for trauma.
- 'Sharps' can be 'entombed' by immersing them in a mixture of sodium chloride and dental plaster in a plas-tic container. The heat from the chemical reaction acts as a disinfectant and the plaster protects against injury.
- Melting the 'sharps' will destroy all infective material and change the shape of the needles to a less hazardous form. An oxyacetylene blowtorch can heat the stainless steel to its melting point of 1600–1700°C; however, some frag-ments of the needle shafts are likely to remain intact and fumes from melting the plastic hubs present a problem.

Noise

Excessive noise can result in tinnitus, irritability, hearing impairment and headaches. Noise affects the inner ear, specifically the receptor hair cells of the organ of Corti within the cochlea. The microscopic hair cells undergo initial reversible damage with the actual destruction of the hairs occurring later. The impairment may then be permanent, ranging from a slight hearing loss for specific frequency ranges and tinnitus, to severe hearing impairment.

Noise in the dental environment arises primarily from high-speed handpieces. Early models produced sound at an intensity sufficient to cause permanent hearing loss in the audible range. Now, noise output is influenced mainly by handpiece wear. Hearing levels for dentists are not signif-icantly different from the general population. However, individual dentists may show significant impairment.

Recommended noise reduction measures include:

- optimal maintenance of handpieces
- reduction of noise levels in the surgery by soundproof-ing with acoustic ceilings
- the use of earplugs for individuals at risk.

FURTHER READING

Bergman M. Side-effects of amalgam and its alternatives: local, systemic and environmental. *Int Dent J* 1990; **40**:4–10.

Council on Dental Materials, Instruments and Equipment. Council on Dental Therapeutics. Safety of dental amalgam – an update. *J Am Dent Assoc* 1989; **119**:204–5.

Department of Health and Human Services. *Dental amalgam: a scientific review and recommended public health service strategy for research, education and regulation.* Washington, DC: Public Health Service; 1993.

Dodes JE. Amalgam toxicity: a review of the literature. *Oper Dent* 1988; **13**:32–6.

Eley BM. *Dental amalgam; a review of safety [Occasional paper, issue 3].* London: British Dental Association; 1993.

Eley BM. The future of dental amalgam: a review of the literature. Part 2: Mercury exposure in dental practice. *Br Dent J* 1997; **182**:293–7.

Eley BM, Cox SW. Mercury poisoning from dental amalgam: an examination of the evidence. *J Dent* 1988; **16**:90–5.

Recommendations on dental mercury hygiene. Revision of FDI technical report number 7. *Int Dent J* 1988; **38**:191–2.

Safadi GS, Safadi TJ, Terezhalmy GT, Taylor JS, Battistio JR, Melton AL. Latex hypersensitivity: its prevalence among dental professionals. *J Am Dent Assoc* 1996; **127**:83–8.

Snapp KR, Boyer DB, Peterson LC, Svare CW. The contribution of dental amalgam to mercury in blood. *J Dent Res* 1989; **68**:780–5.

Appendix two

Infection control

T.M. Gerzina

Dental care personnel have a higher incidence of blood-borne infections than other health-care workers. All blood and body fluids should be considered potentially highly infectious and precautions should be consistently undertaken regardless of what is known of the patient's blood-borne infection status. This simple principle is at the centre of infection control in dentistry.

POTENTIAL PATHOGENS

Herpes virus, hepatitis virus and human immunodeficiency virus are the principal organisms of concern because they can all be life threatening. However, there are many other agents which can be transferred within the confines of a dental practice. The sexually transmitted diseases such as *Neisseria gonorrhoeae* and syphilis (*Treponema pallidum*) are transmissible; so too is *Mycobacterium tuberculosis*. There are a variety of other organisms of lesser gravity, all the way down to influenza, that can be passed on to patients and staff, none of which should be taken lightly.

Paths of transmission

! Be aware

Infection control

All instruments and all surfaces can transmit infection

The dental surgery presents a very wide array of methods of transmission.

Handpieces

Handpieces present a unique challenge because of their internal surfaces and the fragility of some parts. Most can be sterilised by heat. Those that cannot should be thoroughly scrubbed clean under running water using a liquid iodophor and disassembled for internal cleaning and disinfection.

Instruments

All instruments used within the oral cavity will collect contaminated debris and, although the source of infection will not always be obvious, they should always be carefully scrubbed before sterilisation.

Surfaces

All flat surfaces within the surgery, such as bracket table and bench tops, can readily become contaminated with saliva transmitted by hands and aerosol spray. Disciplined infection control procedures are required to minimise the risk. Some viruses do not survive well outside the body, but the hepatitis B virus may survive on bench surfaces for weeks.

Items transferred from the surgery

✦ Summary

Prosthetic items must be sterilised before dispatch to the laboratory

The transfer to a dental laboratory of impressions, records, stone casts, dentures and other articles that have been in a patient's mouth can place laboratory personnel at risk. It is the dentist's responsibility to ensure that all such items are decontaminated.

An impression or intra-oral record should be immediately thoroughly washed under running water to remove saliva, blood and debris. It is possible to disinfect the surface of most of the items used, including elastomeric impression materials, by immersion for 10 minutes in one of the following before sending to the laboratory.
- Chlorine compounds.
- Glutaraldehyde/phenol compounds.
- Glutaraldehyde 2%.

Alginate impressions should be cleaned by spraying with an iodophor and then stored in a sealed plastic bag before delivery.

Prosthetic appliances such as dentures should be washed, soaked for 5 minutes in full-strength sodium hypochlorite and then washed again before delivery.

METHODS OF INFECTION CONTROL

Heat

Notes

Sterilisation by moist heat
- Time – 10 minutes
- Temperature – 134°C
- Pressure – 203 kPa (2 atm)

Precleaning of instruments by careful washing and ultrasonic treatment should be routine practice, followed by either wet or dry heat sterilisation. Cleaning can be achieved by submerging the instruments in an ultrasonic bath operating at 40°C and 35 kHz, for 3–5 minutes using a matched disinfectant. It is recommended that only clean instruments are sterilised.

Moist heat sterilisation (autoclaving)

The most effective conditions are 121°C at a pressure of 1 atm (101 kPa or 15 lbf/in^2) for 20 minutes or 134°C at 2 atm (203 kPa or 28 lbf/in^2) for 10 minutes.

Dry heat sterilisation

To be effective, the minimum requirements are 160°C for 1 hour or 180°C for 30 minutes.

Chemical agents

Instruments and equipment used in the dental surgery which do not contact infectious fluids can be 'cold sterilised' by careful cleaning, followed by exposure to disinfectants for 10–15 minutes. This is not a recommended alternative to autoclaving when appropriate and possible.

Notes

Chemical disinfection
- Agents – various
- Time – 15 minutes minimum
- Concentration – high

Recommended chemical agents include the following compounds.

Alcohols
Both ethyl alcohol 70% and isopropyl alcohol 70% act as denaturants, but are not adequate as disinfectants or surface and skin cleansers.

Phenols
Aqueous solutions of phenols (1–2%) are active against a wide range of bacteria; 0.25% solutions are useful for cleaning and disinfecting suction equipment. The limitations of these agents are as follows.
- They are not sporacidal.
- They exhibit irregular virucidal activity.
- They are ineffective against hydrophilic viruses such as hepatitis B virus.
- They may be inactivated by bioburden.
- They can damage plastic instruments.

Oxidising agents
Hypochlorite and iodine are suitable for surface, immersion and high level disinfection. A 1.5% solution of hypochlorite is highly effective for disinfection of surfaces. Their limitations are as follows.
- They may discolour some surfaces.
- They lose activity and effectiveness over time.

Alkylating agents
Formaldehyde, ethylene oxide and glutaraldehyde are effective chemical sterilising agents when used for prolonged periods. Up to 10 hours, exposure is required for either an 8% aqueous formaldehyde solution or a 70% solution in alcohol. Glutaraldehyde 2% or alkaline glutaraldehyde 2% are also effective and so is a gaseous ethylene oxide. There are some minor risks with the use of glutaraldehyde, particularly with inhalation of fumes, and good ventilation is essential.

Detergents and soaps
Detergents remove residues from instruments and surfaces and can be used for cleaning suction equipment. Hand washes and soaps containing 2,4,4-trichlor-2-hydroxyl-diphenyl ester, povidone iodine or chlorhexidene are effective antibacterial cleansers.

PERSONAL PROTECTION

Summary

Personal protection is for:
- operator
- staff
- laboratory staff
- patients

Clothing
Protective clothing, masks, glasses and gloves should be simple in design, easily cleaned and comfortable. Soiled laundry should be washed in hot diluted laundry bleach. Individual articles should be sterilised before transport to a laundry if contaminated by blood. All protective clothing should be worn only within the surgery and removed on leaving the area.

Hands
Before gloving, hands should be washed with a reliable surgical soap and dried well. The most reliable hand wash is a 4% chlorhexidene gluconate, which exhibits high microbe reduction and residual action. Iodine solutions can be used for individuals who are hypersensitive to chlorhexidene.

Gloves
Gloves are a reasonably reliable form of barrier technique and vinyl, natural and artificial latex are the common types available. Single-use examining gloves are recommended for routine dental procedures. Full surgical gloves are the choice if the clinician has unusually proportioned hands, if there is a record of highly infectious disease or if the practice cares for many patients from a high-risk group. Double gloving is another alternative.

Face masks
Face masks, for routine clinical use, should generally be free of fibreglass and provide high filtration efficiency but, like gloves, they cannot be relied upon for extended protection throughout the clinical day without regular replacement. Generally, 1 hour is a maximum for use of a high filtration mask in a humid atmosphere.

Gowns
Disposable gowns are a protective measure; they may be used when treating the known infectious patient and certainly contribute to convenient clothing protection.

FURTHER READING

Albion Street AIDS Centre, Sydney. *The AIDS manual. A comprehensive reference on the Human Immunodeficiency Virus (HIV)*. Sydney: State Print Publishers Ultimo; 1988.

Christensen RP, Robinson RA, Robinson DF, Ploeger BJ, Leavitt RW, Bodily HL. Antimicrobial activity of environmental surface disinfectants in the absence and presence of bioburden. *J Am Dent Assoc* 1989; **119**:493–505.

Cottone JA. Recent developments in hepatitis: new virus, vaccine and dosage recommendations. *J Am Dent Assoc* 1990; **120**:501–08.

Drennon DG, Johnson GH. The effect of immersion disinfection of elastomeric impressions on the surface detail reproduction of improved gypsum casts. *J Prosthet Dent* 1990; **63**:233–41.

Glick M. Clinical protocol for treating patients with HIV disease. *Gen Dent* 1990; (Nov/Dec):418–25.

Langenwalter EM, Aquilino SA, Turner KA. The dimensional stability of elastomeric impression materials following disinfection. *J Prosthet Dent* 1990; **63**:270–6.

Merchant VA, Molinari JA. Evacuation system lines and solid waste filter traps: associated flora and infection control. *Gen Dent* 1990; (May/Jun):189–93.

Otis LL, Cottone JA. Prevalence of perforations in disposable latex gloves during routine dental treatment. *J Am Dent Assoc* 1991; **118**:321–3.

Schaefer ME. Infection control, OSHA and a hazards communication program. *J Calif Dent Assoc* 1990; **18**:53–8.

Woods RG. *Infection control* [Booklet]. Sydney: Australian Dental Association; 1987.

Index